By examining German university medicine this book presents a new interpretation of the emergence of modern medical science. It demonstrates that the development of modern medicine as a profession linking theory and practice did not emerge suddenly from the revolutionary transformation of Europe at the opening of the nineteenth century, as Foucault and others have argued. Instead, Thomas H. Broman points to cultural and institutional changes occurring during the second half of the eighteenth century as reshaping both medical theory and the physician's professional identity.

Among the most important of these factors was the emergence of a literary public sphere in Germany between 1750 and 1800, a development that exposed medical writing to new discourses such as Jena Romanticism, and created the stage on which would be played out the bitter medical controversies of the 1790s. Entrance into the public sphere also offered physicians the opportunity to create new social roles for themselves as writers and journalists.

Professor Broman's study offers a new perspective on the historical origins of the modern medical profession by using its case study to call into question the standard model of "professionalization," the historical process by which it is commonly understood that professions acquired their modern form. In providing this new perspective, he casts light upon and re-examines certain assumptions about what a profession is that have guided not only histories of professionalization, but also much of the recent writing in social history of medicine.

The transformation of German academic medicine, 1750–1820

Cambridge History of Medicine

Edited by

CHARLES ROSENBERG, Professor of History and Sociology of Science, University of Pennsylvania

Other titles in the Series:

Health, medicine and morality in the sixteenth century EDITED BY
CHARLES WEBSTER

The Renaissance notion of woman: A study in the fortunes of scholasticism and medical science in European intellectual life IAN MACLEAN

Mystical Bedlam: Madness, anxiety and healing in sixteenth-century England
MICHAEL MACDONALD

From medical chemistry to biochemistry: The making of a biomedical discipline
ROBERT E. KOHLER

Joan Baptista Van Helmont: Reformer of science and medicine
WALTER PAGEL

A generous confidence: Thomas Story Kirkbride and the art of asylum-keeping, 1840–1883 NANCY TOMES

The cultural meaning of popular science: Phrenology and the organization of consent in nineteenth-century Britain ROGER COOTER

Madness, morality and medicine: A study of the York Retreat, 1796–1914
ANNE DIGBY

Patients and practitioners: Lay perceptions of medicine in pre-industrial society
EDITED BY ROY PORTER

Hospital life in Enlightenment Scotland: Care and teaching at the Royal Infirmary of Edinburgh GUENTER B. RISSE

Plague and the poor in Renaissance Florence ANNE G. CARMICHAEL

Victorian lunacy: Richard M. Bucke and the practice of late nineteenth-century psychiatry S. E. D. SHORTT

Medicine and society in Wakefield and Huddersfield, 1780–1870
HILARY MARLAND

Ordered to care: The dilemma of American nursing, 1850–1945
SUSAN M. REVERBY

Morbid appearances: The anatomy of pathology in the early nineteenth century
RUSSELL C. MAULITZ

Professional and popular medicine in France, 1770–1830: The social world of medical practice MATTHEW RAMSEY

Abortion, doctors and the law: Some aspects of the legal regulation of abortion in England, 1884–1984 DONALD DENOON

Health, race and German politics between national unification and Nazism, 1870–1945 PAUL WEINDLING

The physician–legislators of France: Medicine and politics in the Early Third Republic, 1870–1914 JACK D. ELLIS

Continued on page following the Index

The transformation of
German academic medicine
1750–1820

THOMAS H. BROMAN
University of Wisconsin, Madison

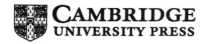

CAMBRIDGE
UNIVERSITY PRESS

PUBLISHED BY THE PRESS SYNDICATE OF THE UNIVERSITY OF CAMBRIDGE
The Pitt Building, Trumpington Street, Cambridge, United Kingdom

CAMBRIDGE UNIVERSITY PRESS
The Edinburgh Building, Cambridge CB2 2RU, UK
40 West 20th Street, New York NY 10011–4211, USA
477 Williamstown Road, Port Melbourne, VIC 3207, Australia
Ruiz de Alarcón 13, 28014 Madrid, Spain
Dock House, The Waterfront, Cape Town 8001, South Africa

http://www.cambridge.org

© Cambridge University Press 1996

This book is in copyright. Subject to statutory exception
and to the provisions of relevant collective licensing agreements,
no reproduction of any part may take place without
the written permission of Cambridge University Press.

First published 1996
First paperback edition 2002

Typeface Bembo.

A catalogue record for this book is available from the British Library

Library of Congress Cataloguing in Publication data
Broman, Thomas Hoyt.
The transformation of German academic medicine, 1750–1820 / Thomas
H. Broman.
        p.   cm. – (Cambridge history of medicine)
Includes bibliographical references and index.
ISBN 0 521 55231 1 (hardcover)
1. Medicine – Germany – History – 18th century.   2. Medicine –
Germany – History – 19th century.   3. Physicians – Germany –
History – 18th century.   4. Physicians – Germany – History – 19th
century.   I. Title.   II. Series.
R510.B76   1996
610′.943′09033–dc20   95-48292   CIP

ISBN 0 521 55231 1 hardback
ISBN 0 521 52457 1 paperback

Meinen verehrten Doktorväter

Geison, Grafton, and Turner,
and
in memory of my real father,
who loved history
but preferred his with a little more action

CONTENTS

Acknowledgments   *page* ix

Introduction   1
1   Physicians in eighteenth-century Germany   13
2   Fractures and new alignments   42
3   Physicians and writers: Medical theory and the
    emergence of the public sphere   73
4   The art of healing   102
5   Breaking the shackles of history: The Brunonian
    revolution in Germany   128
6   German academic medicine during the reform era   159
Conclusion: Disciplines, professions, and the public
sphere   193

Index   203

ACKNOWLEDGMENTS

The completion of a book is the occasion for such an outpouring of relief and gratitude that an author can scarcely resist the temptation to rattle on and on, much like an Oscar winner at the Academy Awards. Fortunately, there is little reason to resist, because the author's friends will eagerly search these lines for proper recognition, and even readers who do not know the author personally will be likely to take a look in search of clues to the author's scholarly alliances and antipathies. In this respect, a book's acknowledgments can be scrutinized much as scholars of Soviet politics used to hunch over photos of the Politburo taken at the annual May Day parade. On then with the show.

This book began a very long time ago, back in 1981 at Princeton University, with a seminar on science in the German universities offered by R. Steven Turner. The impetus to study German science and medicine came not just from the topic's intrinsic interest, but also from Steve's detailed knowledge, critical judgment, and humorous compassion. A second impetus came from Gerry Geison's suggestion that I work on the conflict between clinical and scientific medicine, a suggestion that has borne much fruit and continues even today to test my resourcefulness. Tony Grafton added his knowledge of eighteenth-century intellectual history, along with bountiful moral support.

A significant portion of the early research for this book was conducted with a DAAD Fellowship in 1983–4, when I was extended the hospitality of Prof. Heinrich Schipperges and the Institut für Geschichte der Medizin at the University of Heidelberg. Most of the research on the eighteenth-century portions of the book was conducted in 1989–90 while on an NSF Postdoctoral Fellowship at Yale University. There I found a wonderful library collection and stimulating conversation with Larry Holmes and John Warner, both of whom I am privileged to number among my most valued colleagues. Finally, an Extramural Grant from the National Library of Medicine (Number 5 R01 LM05409-02) for the summers of 1992 and 1993 allowed me to complete my archival research in Germany and finish preparing the manuscript for submission.

A number of friends and colleagues have contributed substantially to this book. Mary Lindemann and Mimi Wessling have given generously of their knowledge of the social history of medicine in eighteenth-century Germany, and I have profited immeasurably from it. I have similarly profited from Lynn Nyhart and Arleen Tuchman with respect to science and medicine in nineteenth-century Germany. Judith Norman, Stuart Strickland, and Maria Trumpler came along at a time in my life when I thought I would never see my way through the murky depths of *Naturphilosophie* and gave me heart to persevere. Louise Robbins read through the completed manuscript and made numerous stylistic improvements. Finally, it will be evident to anyone who reads this book how deeply indebted I am to the work of Anthony La Vopa, whose portrait of students trying to make their way in clerical careers crystallized my own dim understanding of what *Beruf* meant in early modern Germany. I have never met Tony La Vopa, but more than any single person he has shaped my thinking about the medical profession in the eighteenth century.

One of the pleasures of working in Madison is the abundance of stimulating colleagues found here. I mention most especially Klaus Berghahn and Nancy Kaiser in the German Department, Suzanne Desan and David Sorkin in History, and Michael Shank and Harold Cook in my own department, History of Science. Hal Cook deserves special mention for having patiently endured many hours of my pestering him for his thoughts about the early modern medical profession, and I gratefully acknowledge his contributions. Hal would not endorse everything I say here about the professions, I suspect, but my thinking about physicians in early modern Europe has benefitted greatly from his work.

When I began my graduate study in history of science, I encountered two people who are both personal friends and stimulating colleagues. John Carson is sui generis, as anyone who knows him can attest. Possessed of the sharpest critical faculty I have ever encountered, John is at the same time a kind and compassionate person. He makes the scholarly life both provocative and comfortable. Peter Dear recently described me affectionately as a thorn in his side; here I happily return the compliment. After all, it was after an argument with Peter about Kuhn's *Structure of Scientific Revolutions* that I was first convinced to go to Princeton. Since then I continued to profit from Peter's insight and ability to wear simultaneously the hats of historian, philosopher, and sociologist of knowledge. Many people talk about integrated science studies, or "cultural studies" of science, to use the currently fashionable term: Peter is one of the few to actually produce such a thing.

Many people have patiently endured the slow metamorphosis of my dissertation into this book, but none more patiently than Lynn Nyhart. Her task has been a difficult one, as colleague, critic, and partner, but Lynn has accomplished it with deep reserves of intelligence and affection. Most marvelous of all has been her willingness to continue reading my prose and criticize it honestly and effectively, even though she knew that what I wanted to be told was that it was perfect. Treacherous work indeed, but she has done it and created a protected space where doubt and despair found no entrance.

INTRODUCTION

In recent years, the professions have been a subject of growing fascination for historians and sociologists. The reasons are not difficult to find. Talcott Parsons may have overstated the centrality of the professions when he claimed in 1968 that they were "the most important single component" in modern society,[1] but there is no denying the prominent position occupied by professional "experts" of various stripes. One has only to take in the nightly news broadcast on public television, where it seems that nearly every matter of current interest is rendered as a debate between experts, to appreciate the role they play in our world. Or consider that in 1993, when Hillary Rodham Clinton began putting together a proposal for reforming America's health care system, her first act was to gather together a group of professional experts on various aspects of health care to discuss the framework of such a plan. It is not that fundamental political and ideological issues – such as the desirability of guaranteeing medical care to every citizen – were thereby rendered meaningless or unimportant in the face of such consultations. But the political questions were shaped in significant ways by what those experts had to say about the way the world is.

The reference to medicine is an appropriate one, because in one sense this book is about the origins of the modern medical profession. Put that way, of course, the project sounds a little grandiose. I do not pretend that this book will represent a synthesis of the kind offered by Paul Starr's *The Social Transformation of American Medicine* (1982), or Magali Sarfatti Larson's *The Rise of Professionalism* (1977). Mine is a more modest study of medicine in Germany from 1750 to 1820, with special emphasis on the role of universities in constituting professional identity. Yet I believe this book does offer a new perspective on the historical origins of the modern medical profession by using its case study to call into question the standard model of "professionalization," the historical process by which it is commonly understood that professions acquired their modern form. In providing this new perspective, I want to throw light upon and reexamine certain assumptions about

---

1 Gerald L. Geison, "Introduction," in *Professions and the French State, 1700–1900*, ed. Gerald L. Geison (Philadelphia, 1984), p. 2.

what a profession is that have guided not only histories of professionalization, but also much of the recent writing in social history of medicine. Thus, instead of presenting Germany as an alternative to France or somewhere else as the well-spring of the modern medical profession, I seek to ask some more basic questions about what a "modern" profession actually is and how it came into being.

In its general outline, the usual story of the professionalization of medicine runs like this: prior to some time in the nineteenth century, physicians – which for my purposes means exclusively holders of the doctor of medicine degree – were an occupational group hard pressed to establish themselves comfortably in society. Besieged by a host of competitors, such as surgeons, midwives, apothecaries, and anybody else who treated illness for remuneration, and hampered by their lack of the modern scientific tools of diagnosis and treatment, physicians represented a minor and not particularly well-respected group of healers. However, three important nineteenth-century developments would change this situation. First, the growth of the modern bureaucratic state created an authority to which physicians and other professional groups could appeal for effective legal sanctions against unlicensed practice. Such sanctions, of course, had filled legal codices since the Middle Ages, but only after 1800 did states begin to develop the enforcement apparatus that would make them effective to any considerable degree. Second, the advance of industrialization and the consequent growth of urban centers in a host of countries disrupted traditional patterns of community life that had supported the kinds of medical practice so characteristic of early modern society. In place of the trust and personal acquaintance that had been the mainstays of the exchange of services in the preindustrial world, people came to rely ever more on experts, creatures whose legitimacy depended on institutions (such as universities and licensing boards) empowered by government and society to create such beings. Third, the rapid advance of scientific knowledge during the nineteenth century increased physicians' efficacy at the bedside, which lent them new prestige and authority.[2]

In each of its guiding themes – the growth of state power, the processes of urbanization and industrialization, and the expansion of scientific knowledge – the standard history of professionalization reveals its deep affinity with stories about the emergence of "modernity" in the nineteenth century. As a story about modernization, professionalization requires the existence of a social structure resembling the one we now know. Thus modernization often begins (in Europe) with the French Revolution, which conventionally is taken to have wiped away much of the residue of an older social order. The extent to which the Revolution failed to accomplish this in Germany, of course, becomes the basis for explaining why Germany strayed off the path to modernity and onto the road leading to totalitarianism and national socialism. It also becomes the basis for assessing the

2 It goes almost without saying that national variations from this standard narrative can be considerable. But even those countries that deviate the most from it in terms of when various stages were reached nonetheless display a considerable conformity with the basic pattern.

"delayed" modernization of German science and medicine. But as has been argued most powerfully by Blackbourn and Eley, models of modernization are not terribly informative in studying German history.[3] And as I hope to show here, the "peculiarities" of the German situation gave rise to their own dynamic of professional change.

In any case, one problem with casting the history of professions as a modernization story is that the telos that shapes the story can be read back into history as a kind of unseen hand that motivates the action. Thus when historians have reached back beyond the French Revolution to study the eighteenth-century professions, they have often carried assumptions about the modern professions back into the earlier era. The most important of these assumptions is what I call a "functionalist" conception of the professions. By this I mean that the professions are described essentially as a kind of work, healing in the case of medicine, and the major features of interest are the institutions, legal structures, and social rewards that attend such work. This kind of approach is quite prominent among sociologists of the professions. Eliot Freidson, whose work on the sociology of medicine has more or less defined the field for a quarter century, invoked this occupational frame of reference when he described contemporary Anglo-American professions as groups whose social prestige depends on "their training and identity as particular, corporately organized occupations to which specialized knowledge, ethicality and importance to society are imputed, and for which privilege is claimed."[4] Freidson's definition, while placing professions in a complex fabric of the social organization of work as well as intellectual and cultural beliefs, nonetheless treats them functionally as parts of a particular kind of social mechanism or system.[5]

Historians of medicine, too, have paid considerable attention to healing as social practice. This interpretive angle became a self-conscious historiographic program in the late 1970s, in reaction against a medical historiography attacked by critics as self-serving and too centered on the triumphal progress of medical science.[6] Charles Webster and Margaret Pelling, in discussing the history of medicine in Britain, called for studies of the social dynamics of health care that would encompass the entire scope of such services and ignore polemical or self-interested distinctions between "legitimate" practitioners and "quacks" or "charlatans."[7]

---

3 David Blackbourn and Geoff Eley, *The Peculiarities of German History* (Oxford, 1984).
4 Eliot Freidson, "The Theory of Professions: State of the Art," in *The Sociology of the Professions*, ed. Robert Dingwall and Philip Lewis (New York, 1983), p. 25.
5 For other recent work on the sociology of the professions, see Andrew Abbott, *The System of Professions* (Chicago, 1988); Rolf Torstendahl and Michael Burrage (eds.), *The Formation of Professions: Knowledge, State and Strategy* (London, 1990); Rolf Torstendahl and Michael Burrage (eds.), *The Professions in History and Theory* (London, 1990); and Thomas L. Haskell (ed.), *The Authority of Experts: Studies in History and Theory* (Bloomington, Ind., 1984).
6 For a particularly vigorous statement of this position, see John Woodward and David Richards, "Towards a Social History of Medicine," in *Health Care and Popular Medicine in Nineteenth Century England*, ed. John Woodward and David Richards (London, 1977), pp. 15–55.
7 Margaret Pelling and Charles Webster, "Medical Practitioners," in *Health, Medicine and Mortality in the Sixteenth Century*, ed. Charles Webster (Cambridge, 1979), pp. 165–235.

From a similar perspective, Susan Reverby and David Rosner called for the historiography of American medicine to move away from the history of great doctors and their discoveries. Deliberately allying themselves with Henry Sigerist's socialist politics – while conveniently downplaying Sigerist's own considerable attachment to a triumphalist history of medical science – Reverby and Rosner called for attention to "the social and political responses to disease, the social epidemiology of health and illness, the changing legitimation and importance of professionalism, the ideological and social control aspects of medicine, and the social role of health care institutions."[8] A short time thereafter, Roy Porter began popularizing the metaphor of early modern health care as a consumer-driven marketplace overflowing with providers competing for economic advantage (or mere survival).[9]

The first German scholars to adopt this approach came from outside the traditional domain of medical history. In the early 1980s, two doctoral students at the University of Bielefeld, Claudia Huerkamp and Ute Frevert, wrote dissertations on the history of medicine that broke significant new ground. Influenced by Jürgen Kocka, whose own interests centered on the social history of the educated middle class (*Bildungsbürgertum*), both Frevert and Huerkamp treated their subject as case studies in the history of the *Bildungsbürgertum*. Frevert's study dealt with the "politicization" of health and illness in the late eighteenth and nineteenth centuries, a process she illustrated with examinations of the "medicalization" of poverty at the end of the eighteenth century and the introduction of health insurance in the second half of the nineteenth century.[10] Huerkamp's book based itself more self-consciously on the Anglo-American literature on professionalization, and told the story of the formation of a modern medical profession in Prussia in the nineteenth century.[11] More recently, scholars such as Sabine Sander, Robert Jütte,

8 Susan Reverby and David Rosner (eds.), *Health Care in America: Essays in Social History* (Philadelphia, 1979), quoted on pp. 3–4. It should be noted that Reverby and Rosner's polemics came at a time when there already existed a considerable literature on the "social history" of American medicine, broadly construed. For a discussion see Ronald L. Numbers, "The History of American Medicine: A Field in Ferment," *Reviews in American History* 10 (1982): 245–63.

9 Roy Porter, "William Hunter: A Surgeon and a Gentleman," in *William Hunter and the Eighteenth-Century Medical World*, ed. W. F. Bynum and Roy Porter (Cambridge, 1988), pp. 7–34; Dorothy Porter and Roy Porter, *Patient's Progress: Doctors and Doctoring in Eighteenth-Century England* (Stanford, Calif., 1989), pp. 16–22; and Roy Porter, *Health for Sale: Quackery in England 1660–1850* (Manchester, 1989).

10 Ute Frevert, *Krankheit als politisches Problem 1770–1830. Soziale Unterschichten in Preußen zwischen medizinischer Polizei und staatlicher Sozialversicherung* (Göttingen, 1984). For an extensive critique of Frevert, see Francisca Loetz, *Vom Kranken zum Patienten: "Medikalisierung" und medizinische Vergesellschaftung am Beispiel Badens 1750–1850* (Stuttgart, 1993), esp. chap. 1. Loetz argues (correctly, I think) that Frevert's treatment of "medicalization," which draws heavily upon the work of Michel Foucault and Jean-Pierre Goubert, misconstrues medicalization as fundamentally a process of state-sponsored professional control.

11 Claudia Huerkamp, *Der Aufstieg der Ärzte im 19. Jahrhundert. Vom gelehrten Stand zum professionellen Experten: Das Beispiel Preußens* (Göttingen, 1985). See also Huerkamp, "Ärzte und Professionalisierung in Deutschland. Überlegungen zum Wandel des Arztberufs im 19. Jahrhundert," *Geschichte und*

and Francisca Loetz have followed a line more closely resembling the English-language historiography. Their work is less concerned with social theory than it is with presenting detailed studies of health care at the local level.[12]

This approach to the social history of medicine has opened vast new areas of historical experience to scholars. At its best, for example in Hilary Marland's description of the institutions and providers of health care in the two English towns of Huddersfield and Wakefield between 1780 and 1870, or in Irvine Loudon's monograph on the "general practitioner" in England, it can present detailed analyses in a richly elaborated social context.[13] Sander's study of surgeons in Württemberg has the same virtues, and it is hardly an exaggeration to say that Frevert's and Huerkamp's books have powerfully influenced the historiography of German medicine. Yet when historians have turned to study of the medical professions as an early modern social category, they have fashioned an image deeply colored by their functionalist assumptions about what a profession is. For example, Pelling surely exaggerated the case when she dismissed early modern English doctors of medicine as a "small group" of healers whose importance had been vastly inflated by a whiggish historiographic tradition.[14] Physicians may indeed have been unimportant in terms of the overall performance of healing in English society. But if physicians were really so indistinguishable from other healers, as Pelling wants to argue, then we might well wonder that anyone could be so dull as to spend so much time and money acquiring what amounted to a worthless degree. Questions such as these open the door to the complex problem of what professional identity meant in early modern Europe.[15]

In the newer German historiography, meanwhile, an even stronger functionalist mentality has ruled. Frevert's bleak portrait of physicians deliberately seeking to professionalize as a means of gaining authority over their patron-patients and eliminating economic competition from other healers has become the unquestioned standard for describing the profession's situation at the end of the eigh-

Gesellschaft 6 (1980): 349–82, which illustrates her reliance on the work of Anglo-American sociologists such as Eliot Freidson and Magali Sarfatti Larson. For an English-language synopsis, see Huerkamp, "The Making of the Medical Profession, 1800–1914: Prussian Doctors in the Nineteenth Century," in German Professions, 1800–1950, ed. Geoffrey Cocks and Konrad Jarausch (Oxford, 1990), pp. 66–84.

12 Sabine Sander, Handwerkschirurgen: Sozialgeschichte einer verdrängten Berufsgruppe (Göttingen, 1989); Robert Jütte, Ärzte, Heiler und Patienten: Medizinischer Alltag in der frühen Neuzeit (Munich, 1991); and Loetz, Vom Kranken zum Patienten. Loetz's book represents a middle position between Sander and Frevert. It attempts both to offer a detailed social history and to interpret the narrative in terms of a revised understanding of medicalization.

13 Hilary Marland, Medicine and Society in Wakefield and Huddersfield 1780–1870 (Cambridge, 1987); and Irvine Loudon, Medical Care and the General Practitioner, 1750–1850 (Oxford, 1986).

14 Margaret Pelling, "Medical Practice in Early Modern England: Trade or Profession?" in The Professions in Early Modern England, ed. Wilfred Prest (London, 1987), pp. 90–128.

15 Even in England, Lisa Rosner has argued, university credentials and other kinds of official recognition made a difference to medical practitioners and patients. See Lisa Rosner, Medical Education in the Age of Improvement: Edinburgh Students and Apprentices 1760–1826 (Edinburgh, 1991), p. 22.

teenth century.[16] According to this view, physicians attempted to broaden the market for their services by using the new periodical media to offer a range of expert advice. At the same time, their advocacy of increased government involvement in medical police worked toward the elimination of the profession's competitors.[17] This picture is deeply misleading on two grounds. First, it paints an excessively negative picture of physicians' situation. It is certainly true that physicians complained loudly and repeatedly about the handicaps they faced. But if we pay attention to aspects of professional life other than bedside practice, their situation looks brighter by several degrees. Second, Frevert's picture misrepresents what physicians *did* want changed. To conclude that their programmatics amounted to a call for "professionalization" is nothing less than to import a distinctively modern sensibility into the minds of people who lived in different circumstances from those of modern professions.[18]

It seems to me that both Pelling's and Frevert's claims about early modern physicians arise from the same problem: the inappropriateness of applying the criteria of modern professionalism to its early modern version.[19] One response to this difficulty would be simply to deny that a medical "profession" existed before the nineteenth century, a position taken by Freidson.[20] Pelling seems to hold a similar view: Although there may indeed have been something called a "profession of medicine" in sixteenth- and seventeenth-century England, it was not an especially significant category in terms of what that society looked like and how health care was provided. But there is another way to approach the issue. Instead of letting the characteristics of modern professions be the grounds for denying the existence or the importance of early modern professions, we might ask instead what the early modern professions *were* and how they thought of themselves and were thought of by their contemporaries.

One widely agreed-upon criterion of professionalism in the early modern period has been that of gentility. Writing about English professions, Wilfred Prest described them as "all nonmercantile occupations followed by persons claiming gentility," a definition broadly similar to the one used by Geoffrey Holmes in his

---

16 Frevert, *Krankheit als politisches Problem*, pp. 36–44; Huerkamp, *Der Aufstieg der Ärzte*, pp. 22–34; and Nelly Tsouyopoulos, "The Influence of John Brown's Ideas in Germany," in *Brunonianism in Britain and Europe*, ed. W. F. Bynum and Roy Porter (London 1988), p. 63–74.
17 Despite her vigorous criticism of Frevert on other points, Loetz agrees with her in this respect. See Loetz, *Vom Kranken zum Patienten*, pp. 73–87.
18 For a more nuanced presentation of the professional situation of M.D.s in early modern Germany, see Mary Lindemann, *Health and Healing in Eighteenth-Century Germany* (forthcoming fall 1996, Johns Hopkins Univ. Press).
19 A list of those criteria usually runs: (1) specialized and advanced education, (2) a code of conduct or ethics, (3) competency tests leading to licensing, (4) high social prestige in comparison to manual labor, (5) monopolization of the market in services, and (6) considerable autonomy in conduct of professional affairs.
20 Eliot Freidson, *Profession of Medicine: A Study of the Sociology of Applied Knowledge* (New York, 1970), pp. 3–12. Freidson, it must be noted, was not attempting to provide a history of the medical profession or an account of professionalization. Rather he was using medicine's past to highlight certain aspects of the contemporary profession.

study of professions in Augustan England.[21] This, however, makes the category of "profession" a very broad one indeed. Prest himself acknowledged as much, pointing out that such professions in England "would include (just to begin with the letter 'a') accountants, actuaries, and architects."[22] Although agreeing that gentility was crucial to professional stature, I would like to narrow the range of professions considerably by tying professional status to possession of a degree from one of the university faculties of theology, law, or medicine. This very minimalist definition, comprising only the hoary trinity of medieval professions, can certainly be criticized as too narrow. But it has at least two virtues. First, it throws a spotlight on the meaning of a university degree and universities as institutions in the constitution of professional identity and authority. Moreover, for those who are weary of wrangling over just which groups were or were not professions, it has the advantage of calling "professions" only those occupations that nearly everyone would agree belong in the category.

By emphasizing the importance of a university degree in conferring professional status, we have already begun moving away from a functionalist view of the professions to one that I believe better captures physicians' place in early modern society. Put succinctly, I would argue that belonging to a profession like medicine in early modern Europe did not so much define a particular kind of *work* as it characterized a particular kind of *person*. As Steven Turner has written with respect to the learned professions in eighteenth-century Germany, possession of a university degree allowed its holder to claim membership in a social elite of learned gentlemen (*Gelehrtenstand*). It is essential to understand that such claims by the *Gelehrtenstand* to social distinction did not rest primarily upon their store of expert knowledge or its application in socially useful work.[23] It depended rather on the professional man's immersion in ancient literature, his Latin eloquence, and the broad erudition that defined him as an educated man in the humanist culture shared by himself and his patrons and patients. Harold Cook's work on the English medical profession in the seventeenth century has similarly emphasized the physician's gentlemanly character and his position as learned advisor to his patients.[24]

In this world, one of the crucial determinants of social position was a person's proximity to the center of authority. Patronage therefore mattered a great deal to making a successful professional career. And it is precisely here, when talking

21 Wilfred Prest, "Introduction: The Professions and Society in Early Modern England," in Prest, *Professions*, pp. 1–24, quoted on p. 17; Geoffrey Holmes, *Augustan England: Professions, State and Society, 1680–1730* (London, 1982), pp. 7–8.
22 Prest, "Introduction," pp. 14–15. Prest might have included with his "a's" army officers, a profession described at length by Holmes.
23 R. Steven Turner, "The *Bildungsbürgertum* and the Learned Professions in Prussia, 1770–1830: The Origins of a Class," *Social History/Histoire Sociale* 18 (1980): 105–35.
24 Harold J. Cook, "Good Advice and Little Medicine: The Professional Authority of Early Modern English Physicians," *Journal of British Studies* 33 (1994): 1–31; and idem, "The New Philosophy and Medicine in Seventeenth-Century England," in *Reappraisals of the Scientific Revolution*, ed. David C. Lindberg and Robert S. Westman (Cambridge, 1990), pp. 397–436.

about patronage, that we face the greatest danger of falling into an overly functionalist view of the professions. Patronage was neither a necessary evil with which
physicians as protoscientific experts had to contend, nor was it dependent primarily on the physician's skills as a healer.[25] To be sure, the care and healing of a
suitably influential patient often turned out to have happy consequences for the
physician as well. But patronage could be extended for a host of other reasons too:
reward for personal service or established family loyalty, displays of courtly majesty
and munificence, even simple bribery. As Colin Jones has written in his wonderful
account of the *médecins du roi* in France at the end of the old regime, "neither
scientific standing nor even prowess as a practitioner" were necessary for appointment as the king's *premier médecin,* nor, one would assume, for any of the other
several dozen medical posts in the royal household.[26] Of course these physicians
were installed to function as healers. But they also were simply *there* as part of the
spectacle of royal display. Court physicians functioned in other interesting ways as
well. As described recently by Bruce Moran and Pamela Smith, German princes
often extended patronage to physicians who doubled as ambassadors or administrators, or whose alchemical skills or commercial acumen promised monetary reward.[27]

If this brief portrait accurately captures the early modern medical profession,
then we now must ask what happened to transform this assortment of gentlemanly
erudits, advisors, scholars, court favorites, alchemists, hangers-on, and yes, healers,
into the modern scientific experts we know today. The "early modern" and
"modern" professions appear to be facing each other across a great chronological

25 It has become common currency among historians and sociologists that members of professions
chafed under the system of social deference and patronage in which they lived and worked.
Physicians, it is said, resented the fact that socially superior patients "dominated" their relationship
over the more technically expert physicians, and therefore the latter sought to professionalize as a
way of reversing this situation. An extremely influential version of this thesis stressing the role of
hospitals in changing the doctor/patient relationship is Ivan Waddington, "The Role of the
Hospital in the Development of Modern Medicine: A Sociological Analysis," *Sociology* 7 (1973):
211–24. Although physicians did complain repeatedly about patients' unwillingness to cooperate in
carrying out prescribed treatments and patients' demands that the physician "do something," such
complaints do not obviously reflect social resentments or a desire on the part of physicians for
"liberation" from deference. At least in German Central Europe, the world of eighteenth-century
physicians was so deeply structured by social hierarchy – and indeed their ambitions were so
thoroughly intertwined with those same hierarchies – that we must be careful about treating this
form of social organization as an obstacle in the path of professional progress.
26 Colin Jones, "The *Médecins du Roi* at the End of the *Ancien Régime* and in the French Revolution,"
in *Medicine at the Courts of Europe,* ed. Vivian Nutton (London, 1990), pp. 209–61, quoted on p.
217.
27 Bruce T. Moran, *The Alchemical World of the German Court: Occult Philosophy and Chemical Medicine
in the Circle of Moritz of Hessen (1572–1632),* Sudhoffs Archiv Beihefte, Heft 29 (Stuttgart, 1991);
idem, "Prince-Practitioning and the Direction of Medical Roles at the German Court: Maurice of
Hesse-Kassel and his Physicians," in Nutton, *Medicine at the Courts of Europe,* pp. 95–116; and idem,
"Patronage and Institutions: Courts, Universities, and Academies in Germany; an Overview: 1550–
1750," in *Patronage and Institutions: Science, Technology, and Medicine at the European Court 1500–1750,*
ed. Bruce T. Moran (Rochester, N.Y., 1991), pp. 169–183; Pamela H. Smith, "Alchemy as a
Language of Mediation at the Habsburg Court," *Isis* 85 (1994): 1–25.

and conceptual chasm, a chasm effectively accepted as real by much recent historiography. Historians of French medicine, most recently Toby Gelfand and Matthew Ramsey, have taken the structural upheavals of the French Revolution as providing a clean break from which a modern profession would emerge.[28] The passage of the Apothecaries Act (1815) does the same kind of work in Great Britain, effectively "depriviling" academically trained physicians by licensing surgeon-apothecaries for general practice, and creating the conditions in which a new profession could develop.[29] Finally, in Germany the breakup of the Holy Roman Empire in 1806 and the creation of the new "Humboldtian" university of Berlin in 1810 performs the same historiographic service.

This book treats the question of how the "older" medical profession changed into the "modern" one not as a problem of discontinuity, but rather as the transformation of a continuously existing elite. My central point is that the modern profession did not arise from the ruins of the old regime. Instead, it developed out of the adaptation of an established elite to new circumstances. To make this case, I will first locate university-educated physicians in their social and cultural context, a world in which bedside practice was but one facet of a complex identity (Chapter 1). The first crucial step in changing that world took place with the introduction of Enlightenment ideology during the second half of the eighteenth century, an ideology of utilitarian knowledge that began to break down physicians' corporate identity, forcing them to articulate a new vision of professionalism (Chapter 2). This movement toward a new professional identity was a long and not particularly placid process, as will be obvious when we turn to *Naturphilosophie* and Brunonianism, two contentious intellectual programs of the 1790s. The disagreements surrounding those two movements lent professional discourse a considerable measure of heat during the 1790s and 1800s, and in those disputes we can detect a profession attempting to find its place in the new political and cultural order of the dawning nineteenth century (Chapters 3–5). By the 1820s, when my story ends, that process of constructing a new professional identity had by no means ended. As we will see, however, some of its crucial foundations had been laid (Chapter 6).

This development in professional identity will be traced from a number of perspectives, but for my purposes two stand out as especially significant. The first of these is the emergence of a discourse of theory and practice. In my view, the

28 Matthew Ramsey, *Professional and Popular Medicine in France, 1770–1830* (Cambridge, 1988), pp. 71–125; and Toby Gelfand, *Professionalizing Modern Medicine: Paris Surgeons and Medical Science and Institutions in the Eighteenth Century* (Westport, Conn., 1980). Still enormously influential, too, are Michel Foucault, *The Birth of the Clinic*, trans. A. M. Sheridan Smith (New York, 1975); and Erwin Ackerknecht, *Medicine at the Paris Hospital, 1794–1848* (Baltimore, 1967), both of which argue the case for radical discontinuity.

29 Porter, "William Hunter"; Ivan Waddington, *The Medical Profession in the Industrial Revolution* (Dublin, 1984), pp. 9–28; and M. Jeanne Peterson, *The Medical Profession in Mid-Victorian London* (Berkeley, 1978), pp. 5–30, which invokes the traditional hierarchical division of the "medical profession" between physicians, surgeons, and apothecaries, but nonetheless describes the breakdown of this hierarchy during the early nineteenth century.

essential characteristic of the modern professions is not their legal monopolies over prescribed forms of social practice, nor their requirement for advanced education, nor their largely self-regulating structures. More than anything else, modern professions such as medicine are distinguished by their possession of scientifically validated theory from which they claim to derive concrete practices.[30] What allows those professionals to speak and practice as "experts" is nothing other than the explicit or implicit reference of their statements or actions to a coherent body of theoretical doctrine validated according to the norms of scientific practice.

The relationship between knowledge and the kind of power manifested in professional practices has been analyzed by a number of scholars, most famously by Michel Foucault in *Discipline and Punish*.[31] But Foucault did not translate his analysis of "discipline" into the social categories of the modern professions, nor did he or more recent commentators indicate the necessity of creating a link between theory and practice *in discourse* as the crucial element of professional identity. Yet I believe the discursive quality of the link is crucial. If modern professions such as medicine have authority and deploy a certain power through their practices, it is not merely because under the glare of critical scrutiny scientific theory turns out to be useful in the exercise of power. The authority and social status of professions derives instead from their deployment of an explicit, discursive linkage between theory and practice, and from the high valuation that our society places on the linkage.[32]

The ubiquity of theory-practice discourse today in medicine and other professions makes it easy for us to overlook the fact that the linkage is of relatively recent invention. German physicians in 1750 did not see themselves as scientific experts, and their education made little attempt to base therapeutic doctrines on theoretical principles. Moreover, when confronted by an Enlightenment ideology demanding a demonstration of the practical utility of their theories, physicians reacted in a complex way. They adopted stances that aligned them with the utilitarian advocates of social progress, but they also defended the social status derived from their command of esoteric and ancient knowledge. Ultimately, the tensions introduced

---

30 Not every profession makes such claims, of course. The law is a striking exception to this general pattern, which deserves more careful scrutiny from a comparative perspective than it has hitherto received. But even allowing for the exceptions provided by the law and other non science-based professions, there are a large number of professions that do claim to have a scientifically validated practice.

31 Michel Foucault, *Discipline and Punish: The Birth of the Prison,* trans. Alan Sheridan (New York, 1977). For commentaries on how Foucault's ideas apply to the professions, see Jan Goldstein, "Foucault among the Sociologists: The 'Disciplines' and the History of the Professions," *History and Theory* 23 (1984): 170–92; and Magali Sarfatti Larson, "In the Matter of Experts and Professionals, or How Impossible It Is to Leave Nothing Unsaid," in Torstendahl and Burrage, *The Formation of the Professions,* pp. 24–50.

32 I have argued this point more extensively in Thomas Broman, "Rethinking Professionalization: Theory, Practice and Professional Identity in Eighteenth-Century German Medicine," *The Journal of Modern History* 67 (1995): 835–72.

into professional identity by Enlightenment ideology were revealed in the 1790s by Brunonianism, a medical movement advocating the radical union of theory and practice. The uproar created by Brunonianism demonstrates beyond any doubt just how novel and threatening theory-practice discourses were at that time.

The second major perspective that informs this story is provided by the public sphere. The last decades of the eighteenth century marked the emergence in German-speaking Europe of what Jürgen Habermas described more than thirty years ago as the bourgeois public sphere, an arena of cultural activity where private individuals sought to speak for a "public" by defining objective standards of reason and taste. One of the most distinctive features of this new public sphere, and one of paramount importance for my story, is the emergence of the peculiarly modern institution of "criticism," embodied in new review periodicals and justified in the Enlightenment's appeal to the universality of reason.[33] Taking their cue from Habermas himself, most scholars of the eighteenth-century public sphere have interpreted criticism as the manifestation of a new kind of political discourse.[34] Yet the ramifications of the public sphere extended well beyond politics. As will become apparent in the discussion of *Naturphilosophie*, the practice of criticism also fundamentally reshaped the way that German intellectuals talked about nature, whether in the guise of natural philosophy or medicine. Furthermore, the creation of the public sphere gave physicians and other intellectuals an opportunity to conceive of their various social roles in new ways. Brunonianism and *Naturphilosophie* were as much debates over the nature of the medical profession and its place in the public sphere as over particular medical and scientific theories.

As I will show in the following narrative, the development of the public sphere played a uniquely important role in the evolution of the medical profession and the German universities between 1750 and 1820. It represented a new level of cultural self-awareness; in fact, it might not be too much of an exaggeration to say that the public sphere introduced the idea of "culture" as such into considerations

33 Jürgen Habermas, *The Structural Transformation of the Public Sphere,* trans. Thomas Burger with Frederick Lawrence (Cambridge, Mass., 1989), esp. pp. 14–56. See also Klaus Berghahn, "From Classicist to Classical Literary Criticism, 1730-1806," in *A History of German Literary Criticism,* ed. Peter Uwe Hohendahl (Lincoln, Neb., 1988), pp. 13–98. The wellspring for scholarship on the emergence of writers and the public sphere is Hans Gerth, *Bürgerliche Intelligenz um 1800: Zur Soziologie des deutschen Frühliberalismus* (Göttingen, 1976), originally published as a doctoral dissertation in 1935. For a recent critical appreciation of Habermas, see Anthony La Vopa, "Conceiving a Public: Ideas and Society in Eighteenth-Century Europe," *The Journal of Modern History* 64 (1992): 79–116.

34 See Keith Michael Baker, "Public Opinion as Political Invention," in idem, *Inventing the French Revolution: Essays on French Political Culture in the Eighteenth Century* (Cambridge, 1990) pp. 167–99; Roger Chartier, "The Public Sphere and Public Opinion," in idem, *The Cultural Origins of the French Revolution,* trans. Lydia G. Cochrane (Durham, N.C., 1991), pp. 20–37; Dena Goodman, *The Republic of Letters: A Cultural History of the French Enlightenment* (Ithaca, N.Y., 1994); and Hans Erich Bödeker, "Journals and Public Opinion: The Politicization of the German Enlightenment in the Second Half of the Eighteenth Century," in *The Transformation of Political Culture: England and Germany in the Eighteenth Century,* ed. Eckhart Hellmuth (Oxford, 1990), pp. 423–45. An excellent collection of essays on the public sphere that emphasizes its function in political discourse is *Habermas and the Public Sphere,* ed. Craig Calhoun (Cambridge, Mass., 1992).

of art, literature, and science.[35] This new understanding of culture would have important consequences for medicine and medical education, as we shall see. But perhaps even more intriguingly, I suspect that the emergence of the public sphere was a necessary condition for the articulation of the theory-practice discourse discussed above. After all, Brunonianism advocated the same vision of medicine as a scientific practice that would become the hallmark of the modern professions, and the debate over Brunonianism was an intensely public one. It would of course be overly simplistic – and certainly premature, based on the evidence presented in this book – to claim that the formation of the public sphere was uniquely or even primarily responsible for such a change. Yet I must confess that I find this possibility enormously attractive, even if the case for it cannot be made fully convincing at present.

35 Speaking about the eighteenth-century public sphere, Habermas claimed that "the fully developed bourgeois public sphere was based on the fictitious identity of the two roles assumed by the privatized individuals who came together to form a public: the role of property owners and the role of human beings pure and simple." As Habermas shows, this identity had two consequences. First, it allowed private individuals to defend their interests as property owners under the guise of speaking for "humanity" in general. Second, the experience of bourgeois family life, which Habermas labeled the "intimate sphere" in contrast to the "sphere of civil society," became the source for many of the values that would inform public debates over culture. Here again, the seeming universality of family life and its separation from the economic transactions of civil society made it possible for private individuals to speak about culture in the public sphere as if speaking for humanity, instead of from a narrowly bourgeois standpoint. Habermas, *Structural Transformation of the Public Sphere*, pp. 43–56.

1

Physicians in eighteenth-century Germany

THE IDEAL DOCTOR

During the eighteenth century, it was standard practice for medical professors to present their subjects as a series of lectures based on textbooks written either by themselves or by other scholars. Many professors preferred to write their own text, no doubt in part for the income they hoped to earn from its purchase by students, but they could just as reasonably select someone else's work if it suited their purposes. Thus one student, who enrolled at the Prussian university of Duisburg in 1763, recalled later that during his first semester he heard one of his professors lecture on surgery "from his own manuscript," and on anatomy "according to Heister's compendium."[1] More remarkable, perhaps, is what the student reported about the other member of the Duisburg medical faculty. From that professor, he wrote, "from 8–9 o'clock I heard physiology according to Boorhaave's [sic] compendium, from 9–10 o'clock pathology, likewise according to Boorhaave, and from 3–4 in the afternoon therapy, again from Boorhaave."[2]

Indolence surely had something to do with this complete reliance on Boerhaave, but the professor's contemporaries could scarcely have faulted his choice of authority, for Herman Boerhaave (1668–1738) was a figure of incomparable stature to eighteenth-century physicians. Time and again they invoked his authority in their writings, exalting him to an honored place in the pantheon of medical immortals. By the hundreds they flocked to the University of Leiden to hear him lecture on medicine, botany, and chemistry. One of those students, Gerard van Swieten (1700–72), under whose leadership the University of Vienna became one of Europe's leading medical centers, wrote that at the great man's funeral "the university, the town, the state, and indeed all men throughout the world were in mourning."[3] Albrecht von Haller (1708–77), himself a scholar of no middling

---

1 Carl Arnold Kortum, *Des Jobsiandichters Carl Arnold Kortum Lebensgeschichte, von ihm selbst erzählt*, ed. Dr. K. Deicke (Dortmund, 1910), p. 33.
2 Ibid., p. 34.
3 "Dum acerbum MAGNI BOERHAAVII funus Academia, Civitas, Respublica, imo per orbem terrarum lugerent omnes boni, . . ." Gerard van Swieten, *Commentaria in Hermanni Boerhaave Aphorismos de Cognoscendis et Curandis Morbis* (Leiden, 1766), Praefatio. Swieten went on to lament that

stature, called Boerhaave in a famous phrase the "teacher of all of Europe" (*communis Europae Praeceptor*), and Haller's own biographer, Johann Georg Zimmermann (1728–95), spoke reverently of the influence exerted by Boerhaave on Haller after the latter's arrival in Leiden in 1725. Above all else, Zimmermann emphasized Boerhaave's devotion to his students, claiming that no reward or inducement could lure him away from his teaching duties. Even Peter the Great, the Russian Czar, was forced to wait patiently an entire night outside Boerhaave's home "so that next morning he could hold a discussion with him on various portions of science before the commencement of [Boerhaave's] public lectures."[4]

Such eulogies could be piled up at will. These men, after all, were educated in the humanist tradition; unrestrained praise came to them as readily as bitter vilification. Yet the traces of Boerhaave's lingering influence on European medicine can be discerned from more than the fulsome words pronounced in his memory. His introductory textbook of medical theory, the *Institutiones medicae,* originally published in 1708, went through thirty-three Latin and twenty vernacular editions, most of them pirated and published in nearly every country in western Europe. Haller and Swieten devoted themselves to reproducing and commenting on different sets of Boerhaave's lectures, Haller in the *Praelectiones academicae, in proprias institutiones rei medicae* (Academic lectures on the particular institutes of medicine), and Swieten in the *Commentaria in Boerhaave aphorismos de cognoscendis et curandis morbis* (Commentary on Boerhaave's aphorisms on diagnosing and curing disease). These publications too were reissued throughout the eighteenth century.[5]

Boerhaave, in short, was one of those extraordinary individuals whom both contemporaries and later generations regarded with unmixed veneration. What can account for such an enormous presence by one man in the consciousness of eighteenth-century European physicians? Boerhaave's was not the talent of a Vesalius or a Harvey; his most prominent modern biographer concedes that he contributed no profound discoveries to science or medicine.[6] Rather what made Boerhaave a living embodiment of the ideal doctor was the astonishing breadth of his learning. He wrote, and wrote insightfully, on natural philosophy, chemistry, botany, physiology, pathology, therapeutics, even theology. Not only was he master of all these subjects, but his erudition comprehended the ancient sources as easily as the moderns. His treatises and textbooks drew upon the entire history of medicine and natural philosophy for their fiber and substance, from which Boerhaave, calling upon his gifts as a writer, fashioned an elegant and lucid prose. This

he had himself "suffered irreparable damage and lost the oracle that I had been able to consult in doubtful cases (*irreparabile damnum fecissem, & perdidissem oraculum, quod in rebus dubiis semper consulere licuit*)."
4 Johann Georg Zimmermann, *Das Leben des Herrn von Haller* (Zurich, 1755), pp. 26–27.
5 Complete publishing histories for Boerhaave's writings are compiled in *Bibliographia Boerhaaviana,* ed. G. A. Lindeboom (Leiden, 1959).
6 G. A. Lindeboom, "Hermann Boerhaave," in *Dictionary of Scientific Biography,* ed. Charles Coulston Gillispie, vol. 2 (New York, 1970), pp. 224–8.

order and clarity of presentation also made Boerhaave a celebrated teacher, but even to separate the qualities of a "scholar" and a "teacher" in this way would have been foreign to his way of thinking, so intimately did the sifting of knowledge find its embodiment and justification in the lecture hall.

Finally, in addition to Boerhaave's scholarly talents, he was a renowned practitioner, for whose advice and treatment patients came calling – either in person or by letter – from all over Europe.[7] Nor did his work at the bedside exist in isolation from his teaching, for Boerhaave also instructed students in the practice of medicine. His small teaching clinic in Leiden became a model that two generations of professors would later emulate. In this area too, he left his mark as a writer. His *Aphorismi de cognoscendis et curandis morbis* (Aphorisms on diagnosing and curing disease, 1709), the book on which Swieten's *Commentaria* would later be based, was published in more than forty Latin and vernacular editions.[8]

The esteem accorded Boerhaave by his fellow physicians tells us much about what they saw in themselves. Boerhaave was hailed for his scholarly erudition and literary elegance because erudition and elegance were the marks of the physician and the gentleman. Learnedness provided the badge by which physicians could recognize themselves in a society crowded with people who undertook to heal ailments. Boerhaave earned praise as a teacher because universities and the education they offered were the indispensable foundation for the existence of physicians as a professional group. Possession of a university degree validated an individual's claims to learnedness, and conferred upon the bearer right of entry into one of the three professions of theology, law, or medicine. Lastly, Boerhaave was celebrated as a healer and teacher of healing because what distinguished the physician from other learned men was partly built up from the bedside encounter between doctor and patient. The doctor of medicine was not only a scholar and teacher in the original Latin meaning of the word "doctor," but also a healer in our contemporary connotation.

Nowhere did the attachment of physicians to a scholarly ideal find its expression more distinctly than in a collection of medical biographies published between 1749 and 1753 by Friedrich Boerner (1723–60). Boerner, a medical professor at the University of Leipzig, used his *Nachrichten von den vornehmsten Lebensumständen und Schriften jetztlebender berühmter Aerzte und Naturforscher in und um Deutschland* (Reports on the foremost circumstances and writings of currently living, renowned physicians and natural philosophers in and around Germany) to celebrate the piety, virtue, and most of all the learnedness of his contemporaries. The biographies consisted of two portions, both of which underscored the scholarly achievements of Boerner's subjects. First, he presented a sketch of the person's education and career, which was based upon information solicited from the subject. To that description, which could be quite detailed, he then appended a

7 G. A. Lindeboom, *Herman Boerhaave. The Man and His Work* (London, 1968), pp. 306–9.
8 Lindeboom, *Bibliographia Boerhaaviana*, pp. 41–7.

comprehensive bibliography of the individual's publications, a list from which no writing, no matter how minor, was excluded.

The remarkable thing about the *Nachrichten* is the way Boerner shaped the information provided him to construct essentially the same story about each person's life. As a child, the subject was raised by parents who invariably took care to inculcate the deepest piety in him. Upon entering school, the child encountered talented teachers who provided him with the basic tools of higher studies and who awakened in him a desire for immersion in medicine, natural philosophy or, in some cases, theology (Boerner's subjects rarely displayed an interest in law). At somewhat greater length, Boerner then detailed the influence of the teachers who guided the young man during his time at university. No school was too inadequate, no diploma mill too disreputable, that he could not find something praiseworthy about it. In Boerner's hands, every university became a center of inspired teaching and profound scholarship.

Travel played a substantial role in these standard biographies. First, Boerner's subjects – along with many other students of the period – routinely divided their university studies between two or more schools. In his biography of Emanuel Christian Löber (1696–1763), for example, Boerner wrote that Löber began his medical education at the University of Jena in 1714, and moved over to the University of Halle in 1718, where he stayed one year "not without benefit," studying with the famous physicians Friedrich Hoffmann (1660–1742) and Georg Ernst Stahl (1660–1734), and with the philosopher Christian Friedrich Wolff (1679–1734). Then Löber, prompted by the writings of Boerhaave, took himself off to Leiden, where, Boerner assures us, the teachings of the great doctor "pushed deep roots into his heart." Löber next returned home (still without his doctoral degree) to begin his medical practice, but in 1721 he returned to Leiden to sit once more at the feet of the "Dutch Hippocrates." Finally, in 1722, Löber returned to Halle, finished the requirements for his degree, and began his career after eight years of study.[9]

A second type of travel consisted of tours undertaken by students at the end of their formal education. Boerner took pains to distinguish the scholarly aims of his subjects' travels from the "grand tours" conducted by aristocrats and countless other young men of means. "Scholars do not travel just to have traveled," he explained at one point, "they travel for the benefit of their fatherland and for the benefit of the science to which they have dedicated themselves."[10] Although tours of this sort commonly took place after graduation, they often included more or less formal courses of study with individual scholars, along with other contacts.

9 Friedrich Boerner, *Nachrichten von den vornehmsten Lebensumständen und Schriften jetztlebender berühmter Aerzte und Naturforscher in und um Deutschland*, Bd. 1 (Wolfenbüttel, 1749), pp. 667–9. Eight years was an unusually long time to spend on a medical degree. Many students were graduated with an M.D. within four years of first enrolling at a university.
10 Ibid., p. 627. For two accounts of the social and cultural functions of the Grand Tour, see Jeremy Black, *The British and the Grand Tour* (London, 1985); and William Edward Mead, *The Grand Tour in the Eighteenth Century* (1972 repr. of Boston, 1914).

One of Boerner's more luxuriant travel narratives tells the story of Christian Ludwig Mögling (1715–62), who began an extensive tour in 1735.[11] Armed with letters of introduction from his prince, the Duke of Württemberg, and from other notables, Mögling first visited the universities of Giessen and Marburg. At the latter school, he made the acquaintance of Christian Friedrich Wolff, who since Löber's time had been driven out of Halle because of questions over his religious orthodoxy. Mögling then continued north to Leiden – an absolutely *de rigueur* station before Boerhaave's death in 1738 – where he attended lectures and where he also came into contact with Linnaeus and Swieten. Mögling next journeyed to Paris, where, Boerner reports, he found attractions aplenty: "exquisite gardens, magnificent royal palaces there and in the neighboring region, [and] beautiful collections of curiosities from nature and art."[12] It must have all been most impressive to a young man from the Germanic provinces, for he stayed in Paris a full year. Aside from gawking at tourist attractions, he pursued more serious business with the city's renowned scientific and medical figures. According to Boerner, he studied chemistry with Lémery, botany with Jussieu, anatomy with Winslow, and surgery at the hospitals of the Charité and the Hotel Dieu. Meanwhile, the letters he had brought along gained him entry to the most elite salons, where among others he met the Cardinal de Polignac, President of the Académie Royale des Sciences, who offered Mögling an associate membership in that prestigious body. Mögling, feeling bound to his prince, declined, but did secure a letter of introduction from Polignac for use in Italy, his next destination. Traveling southward through the Rhone valley, Mögling paused briefly in Lyon, where he was made an honorary member of the local academy of science. In Italy, he visited Turin, Bologna, and Florence, where he met local scholars, inspected natural history cabinets, and marveled at the art. He next established himself in Rome, during which time he was presented to the Pope, Clement XII, and took a side trip to Naples, where he scaled Mt. Vesuvius. Upon leaving Rome he once again journeyed to Bologna, where he attended a public dissection, and then to Venice and Padua.[13] Finally, in March 1738, he arrived home in Württemberg, "happy and learned."

Descriptions such as this one occupied a central place in Boerner's *Nachrichten,* because travel figured crucially in the formation of a scholar. If learnedness consisted of the broad erudition exemplified by Boerhaave, then by what better means could a young man acquire such knowledge than through personal experience of extraordinary objects and places? It is noteworthy, however, that what counted most about travel was its presumed contribution to later scholarship. While Boerner did mention that Mögling studied surgery in Paris, the role of physicians as healers was scarcely visible in most of his biographies. No doubt this

---

11 Boerner, *Nachrichten,* Bd. 1, pp. 723–8.
12 Ibid., p. 723.
13 Boerner, perhaps by now short of breath, merely reports "in all these just-named places he found great scholars and noteworthy objects." Ibid., p. 128.

reflected the scholarly audience for whom they were primarily intended, but even in other writings directed at the broader public physicians emphasized their scholarly virtues. One sees this, for example, in *Der Arzt. Eine medicinische Wochenschrift* (The physician, a medical weekly), a journal of popular medical enlightenment published between 1759 and 1761 by a Hamburg physician, Johann August Unzer (1727–99). One of Unzer's primary concerns in his publication was to educate readers in making sound judgments about their health and about those who offered themselves as healers. To that end, he described how to distinguish a true doctor from a false one. A true doctor, he wrote, is someone who possesses three qualities: a great heart, a good faculty of reason, and the appropriate learnedness.[14]

The term used by Unzer to designate the learnedness of the true physician, *Gelehrsamkeit,* was the word most commonly used to denote those qualities attributed to Boerhaave and the subjects of Boerner's *Nachrichten.* Learnedness alone did not make the practitioner, however, and Unzer cautioned readers not to allow the possession of degrees and other testimonials to deceive them about someone's ability to treat illness effectively. A practitioner who could not reason well – and by "reason" (*Vernunft*) he was referring to the ability to apply general principles to particular cases, what was called "practical reason" – could have all the *Gelehrsamkeit* in the world and still not be able to do anything at the bedside. Yet *Gelehrsamkeit* was indispensable to the physician, for it provided him with the tools for penetrating to the true causes of an ailment and eliminating those causes. There were plenty of healers around who could set a broken bone, cauterize a wound, or assist at a birth. But only the learned doctor possessed those deep insights into nature that permitted him to understand the origins and development of the more complicated ailments of humanity.

Whether presenting themselves to other well-educated people or to a wider slice of the literate public, physicians rarely failed to cloak themselves in the mantle of *Gelehrsamkeit.* That they should do so is hardly surprising, for these physicians lived at a time when both they and their patrons had been thoroughly schooled in the humanist values of eloquence and erudition. The self-image that physicians sought to cultivate did not depend particularly on picturing themselves as experts, for anyone professing such a thing would have seemed narrow and crude. To the extent doctors did claim expertise – and they could scarcely have dispensed with it entirely – they based that claim not so much on any specious scientific "rigor," but instead on an intensive engagement with the subject of health and illness, which produced both breadth and depth of experience.

If physicians were unable to claim nobility of birth, the professional image they held attempted to substitute the next best thing: a nobility of books. Their dignity rested on the authority they held over a portion of the European cultural tradition,

14 "Von dem Charakter der wahren und falschen Aerzte," *Der Arzt. Eine medicinische Wochenschrift,* Neue Auflage, Teil 1, Stück 1 (Hamburg, 1767), pp. 3–16, esp. 9–11.

a tradition of writings that linked the eighteenth century to a fabulous yet palpably real Golden Age of antiquity. With this description in mind, then, we must now situate it in some real historical circumstances, by addressing two problems. First, what currency did this image hold? Did physicians' presentation of themselves correspond to a position of respect and authority in society? What kind of authority was it? Second, how was this professional image cultivated and transmitted? How did medical faculties – the institutions charged with this task – perform their function? These questions will occupy us for the rest of the chapter.

PHYSICIANS IN SOCIETY

The eighteenth-century healing business suffered no lack of willing participants. No matter where he lived, a doctor was likely to find himself surrounded by all kinds of people who took it upon themselves to render advice on health matters. A number of occupations in early modern Europe were directly tied to some aspect of healing: surgeons, barbers, midwives, the operators of bathing establishments, and apothecaries. These people not only practiced their particular specialty, but also frequently ventured outside it, as numerous legal complaints attest. Alongside these regular healers, there existed a more shadowy – or shady – group of urine-gazers, stone cutters, drug peddlers, and charlatans of various stripes, itinerant both by trade and/or necessity, frequenters of local fairs and markets, who provided reformers with a politically painless target for their indignation. Finally, there existed one final group, poorly understood by historians, whose healing activities comprised the routine occurrences of community life: wise women and men possessed of quasimagical powers, wives, mothers, and other relatives and neighbors, who often administered care during the initial stages of an illness and who supervised it after outsiders were summoned to help.[15]

Amidst this plethora of healers the physician had to make his living, and often it was not easy. The credentials which he brought with him, his university degree, his erudition and command of Latin, meant little to the large majority of the population. It was not merely that rural peasants had enjoyed little or none of the formal schooling that would permit them to appreciate the physician's gifts, but they possessed their own culture and world view, one somewhat at variance with the physician's own beliefs.[16] Although this does not mean that physicians were

---

15 For two superb portraits of medical practice in eighteenth-century Germany, see Barbara Duden, *Geschichte unter der Haut: Ein Eisenacher Arzt und seine Patientinnen um 1730* (Stuttgart, 1987); and Mary Lindemann, *Health and Healing in Eighteenth-Century Germany* (forthcoming fall 1996, Johns Hopkins Univ. Press). See also Robert Jütte, *Ärzte, Heiler, und Patienten: Medizinischer Alltag in der frühen Neuzeit* (Munich, 1991); and for France, Matthew Ramsey, *Professional and Popular Medicine in France, 1770–1830* (Cambridge, 1988), esp. pp. 229–276.

16 Not too long ago, historians favored the model of two mostly distinct cultures in the early modern world, an attitude represented by Ramsey, *Professional and Popular Medicine in France*; Robert Muchembled, *Popular Culture and Elite Culture in France, 1400–1750* trans. Lydia Cochrane (Baton Rouge, La., 1985); David Sabean, *Power in the Blood: Popular Culture and Village Discourse in Early*

shut out from practicing among the peasantry, it does suggest the physician's dependence upon the thin stratum of society that shared his education: princes and their entourage of courtiers, government bureaucrats, churchmen, lawyers, educated businessmen and town officials. Even here the way was not easy. A few unsuccessful cases, especially at the beginning of a career, could cause a doctor to lose favor among his patrons, and trust once lost was difficult to regain.

The most difficult times came when a newly graduated doctor was just starting out. A young physician could not just hang out his shingle anywhere; towns in early modern Germany were little enclaves exceptionally closed to outsiders. While towns might welcome journeymen craftsmen to their workshops and tradesmen to their fairs, the former were expected to be under the watchful eye of local guild masters, and both journeymen and tradesmen were expected to disappear when their allotted time in the town had run out. Fearing another addition to the welfare rolls, town elders cast a suspicious eye on any stranger who arrived and proclaimed his intention of staying.[17] Even without run-ins with municipal elders, strangers faced obstacles to making a living, for residents were often unwilling to lend their trust and health to someone they did not know, someone who had not been chased from their gardens as a child and whose confirmation they had not attended.

For this reason, a young doctor often began practicing in his home town, although even there it was likely to be trying. When Friedrich von Hoven (1759–1838) returned home to the town of Ludwigsburg soon after taking his M.D. at the University of Stuttgart in early 1781, he found the available patients had largely been divided between the two established doctors. For a beginner, he wrote years later in his autobiography, "there remained nothing but the poor, who pay a doctor solely with their praise, as well as patients given up on by the others," who in desperation turn to the nearest available doctor.[18] Try as he might, Hoven was unable to make much progress and his practice remained confined largely to the poor. Even there, he reported, it grew slowly, "since the very first patient I received suffered from a typhoid-type fever and died shortly thereafter, along with several others."[19] Only four years later, in 1785, would Hoven's fortunes begin to

---

Modern Germany (Cambridge, 1984); Carlo Ginzburg, *The Cheese and the Worms*, trans. John and Anna Tedeschi (Baltimore, 1980); Peter Burke, *Popular Culture in Early Modern Europe* (New York, 1978); Natalie Zemon Davis, *Society and Culture in Early Modern Europe* (Stanford, Calif., 1975); and Keith Thomas, *Religion and the Decline of Magic* (New York, 1971). Working from the perspective of how medicine was practiced, this separation has been vigorously criticized by Roy Porter's, *Health for Sale: Quackery in England 1660–1850* (Manchester, 1989); and Lindemann, *Health and Healing in Eighteenth-Century Germany*, esp. chaps. 4 and 5. My own position is somewhat middling. I accept the overwhelming evidence amassed by Lindemann discounting the rigidity of the boundary between "elite" and "popular" medical cultures, yet I remain convinced that the ongoing academic medical tradition gave university-trained physicians a sense of their practice that did not necessarily resonate widely in society.

17 Mack Walker, *German Home Towns: Community, State, and the General Estate 1648–1871* (Ithaca, N.Y., 1971), pp. 77–92, 102–7.

18 Friedrich von Hoven, *Lebenserinnerungen* (Berlin, 1984), p. 82.

19 Ibid.

change. In the meantime, he pursued further scientific studies and began writing a treatise on fevers that would be published in 1789.

In the face of the kind of obstacles encountered by Hoven, it is not surprising that many doctors were the sons or grandsons of doctors. Even the most learned beginner, Hoven wrote, must have a doctor for a father, or he must have close ties to the leading families in town, or marry into one of them. In his own case, however, none of these situations prevailed. His father was a junior officer in the Württemberg army, with no useful connections.[20] And indeed, his practice began to grow only when he received a crucial endorsement. One day, a certain "prominent and wealthy gentleman" in Ludwisgburg fell ill and, as was his custom, summoned from nearby Stuttgart one of the leading doctors, a personal physician to the Duke of Württemberg and professor at the University. This doctor, named Hopfengärtner, had been one of Hoven's teachers and was a special mentor of his. After visiting the patient two or three times, Hopfengärtner decided he was no longer in any danger, and recommended that Hoven be called in to supervise the rest of the recovery. On this basis Hoven was engaged, and when the patient recovered he continued on as the family's doctor. "From the [subsequent] growth of my practice," Hoven recalled, "I soon realized what the recommendation of a physician so highly regarded in Ludwigsburg had accomplished for me."[21]

In many ways, medical practice seen at the local level had a distinctly guild-like quality to it. Formal guilds existed, of course, for certain healers, such as surgeons, barbers, and apothecaries. But doctors of medicine too seemed to exhibit a guild mentality in the way sons could claim the family business as their birthright, and in the acceptance by physicians of the diversity of healers. Rather than seeking to gain an economic advantage at the expense of other groups, physicians chose social stability over competition. At no time during the eighteenth century does one hear German physicians calling for elimination of other healers or restriction on their rightful activities.

The key word here is "rightful," for doctors complained bitterly and unceasingly about infringements by other healers against the ordained spheres of action. They denounced such healers as *Pfuscher*, a term so enmeshed in its social and cultural context that it is untranslatable. The modern dictionary rendering of *Pfuscher* is "bungler," and indeed eighteenth-century writers meant to portray *Pfuscher* as incompetent. But the incompetence of a *Pfuscher* derived not from an inherent lack of ability or knowledge but from the fact that he or she was an interloper, a transgressor.[22] An apothecary may be skilled at concocting medicaments, but becomes a *Pfuscher* when attempting to prescribe them, just as a master wheelwright is not qualified to be a carpenter. In fact, writers readily

20 Ibid., p. 91.
21 Ibid., p. 92.
22 The definitive account of *Pfuscherey* is Lindemann, *Health and Healing in Eighteenth-Century Germany*, chap. 3; see also Manfred Stürzbecher, *Beiträge zur Berliner Medizingeschichte* (Berlin, 1966), pp. 134–8.

acknowledged that physicians could be *Pfuscher* as well by undertaking healing activities not proper to them.[23] The learnedness or *Gelehrsamkeit* of a physician therefore was not a claim to monopolization of the healing market, as the claim to science (*Wissenschaft*) would become in the nineteenth century.[24]

Despite the outcry raised by physicians against *Pfuscherey*, transgressions of perceived boundaries in the healing market occurred regularly, and given the structure of society most of these worked to the disadvantage of physicians. When the circumstances of medical practice are taken together, it is easy to see why physicians were not a very numerous group in the early modern world. The market for healing was highly fragmented, the potential clientele for physicians among wealthy or well-educated people was narrow, and the establishment of trust among the population was laborious where it was not short-circuited by family tradition or connections. We may well wonder, therefore, that anyone would take the trouble to obtain an M.D. when making a living from it appeared to be so precarious. The answer is that possession of an M.D., while perhaps of only limited value at the bedside, opened the door to a series of paid official positions that were the domain of physicians alone. These offices comprised a hierarchy of governmental service that began at the lowest levels with the town or district doctor, or *Physicus,* and the official doctor to the local army garrison.[25] At somewhat higher levels, a physician could aspire to appointment as court physician (*Hofmedicus*) to a prince or church prelate, or installation as personal physician (*Leibarzt*) to a lower member of the nobility. Next came appointment as professor of medicine at a university, and at the top stood the personal physicians to the great princes, kings, and prelates of the Empire and professors at the most prestigious universities.[26]

Few of these offices, it should be noted, came with a salary commensurate with

23 In the Palatinate, physicians were prohibited in 1775 from undertaking external cures "without the aid of a surgeon." Eberhard Stübler, *Geschichte der medizinischen Fakultät der Universität Heidelberg 1386–1925* (Heidelberg, 1926), p. 131. See also the comments of an anonymous writer in "Ueber die Münsterschen Medizinalgeseze," *Deutsches Museum,* Bd. 1 (1778), p. 32.

24 Claudia Huerkamp, *Der Aufstieg der Ärzte im 19. Jahrhundert* (Göttingen, 1985), pp. 56–110.

25 As a legal stipulation, positions in the bureaucracy were expressly reserved for doctors of medicine only occasionally, as in the dioceses of Würzburg in 1743 and Münster in 1777. See *Sammlung der hochfürstlich-wirzburgischen Landesverordnungen,* Teil 2 (Würzburg, 1776), p. 355; *Unterricht von dem Kollegium der Aerzten in Münster wie der Unterthanen bey allerhand ihm zustoßenden Krankheiten die sichersten Wege und besten Mittel treffen kann seyne verlohrene Gesundheit wieder zu erhalten nebst den Münsterschen Medizinalgesetzen entworfen* (Münster, 1777), p. 140. In a few other states, laws stipulated that all practitioners of internal healing have an M.D., which by implication applied to *Physici.* "Churfürstlich-Pfälzische Medizinalordnung für die Herzogthümer Julich und Berg," *Archiv der medizinischen Polizey und der gemeinnützigen Arzneikunde* 3 (1785): 28. But as a matter of practice, such positions rarely went to anyone but holders of the M.D., or, in some cases, to holders of another university degree, the license. The difference between these two degrees will be explained below.

26 A few comparable offices did exist for other healers, such as court surgeon, personal surgeon, and court apothecary. But they were far less extensive than the positions available to doctors. Stürzbecher, *Beiträge zur Berliner Medizingeschichte,* pp. 146–7; and Alexander von Hoffmeister, *Das Medizinalwesen im Kurfürstentum Bayern* (Munich, 1975), p. 97. On the general problem of starting out in practice and advancing through the medical hierarchy, see Mary Nagle Wessling, *Medicine and Government in Early Modern Württemberg* (Ph.D. diss., University of Michigan, 1988), pp. 19–23.

the needs of providing for a family. Only those at the top of the pyramid offered incomes sufficient to enable the holder to live as he believed befitted his station. But at all levels an individual could accumulate and combine offices. Thus during the eighteenth century many medical professors also held the office of *Physicus* in their local town or district, and such combinations were sometimes used to recruit faculty members. When the University of Giessen attempted to attract the anatomist August Schaarschmidt (1720–91) to its medical faculty in 1763, for example, it offered him not only a professoriate, but also the positions of *Physicus* and doctor to a local cloister. It was also not unknown for one individual to be *Physicus* for several districts.[27]

Friedrich von Hoven was one such doctor who rose through the medical ranks. Even before he received the crucial recommendation that gained him entry into the homes of prominent families, he had begun to mount the ladder comprising the medical hierarchy. Ludwigsburg, his home town, hired two *Physici* to supervise medical affairs, and at the time Hoven began practicing these positions were filled by the same colleagues who also divided most of the private practice between them. In 1785, however, the more senior of these doctors died, creating a vacancy for town doctor. The surviving *Physicus* advanced into the first and better salaried position, and Hoven, owing no doubt to his familiarity, references, and the fact that he was the only other M.D. in town, was made the second *Physicus*. He had every reason to expect that upon the death of the first *Physicus* he would advance into that office as well, but he was passed over for that position not once but twice.[28] Hoven ultimately did secure that position, and much more, going on to become a professor at the University of Würzburg and still later director of hospitals in Nuremburg.

A somewhat different path was followed by Joseph F. X. Rehmann. Rehmann was born in 1757, in the town of Waldkirch, where his father was *Physicus*. After graduating from the University of Freiburg in 1778 and traveling to Vienna for further clinical study, he received appointments as district and town doctor in the same principality, although not the same town, where he grew up. In 1781, compelled by what he claimed were the impoverished circumstances of his office

---

27 Negotiations with Schaarschmidt are contained in Archiv Universität Giessen, Med K4: *Dozenten der Medizinischen Fakultät*, "Die Wiederbesetzung der professoribus medicinae primariae betreffend." For holders of multiple appointments as *Physicus*, see biographical information provided for Joseph Anton Weltin, Leonhard Edel, Anton Hagg (whose attempt to combine two *Physicus* positions was denied), and Anton Mayer, in Karl Jäck and E. Th. Nauck, *Zur Geschichte des Sanitätswesens im Fürstentum Fürstenberg* (Allensbach, 1951), pp. 74–5, 85, 89, 91. This book is one of the few local studies of health care in early modern Germany to provide biographical information on the holders of official positions. From these biographies it is evident that certain families were able to establish quasi-hereditary claims to medical offices.

28 Hoven, *Lebenserinnerungen*, pp. 83, 92–95. Hoven reported that the first time he was passed over it was probably due to his youth and relative inexperience. The second time, however, the job was given to someone his own age. From unnamed contacts, Hoven learned that this new man had paid the Duke "two hundred *Louis d'ors*" for the preferment. This seems an excessive amount to pay for the position, but perhaps the explanation lies in the town's strategic location. The new man had previously been *Physicus* in an outlying town, and he may have hoped that by moving to Ludwigsburg, one of the Duke's two residences, he could advance in the Württemberg court.

and practice, Rehmann initiated what would become a series of petitions for appointment to the medical faculty at Freiburg, applying first to be appointed professor of veterinary medicine, then in 1783 to be demonstrator (*Prosector*) of anatomy, and finally professor of physiology in 1784. All efforts were fruitless. His prospects improved markedly in 1787, when he was appointed personal physician to the prince of Fürstenberg, but Rehmann's maneuverings for a position at Freiburg were not at an end. In 1792, informed by friends that the way stood open for him to take a vacant professoriate in Freiburg, Rehmann confided to his patron that he would just as soon remain in his service if only he could secure some additional salary. The prince responded appropriately, and Rehmann remained with him until the principality was dissolved by Napoleon in 1806, whereupon he assumed positions in the newly enlarged Duchy of Baden.[29]

The opportunity that physicians had to advance in government service lifted them outside of the local civic and social fabric, but it also placed them in an anomalous position. For if on the one hand a physician dealt with patients as a neighbor and as one healer among the many regular participants in town life, on the other hand by being appointed to office he became a creature of state government, and therefore an intruder and agent of outside powers. To be sure, part of the physician's "otherness" derived from his university education. Holders of university degrees acquired their social position from a source outside of the normal constitution of burger and peasant society. Those tensions became intensified when a doctor assumed an office such as *Physicus*. The origins of the office lay as far back as the plague years of the fourteenth century, when the first doctors were appointed by towns to supervise precautions against epidemics. But not until the devastation and epidemics of the Thirty Years War did the practice of appointing town doctors become widespread.[30] From the beginning the office had two principal duties connected with it, aside from extraordinary periods of epidemic: care for the indigent poor and supervision of other healers. The latter job in particular involved inspection of apothecaries to ensure that they used approved medicaments prepared in a satisfactory manner and were charging a fair price for them.[31]

By the eighteenth century, *Physici* had become in most places agents of territorial, not municipal, authority. Their role as quarantine officers had diminished

29 Jäck and Nauck, *Geschichte des Sanitätswesens*, pp. 76–8. Similar stories about angling for positions as *Physicus* are related by Wessling, *Medicine and Government in Early Modern Württemberg*, pp. 72–103. Wessling emphasizes in particular the role of family connections – including strategic marriages – and political allegiances in awarding of *Physicus* offices.

30 The town of Aachen listed a doctor in the town's pay for the first time in 1346, which was just before the plague struck western Europe. Egon Schmitz-Cliever, *Die Heilkunde in Aachen von römischer Zeit bis zum Anfang des 19. Jahrhunderts*. Sonderdruck aus der Zeitschrift des Aachener Geschichtsvereins, Bd. 74/75 (Aachen, 1963), p. 26. See also Manfred Stürzbecher, "The Physici in German-Speaking Countries from the Middle Ages to the Enlightenment," in *The Town and State Physician in Europe from the Middle Ages to the Enlightenment*, ed. Andrew W. Russell, Wolfenbütteler Forschungen Band 17 (Wolfenbüttel, 1981), pp. 123–30.

31 The town of Baden in the Aargau appointed its first *Stadtmedicus* in 1627. In 1665, the town council developed guidelines for his duties, including: (1) free treatment of the poor; (2) provision

with the receding threat of plague, but new duties had taken their place. This can be seen in the order from 1762 appointing Joseph Daniel Engelberger as *Physicus* for the small landgravate of Baar in southwestern Germany. The order instructed Engelberger first to obey the authority of the prince who appointed him (whose dominion included the landgravate of Baar as one of several territories) and the prince's counselors, as well as to cooperate with local officials in the landgravate. He was further ordered to care for all patients as diligently and cheaply as possible, especially the poor; to inspect apothecaries for the quantity and quality of their wares; to keep a watch on the local surgeons, barbers, and bathkeepers to see that they adhered to their proper responsibilities, and also to examine those who wished to be approved to engage in surgery; to admonish healers who were not operating within prescribed limits and to report those who continued to do so; and finally to instruct and examine midwives in their craft. For all this Engelberger was promised the respectable annual salary of 400 fl (*Gulden*), 24 fl toward rent of a house, 20 cords of wood, along with quantities of oats, hay, and straw toward the upkeep of two horses.[32] Although it was not specified in the order, Engelberger presumably had the right to receive a fee for inspection of apothecary shops and examination of other healers, extra sources of income that were available to *Physici* elsewhere.[33]

The supervisory powers held by *Physici* in theory were extensive, as Engelberger's example attests, but it is doubtful that they translated into practice. Insofar as every *Physicus* was also required to earn his bread by caring for patients and cooperating with other healers and local authorities, it did not pay for him to be too aggressive in enforcing the medical codes or reporting irregularities to the central government. In the small communities where he operated, those apothecaries and midwives whom he attempted to cite were likely to have a brother-in-law or a cousin capable of repaying the *Physicus* for his zeal. For this reason, the increasing demands placed on *Physici* by princely governments during the eighteenth century, without giving them salaries sufficient for independence from bedside practice, put them in the impossible situation of being neither fully bureaucratic agents nor local healers. As we shall see in the next chapter, govern-

of prescriptions to victims during epidemics, although he was not required to visit them ("*jedoch nit schuldig sein, die inficierten zue besuechen*"); and (3) inspection of apothecaries. The council also recommended the appointment of a lower level *Stadtarzt*, whose duties, among other things, would include visiting patients during epidemics. Ida Wehrli, *Das öffentliche Medizinalwesen der Stadt Baden im Aargau von der Gründung des Spitals 1349–1798* (Aarau, 1960), pp. 58–62, which includes a reprint of the 1665 guidelines.

32 The order is reprinted in Jäck and Nauck, *Geschichte des Sanitätswesens*, pp. 111–17.

33 These arrangements were in every way typical of the duties of *Physici* in other parts of Germany. See Wessling, *Medicine and Government in Early Modern Württemberg* for Württemberg; Lindemann, *Health and Healing in Eighteenth-Century Germany*, chap. 2, for Braunschweig-Wolfenbüttel; and von Hoffmeister, *Das Medizinalwesen im Kurfürstentum Bayern*, pp. 52–5, for Bavaria. According to a mandate issued by the Bavarian government in 1756, bathkeepers and apothecaries in towns outside of Munich were to be examined by *Physici*, who were also instructed to examine the wares of anyone desiring to sell remedies at local markets. "Mandat die Aerzte, Apotheker, und Baader betreffend," in *Sammlung der neust und merkwürdigsten Churbaierischen Generalien und Landesordnungen* ed. W. X. A. Kreitmayr (Munich, 1771), pp. 444–6.

ments responded to this situation by creating centralized medical boards that usurped many of the privileges – as well as some of the income – of the town and district doctors.

As representatives of princely government, official physicians may have been in an uncomfortable situation, but they could scarcely have dispensed with the linkages to government entirely. For it was precisely this recognition that made doctors of medicine preeminent among healers. It gave them entry to the highest levels of court life, and it held out the possibility for social position and economic security. Although the full advantages fell to only a few individuals, the profession as a whole was supported by those institutions through which doctors were guaranteed a dominant role in healing, if not monopolistic control over it.

THE UNIVERSITIES AND MEDICAL EDUCATION

As members of a learned profession, physicians were yoked inseparably to the universities. It was a university degree that defined someone as a physician and distinguished him from other healers. At the same time, universities existed primarily – and at many universities, exclusively – to supply state and society with men trained in the professions of theology, law, and medicine. Those additional functions that we associate with modern American universities, such as providing a general liberal education for undergraduates and advancing knowledge through research, received at best a secondary emphasis in the universities of eighteenth-century Germany.

Most young men entered upon medical study between the ages of eighteen and twenty, directly after completing their secondary education. As a formal require-ment, no one was supposed to enroll in one of the three "higher" university faculties without first obtaining a master of arts degree in the philosophical faculty, but students who had received the appropriate training at a respectable secondary school were routinely waived through.[34] The choice of which university to attend was usually a simple one: the local school, if there was one. Aside from obvious considerations such as familiarity with the local customs, religion, and dialect, students could also expect to make contacts at the territorial university that would prove useful in their later careers. Finally, the choice was also influenced by the simple fact that many princes issued decrees ordering their subjects to spend at least a few semesters at the territorial university. Failure to do so would put them at a disadvantage in applying for government offices. Because these offices were the major reason for attending the university in the first place, this was potentially a serious threat.[35]

---

34 This was not so often the case at the Catholic universities, where Jesuit domination of the philosophical faculties insured that most students would be required to take a master's degree first.
35 On the attempts to limit the exodus of students from Prussia, see Reinhold Koser, "Friedrich der Große und die preußischen Universitäten," *Forschungen zur Brandenburgischen und Preußischen Ge-schichte* 17 (1904): 95–155, esp. pp. 131–2. In Bavaria, a decree issued in 1796 reiterated previous

Not enough is known about the social background of most medical students. Nobles clearly did not regard medicine as a suitable career for their sons, but aside from this the picture is sketchy.[36] Obviously, in light of what was said above about the importance of connections in making a career, a large portion of medical students were the sons, nephews, or grandsons of doctors. In Protestant territories, sons of clerics also furnished a significant group of medical students, while lawyers' sons shunned it. Finally, a third major group of medical students had fathers working in other branches of healing, such as surgeons or apothecaries.[37]

decrees of 1777, 1780, and 1792, which prohibited Bavarian students from attending non-Bavarian universities, unless the student had family or a benefactor elsewhere who would provide free room and board. The repetition of the decrees suggests they were not adhered to very scrupulously. On the other hand, graduates of local universities clearly enjoyed some preference, as Ingrao's study of the bureaucracy of Hesse-Kassel demonstrates. See Charles Ingrao, *The Hessian Mercenary State: Ideas, Institutions, and Reform Under Frederick II, 1760–1785* (Cambridge, 1987), p. 29(n).

36 Not only can one scarcely find a "von" among any of the physicians who published something or who otherwise appear in the historical record during the 1700s (apart from those who received an honorific ennoblement for their services), but Charles McClelland's research shows that nobles overwhelmingly preferred law, if they took up professional study at all. See Charles E. McClelland, *State, Society, and University in Germany, 1700–1914* (Cambridge, 1980), pp. 46–57.

37 Martina Beese, *Die medizinische Promotionen in Tübingen 1750–1799* (Tübingen, 1977), p. 57, provides information on 144 students who were awarded degrees during the second half of the eighteenth century. Thirty-eight (26 percent) of the graduates' fathers were physicians, 32 (22 percent) were clerics, and 26 (18 percent) made their living as healers other than physicians. A fourth major group of students (15 percent) were the sons of minor civic officials. Other occupational groups consisted of teachers, government councilors, merchants and tradesmen, and craftsmen and laborers. A survey of the biographies published by Boerner in his *Nachrichten* and by Ernst Gottfried Baldinger in *Biographien jetztlebender Aerzte und Naturforscher in und ausser Deutschland*, 3 Stücke (Jena, 1768–1772) produces the following occupational groups:

Father's occupation	Number of students	%
Clerics (including high church officials)	29	25
Physicians	25	22
Surgeons and apothecaries	17	15
Other professors	9	8
Jurists and high government officials	9	8
Merchants and tradesmen	8	7
Total	97	85

Sample size: 114

Other occupations included innkeeper, chamber musician, shoemaker, butcher, blacksmith, tax collector, and various other minor government officials. The fathers' occupations of twenty subjects were not given and were not included in the sample size. These results from Boerner and Baldinger should be treated with some caution, because they were drawn from elite physicians. Yet the general resemblance to the group described by Beese is unmistakable.

The backgrounds of graduates from the Catholic University of Ingolstadt between 1780 and 1800 are also known, but yield a somewhat different picture. Of this group, only 21 percent were the sons of doctors or other healers. Noteworthy at Ingolstadt is the relatively broad spectrum of occupations, including a large number of students from non-learned backgrounds. There were sons of twelve millers, ten brewers, nine bakers, four butchers, four weavers, and so on. Also remarkable

Medical students were likely to find themselves among a tiny minority in most universities. Outside of large medical faculties at Halle, Leipzig, Jena, and Göttingen, most universities did not have more than a dozen medical students at any one time. In the 1760s, the University of Heidelberg had between seven and ten medical students, approximately the same number as at Tübingen, Erlangen, and Erfurt. The Bavarian University of Ingolstadt did somewhat better, averaging seventeen to twenty students in the 1760s and 1770s. But other schools could not even maintain these modest levels. At the University of Fulda, for example, only four students enrolled in medicine during the entire decade of the 1770s.[38] And then there was the Prussian University of Frankfurt an der Oder. When the government inquired in 1766 why there had been no public medical lectures for several years and accused the professors of indolence, the faculty blandly replied that there had been no lectures because there were no students to hear them.[39]

In most German universities, there was no required curriculum in the higher faculties. There was, however, a widely accepted sequence of courses. Assuming that a student already had taken the necessary preliminaries such as ancient and modern languages, mathematics, and experimental physics, most writers agreed that medical study should begin with anatomy and physiology, together with the required auxiliary sciences of botany and chemistry. At the next level, students would take general and special pathology, two subjects that taught the causes and

were the number of peasants' sons who were graduated as physicians from Ingolstadt. Of 240 graduates, 29 (12 percent) listed their father's occupation as "agricola," "rusticus," or "colonia." Of course, there were no clerics' sons at Ingolstadt, at least none who acknowledged it publicly. Rainer A. Müller, "Studium und Studenten an der Medizinischen Fakultät der Universität Ingolstadt im 18. Jahrhundert," *Sammelblatt des historischen Vereins Ingolstadt* 83 (1974): 187–240, esp. 201–2.

The above data tend to underrepresent the number of students from medical families, because only fathers' occupations are counted. More distant though still significant relatives who could have aided entry into the profession, such as grandfathers and uncles, are thereby left out.

38 According to Franz Eulenberg, 310 medical students matriculated at Halle during the decade 1761–70, whereas Göttingen drew 204 students. Assuming a course of study of three years, the medical student population during the 1760s was about 95 at Halle and 60 at Göttingen. See Franz Eulenberg, "Die Frequenz der deutschen Universitäten von ihrer Gründung bis zur Gegenwart," *Abhandlungen der philologisch-historischen Klasse der königlichen sächsischen Gesellschaft der Wissenschaften* 24, no. 2 (1906): 308–313. Comparable figures for Jena in the 1760s are not available in Eulenberg; however, one source reports that Jena had about 100 medical students during both semesters in the year 1788. Ernst Giese and Benno von Hagen, *Geschichte der medizinischen Fakultät der Friedrich-Schiller-Universität Jena* (Jena, 1958), pp. 325–326. The matriculation lists at Leipzig did not list students according to faculty, but the university did keep records of the number of promotions. Between 1761 and 1770, Leipzig awarded 119 medical degrees. Once again taking an average of three years for the course of study, that yields around 35 medical students at any one time during the decade. The figure for Leipzig is from Ernst Theodor Nauck, "Die Zahl der Medizinstudenten deutscher Hochschulen im 14.-18. Jahrhundert," *Sudhoffs Archiv* 38 (1954): 175–86. Although Tübingen averaged 15–17 medical students during the 1760s, that total declined to 9–11 in the 1770s. Beese, *Die medizinische Promotionen in Tübingen*, p. 47. According to Müller, "Studium und Studenten," p. 197, Ingolstadt maintained an average of 17–20 medical students during the 1760s and 1770s.

39 Undoubtedly the Frankfurt medical faculty overstated the severity of the situation a trifle. That such a claim could be made, however, suggests that students had not flocked to Frankfurt in recent times. Conrad Bornhak, *Geschichte der preußischen Universitätsverwaltung* (Berlin, 1900), p. 133.

classification of disease in general and in particular. Building upon their study of chemistry and botany, students also studied *materia medica* during this second stage, in which they learned about various medicaments and their actions on the body. Taken together, the above courses comprised the "theoretical" branch of medical education, while the third step provided "practical" training. The subjects taken at this level were general and special therapy, clinical practice, the method for writing prescriptions (essential in an age when prescriptions could be exceedingly complicated), and specialized courses such as surgery, obstetrics, and forensic medicine.[40]

The division between "theoretical" and "practical" courses refers to the type of knowledge presented, not to the method of instruction. Even subjects such as anatomy and chemistry were taught at mid-century in many universities only as lecture courses, owing to the lack of proper facilities or in some cases to negligence on the part of the faculties. The teaching of anatomy suffered in particular because the acquisition of cadavers was so difficult. Despite repeated orders by governments that the bodies of executed criminals or recently deceased indigents be turned over to universities for dissection, few schools could claim an adequate supply.[41]

Certainly the absence of facilities for anatomical demonstrations and chemical experiments were recognized by critics as serious drawbacks in medical education. Without "practice in exact observation," declared a critic of the curriculum at the University of Kiel in 1783, "all theoretical knowledge is unclear and does not educate a practical physician."[42] Medical professors acknowledged the problem as

40 This general sequence is described in *Anweisung für diejenigen, die sich der Arzneygelehrsamkeit widmen* (Halle, 1770), which was a pamphlet presented to incoming medical students at the University of Halle. Much of the same sequence was prescribed in the plans of study issued by the Bavarian government in 1774 and 1784. See Müller, "Studium und Studenten," pp. 194–5.

41 Even Göttingen, the most prestigious university at mid-century, and Albrecht von Haller, its renowned anatomist, encountered difficulties in securing cadavers. As a result the Hannoverian government issued a series of decrees in 1744 that attempted to improve the supply. Archiv Universität Göttingen, *Medizinische Fakultät. Dekanats- und Promotionsvorgänge und Urkunden*, 1744. Although the Archbishop of Trier gave anatomy a prominent place in his new directive for Trier's medical faculty in 1768, persistent doubts about the morality of dissection made acquisition of corpses virtually impossible. Finally in 1785 the Archbishop ordered that bodies of executed criminals be turned over to the faculty. See Emil Zenz, *Trier im 18. Jahrhundert* (Trier, 1981), p. 72. In Swedish Pomerania, a general medical ordinance of 1779 provided a typical list of subjects liable to dissection at the University of Greifswald: "cadavers of executed criminals; people who died in work houses or other prisons; brutal (*grober*) criminals of common (*geringer*) estate; common people who because of madness have been locked in public institutions; those who die while sentenced to pulling buggies (*bey Karrenstraffe*); those found dead, or vagabonds who die in hospitals, and finally poor people without support, who otherwise must be buried by the police." Johann Carl Dähnert, *Sammlung gemeiner und besonderer Pommerscher und Rügischer Landes-Urkunden, Gesetze, Privilegien, Verträge, Constitutionen und Ordnungen*. Supplement und Fortsetzung, Bd. 2 (Stralsund, 1786), pp. 555–6. A similar set of "candidates" for anatomy were also described in a decree issued for the University of Kiel in 1769. Elisabeth Dann, *Zur Geschichte des anatomischen Unterrichts an der Universität Kiel 1665–1865* (med. Diss., Kiel, 1969), p. 25.

42 Quoted in Ingeborg Utermann, *Gottlieb Heinrich Kannegießer: ein Gelehrter des 18. Jahrhunderts an der Universität Kiel* (Neumünster, 1967), p. 33.

well. The medical faculty at Marburg surely knew that it was touching a raw nerve when it complained to the government of Hesse-Kassel that students and their money tended to remain at Marburg only a couple of semesters, owing to the lack of a botanical garden, chemical laboratory and an anatomy theater.[43] Progressive educators such as Ernst Gottfried Baldinger (1738–1804) insisted that the doctrines of medical practice ranging from physiology through clinical practice be taught through experiments and personal observation. He wrote: "As no one can boast of a physical knowledge of bodies who has not been taught the forces of bodies through observations and experiments, so is a man completely incapable of practicing medicine who has not been taught the medical disciplines practically."[44]

Although some professors lauded the value of experiment, observation, and practical experience with medical phenomena, the centerpiece of medical education remained the spoken and written word. The doctrines that a student was expected to be acquainted with – be they in physiology, pathology, or therapeutics – were largely communicated through lectures and supplemented by textbooks. Baldinger himself, when describing the duties of the medical professor, harshly criticized professors who neither draw upon the writings of others in constructing their courses, nor prod their students to read widely in the literature.[45] Baldinger especially underscored the utility of studying the ancients, whose writings, he believed, provided both professor and student with a treasury of observations and definitions. His plan for teaching pathology consisted primarily of making digests of the doctrines and observations of both ancient and modern writers, and presenting this material in an ordered sequence in his lectures.[46]

The most conspicuous place (from a modern perspective) where the spoken and written word dominated medical curricula was the teaching of clinical practice. An up-to-date faculty in 1750 required a botanical garden, chemical laboratory, and anatomical theater. It did not demand a clinic. Although Baldinger and a few others urged professors to lead students to the bedside, and a few territories mandated this in university statutes,[47] regular courses of bedside clinical instruction

43 Staatsarchiv Marburg, Bestand 16, Rep. VI, Kl. 16, Nr. 1, "Akten, betr. das anatomische Institut zu Marburg," Bd. 1, fols. 6–8.
44 "Ut enim nemo de physica corporum cognitione gloriari possit, nisi qui per experimenta et observationes edoctus sit vires corporum, sic ineptus omnino ad medicinam faciendam, qui non practice informatus disciplinas medicas." Ernst Gottfried Baldinger, *De professore medico eiusque officiis praecipius* (Jena, 1769), p. 25. Similarly, the Erfurt professor Christoph Andreas Mangold (1719–67) argued for practical demonstration in medicine on psychological grounds that the clearest notions we have are those developed directly from sensory experience and that repeated experiences involving several senses produce the best knowledge. Christoph Andreas Mangold, "Programma de necessitate omnes medicinae partes in academiis practice docendi," in *Opuscula medico-physica*, collegit et edidit Ernestus Godofredus Baldinger (Altenburg, 1769), pp. 335–50.
45 Baldinger, *De professore medico*, pp. 10–11.
46 Ibid., pp. 14–19.
47 The statutes issued in 1731 for the University of Würzburg explicitly directed the professor of practice to take students along on patient consultations, as did the statutes for Heidelberg published in 1743. See Franz Xaver von Wegele, *Geschichte der Universität Wirzburg*, Teil 2 (1969 repr. of Würzburg, 1882), pp. 332–3; Stübler, *Heidelberg*, p. 123.

were neither widespread nor demanded. Only one university, Halle, offered such a clinic, and that one declined markedly when its founder, Johann Juncker (1679–1759), died in 1759. Furthermore, even Juncker's clinic was not required; it was taught *privatissime*, that is, by direct arrangement between Juncker and interested students. Within a few years another clinic would be established in Erfurt by a former student of Juncker's, but not until the 1780s would they become a common feature.[48]

It was not as though the role of clinical practice in medicine was discounted by educators. But the absence of clinics reflected a division of labor between the universities and practitioners. During his time at the university, the student took courses in clinical practice that taught him its guiding principles. The most popular texts for this purpose were Boerhaave's *Aphorisms* or Swieten's *Commentaria,* and of course the seemingly ageless *Aphorisms* of Hippocrates. Then following his graduation, a student was expected to attach himself to a more experienced practitioner to learn the business first-hand. Indeed, several territories made such informal "apprenticeships" mandatory.[49]

Travel to hospitals or clinics also filled the need for bedside instruction, though how adequately it did this might be questioned. Although travel played a prominent role in the careers of the physicians profiled in Boerner's *Nachrichten,* it was not merely the prerogative of the medical elite, for a great many students divided their time between two or more universities. Often what drew them to a particular school was the presence of renowned teachers, or simply the availability of courses that their local university did not offer. In some cases, a famous professor could almost single-handedly raise the enrollment of a faculty, as Baldinger did when he began teaching clinical practice at the University of Marburg in 1785. Similarly, another clinician, Friedrich Wendt (1738–1818), drew a sizeable contingent of students to Erlangen in the 1780s.[50] Beyond intellectual enrichment, what students acquired from their concourse with outstanding teachers was something just as precious to their future careers: testimonials. At the end of each course, the student was not examined on the course material, nor did he receive a grade. Instead, what he secured was a statement from the professor testifying to his diligence in attending the course. When the time came for him to return to his

48 Wolfram Kaiser et al., "Collegium clinicum Halense," in *250 Jahre Collegium Clinicum Halense 1717–1967. Beiträge zur Geschichte der Medizinischen Fakultät der Universität Halle* (Halle, 1967), pp. 9–66. The creation of university teaching clinics will be discussed below in Chapter 2.

49 This stipulation was made in the Palatinate in 1775, and also in Brandenburg-Onolzbach in 1785. See Stübler, *Heidelberg,* p. 131, and "Verordnung, daß junge Doct. Medic. unter der Aufsicht eines Medici practici sich anfangs üben sollen," in *Journal von und für Deutschland* 2, Stück 12 (1785): 512.

50 Friedrich Gedike, in his 1789 report to the Prussian government on the conditions of universities in other parts of Germany, noted the scant number of medical students in Giessen and attributed this to the drawing power of Baldinger in nearby Marburg. Elsewhere, Gedike called the medical enrollment at Erlangen "truly remarkable," and there can be little doubt that he thought Wendt was the primary reason for it. See Richard Fester, 'Der Universitäts-Bereiser' Friedrich Gedike und sein Bericht an Friedrich Wilhelm II," *Archiv für Kulturgeschichte* 1. Ergänzungsheft (1905), pp. 42, 70–3.

home university to graduate (as most students did), the student produced these documents in applying for permission to be promoted to doctor of medicine.[51] Because these testimonials would later be submitted when applying for positions, it mattered a great deal that students secure the patronage of prominent teachers, or at the very least the declaration that the student had remained awake during the lectures.

The final phase of a student's career consisted of his examinations, inaugural disputation, and promotion. The most widely used procedures for examination involved two separate sessions. The first exam, called the *tentamen*, brought the student before the assembled professors for two to three hours of questions covering all areas of medicine. If he performed acceptably in this exam, he was then assigned two subjects to work up for his second exam, the *rigorosum*. One topic came from the area of theory ("transpiration," "hearing," or "the liver" were typical), while the other dealt with a practical matter ("smallpox," or "the medical use of mercury"). A few days later, the student again appeared before the faculty to present formal lectures on these two topics and answer questions.[52]

The crowning demonstration of a student's readiness to take a degree was his inaugural disputation. The disputation was based upon a printed Latin dissertation, which could be written by the student, but which could also be the product of one of his professors. Copies of the dissertation were sent to those invited to attend the disputation, and on the day itself copies were placed on tables for reference by the audience. The ceremony began with a Latin oration by the presiding professor, followed at least in some cases by the student's reading forth of the dissertation. Finally, designated opponents – at some places faculty members, at others students – presented their criticisms of the dissertation's theses, followed by the candidate's defense.[53]

The conclusion of his disputation entitled a student to receive a license to be

---

51 Thus one student who petitioned to graduate from the University of Giessen in 1790 displayed testimonials from several professors at the universities of Halle and Göttingen. Archiv Universität Gießen, Med O2: *Promotionen von Ärzten, 1645–1799*. One testimonial given by the Tübingen medical faculty to a student read in part, "[H]e has passed his time at the university very well, and as long as he has remained here . . . he has combined the most well-bred behavior with all diligence in his studies; he has attended his lectures and exercises alertly and without interruption, and he has devoted every effort to making himself an upright doctor." Transcription of *Dekanatsbuch*, Universitätsarchiv Tübingen 14/14, p. 95. My deepest thanks to Prof. Gerhard Fichtner for sharing his transcription of the *Dekanatsbuch* with me.

52 Stübler, *Heidelberg*, p. 119; Halle also had a *tentamen* and a *rigorosum*, although the latter consisted of a write-up of a medical case history given to the candidate by one of the professors. In 1785, Halle combined these into a single examination. See Wolfram Kaiser and Karl-Heinz Krosch, "Die Statuten der medizinischen Fakultät im 18. Jahrhundert," in *250 Jahre Collegium Clinicum Halense*, p. 89. Topics were obtained from the Tübingen *Dekanatsbuch*. Similar topics were used for the *rigorosum* at Giessen as well. Archiv Universität Gießen, Med C1, Bd. 3: *Annalium Facultatis Medicinae Volumen III (1740–1833)*.

53 Werner Kundert, *Katalog der Helmstedter juristischen Disputationen, Programme und Reden 1574–1810*, Reportorien zur Erforschung der Neuzeit, Bd. 8 (Wiesbaden, 1984), pp. 53–75, provides the best available introduction both to academic dissertations and the ceremonies attending their public defense.

promoted to doctor of medicine. Because the license certified the same academic credentials as the doctorate, many young men were satisfied to enter medical practice as *Licenciaten* without going through the final ceremony to become doctors. This decision was especially encouraged in territories such as Württemberg, where it appeared that a doctoral degree was not absolutely required to receive an appointment as a *Physicus* or court physician. However, in other parts of Germany the doctorate was required for these offices, and everywhere it appeared to be mandatory before someone could assume a professorial chair.[54]

One reason that a candidate might prefer to settle for a license or postpone taking his doctoral degree was that it cost a lot of money. In fact, medical study as a whole was an expensive proposition. To begin with, there were the private lecture courses. Although professors officially received a salary to hold public lectures every semester, which by definition were free to students, they also had the right to advertise and give lectures privately on any subject they chose, and to charge each listener a fee. Another major expense consisted of fees for examinations and for the degree ceremonies (*Promotionen*). The amount and distribution of the payments for exams and promotions were regulated by governmental decrees, as, for example, in 1778 when the statutes for the University of Kiel set the doctoral examination fee at 50 Rthlr (*Reichsthaler*), and the fee for the ceremonial promotion at 120 Rthlr. This was no inconsequential sum, because the salary of the senior professor of medicine at Kiel during the same period was only 500 Rthlr.[55]

The examinations and graduation ceremonies were pies in which it seemed that everyone connected with the university could have a finger. Of the 75 fl (*Gulden*) stipulated for the examination by a Bavarian decree of 1720, the following payments were a portion: 3 fl for wine and sweets; 4 fl 30 kr (*Kreutzer*) for "sugarmoney" (*Zuckergeld*) for the professors' wives; 4 fl 30 kr each for the university vice-chancellor and the notary; and 3 fl for the porter. The promotion cost an additional 155 fl in which were included sums for the diploma; payments to the wives of the notary, the dean of the faculty, and the professor conferring the degree, presumably for the festive meal accompanying the ceremony; as well as payments for a religious service, poetry, drinks, and contributions to the local orphanage, the university library, and the Franciscan order.[56]

54 On the number of licentiates in Württemberg, see Beese, *Die medizinische Promotionen in Tübingen*, pp. 44–5; and Theodor Knapp, "Zur Geschichte der akademischen Würden, vornehmlich an der Universität Tübingen," *Zeitschrift für württembergische Landesgeschichte* 2 (1938): 48–116, esp. p. 81. On the history of academic degrees in general, see Knapp, "Doktor und Magister," *Württembergische Vierteljahrshefte für Landesgeschichte*, Neue Folge 34 (1928): 44–56; Ewald Horn, "Die Disputationen und Promotionen an den deutschen Universitäten vornehmlich seit dem 16. Jahrhundert," *Beihefte zum Centralblatt für Bibliothekswesen* 4 (1893–1894): 1–126; and G. Kaufmann, "Zur Geschichte der akademischen Grade und Disputationen," *Centralblatt für Bibliothekswesen* 11 (1894): 201–25.
55 Heinrich Schipperges, "Geschichte der medizinischen Fakultät," in *Geschichte der Christian-Albrechts-Universität Kiel* Bd. 4, Teil 1 (Kiel, 1967), pp. 77 and 96.
56 Karl von Prantl, *Geschichte der Ludwig-Maximilians-Universität in Ingolstadt, Landshut, München* Bd. 1 (1968 repr. of Munich, 1872), p. 533.

The costs for private lectures, examinations, and promotions made medical study an expensive enterprise. But they were by no means the only expenses borne by students. Beginning with his matriculation, formerly a ceremonious occasion accompanied by the taking of an oath, but of late reduced – in Königsberg, at least – to a "simple handshake" and the payment of "2 Rthlr and a few Groschen,"[57] the student faced a swarm of little fees that slowly but steadily drained his pocketbook. Johann Heinrich Jugler (1758–1812), a medical student at Leipzig in the 1770s, described some typical costs:

> In the lecture halls, . . . one may select either a place on the bench or a seat behind a desk. If the latter is chosen, the student tells this to the professor's assistant, who immediately writes the student's name and the hour of the lecture on the back of the chair. For this he gets 16 gr *Stuhlgeld*. In some classes that are held at night, the assistant receives a little something extra, perhaps 4 gr for so-called *Lichtgeld*. During the winter term, the assistant gets 8 gr *Holzgeld* for heating. . . . And if the student wishes to have a testimonial from his professor and says this to the assistant, the latter gets 8 gr for it.

"From all this," Jugler concluded wryly, "one sees that the assistants are in a good position there, especially with the theologians, jurists, and philosophers."[58] He added that he had never heard of these particular extortions being made upon students of medicine at Leipzig, but if the medical students escaped these payments, others devolved upon them alone. For example, students at Leipzig in Jugler's day had the unusual opportunity to work on cadavers themselves, naturally for a price.

> Whoever wishes to make a preparation of a cadaver makes this known and selects for himself the head or one of the extremities. This costs 5 Thlr each time, from which the professor of anatomy receives 3 Thlr, the demonstrator 1 Thlr 8 gr, and the professor's assistant either 8 gr or 16 gr, depending on whether one borrows from the assistant only the anatomical garments or also a scalpel and forceps.[59]

It should be added that less wealthy students often could receive a waiver from at least some of the multitude of fees. One common device was for two or more students to be promoted to doctor together, thereby splitting the costs.[60] Moreover, at many universities there were stipends to which students could apply for support. Unfortunately, those sources often came with stipulations that rather

57 Johann Friedrich Goldbeck, *Nachrichten von der königlichen Universität zu Königsberg zu Preußen* (Leipzig, 1782), p. 103.
58 [Johann Heinrich Jugler], *Leipzig und seine Universität vor hundert Jahren* (Leipzig, 1879), pp. 54–5.
59 Ibid., pp. 59–60.
60 Beese, *Die medizinischen Promotionen in Tübingen*, pp. 48–9, reports that eight candidates were promoted together at Tübingen in 1777 (of whom only three were actually present for the ceremony). Presumably this came with some allowance for "group rates." The archival records from the medical faculties in Göttingen and Tübingen abound in petitions for remission of fees. For example, see Archiv Universität Göttingen, "Dekanatsakten der Medizinischen Fakultät, 1741"; and Archiv Universität Tübingen 58/1, "Examina, Testimonien, Prüfungsarbeiten."

narrowed the range of eligible applicants. This was the case at Wittenberg, where a stipend containing the considerable sum of 400 Thlr was set aside for a medical student of Hungarian nationality.[61] The existence of such fellowships and waivers made medical study accessible to students from poor families, but in general medicine was a game that only those with money could play. The mathematician Abraham Gotthelf Kästner (1719–1800), who studied at Leipzig in the 1730s, wrote that he found the basic medical sciences of botany, anatomy, and chemistry attractive, and "perhaps I would have devoted myself completely to them, if I could have been sure of the necessary costs."[62] Contemporaries made the point quite bluntly that needy students were not welcome in medicine, as one professor wrote in 1770:

It is a shortcoming of medicine that too many poor students choose this faculty; students who should be discouraged from this, because in fact a physician, if he is to be established, has need of expensive travels, books with engravings, and natural history cabinets. But [poor] students least of all have sufficient means for these things. Most of them must become wretched trade-doctors (*Brod-Doctors*), who consequently make themselves contemptible, along with those who have spent much on themselves and learned something.[63]

The argument made by this writer and others against allowing poor students into medicine reflected considerably more than an economic calculation of the costs of medical study and practice. It reflected as well a set of values that held the professions to be an honorable estate, an estate worthy of special dignity in society, requiring a proper background and upbringing no less than a series of university courses to enter. We have already encountered one facet of these values in the standardized biographies published by Boerner. While medicine and other professions may have been open to the occasional impoverished student of exceptional talent – Johann Juncker, the Halle clinician, was one example – for the most part no amount of study could substitute for the bearing and, well, *polish* that poor students supposedly lacked.[64] Although the professions may not have constituted a formal hierarchy of birth, as did the aristocracy, they were anything but an open elite.

61 Rudolf Disselhorst, "Die medizinische Fakultät der Universität Wittenberg und ihre Vertreter von 1503–1816," *Leopoldina*, Neue Folge 5 (1929): 99. On the role played by the *Stiftungen* in opening some degree of social mobility to poor students especially in theology, see Hermann Mitgau, "Soziale Herkunft der deutschen Studenten bis 1900," in *Universität und Gelehrtenstand 1400–1800*, ed. Hellmuth Rössler and Gunther Franz (Limburg, 1970), pp. 233–68.

62 Kästner's autobiographical statement was published in Baldinger, *Biographien jetztlebender Aerzte und Naturforscher*, Stück 1, p. 54.

63 Quoted in Walter Jens, *Eine deutsche Universität. 500 Jahre Tübinger Gelehrtenrepublik* (Munich, 1977), p. 190.

64 For an outstanding description of this corporate ideal with respect to the Protestant clergy, see Anthony J. La Vopa, *Grace, Talent, and Merit: Poor Students, Clerical Careers, and Professional Ideology in Eighteenth-Century Germany* (Cambridge, 1988), pp. 46–57.

THE MEDICAL FACULTIES

Up to this point, we have considered university medicine as the students would have encountered it shortly after mid-century: courses to be taken, formal hurdles to be cleared, expenses to be paid. Yet the faculties where students obtained their education were more than just a collection of teachers. Teaching, of course, was the foundation for the faculties' existence, but alongside that professors performed a variety of functions of an advisory and supervisory nature. This made the German medical faculties rather diffuse institutions. This point is quite significant for our story, because during the second half of the 1700s the faculties' mission would become considerably more focused on pedagogy.

One element of this characteristic diffuseness is shown by the faculties' structure and the way professors were recruited into their ranks. The standard German medical faculty in the eighteenth century was built around three full professors, each known as an *Ordinarius*, who among themselves divided up the domain of medical knowledge. The senior member of the trio in terms of tenure, called the *Primarius*, commonly taught clinical practice, either by reciting some handbook to his students, or by taking them along on visits to his patients, or both. To this he might add associated courses in materia medica, botany, or forensic medicine. The second oldest member of the faculty, the *Secundarius*, lectured on pathology, therapy, chemistry, and anatomy. Whereas the areas covered by the two senior professors showed considerable variability from one university to another, the duties of the youngest member of the faculty usually involved teaching the group of theoretical "basic sciences" known as the *institutiones:* physiology, pathology, therapeutics, semiotics, and dietetics.[65]

This structure had two noteworthy aspects. First, salary was almost invariably tied to seniority. Whoever occupied the position as *Primarius* received the largest regular salary, with gradations for the other full professors. The gradation of salary according to seniority contributed to a second, even more remarkable feature: at the majority of universities professors advanced into the next most senior position when a vacancy occurred, and they assumed the subjects associated with that chair. This process, known as *Aufrücken* (literally, "climbing up"), meant that over the course of a relatively long career a professor would quite possibly teach the entire range of medical subjects, a task for which he was well prepared by an education that familiarized him with the standard authorities in each area. He in turn would teach that same canonical curriculum (regardless of whether it actually contained the same books) to the next generation of students.

Aufrücken was a system that embodied all the values of broad learning that we examined previously. These same values, as well as the lack of a clear occupational boundary between professors and practitioners, can be seen in the way that new

---

65 These teaching assignments come from the 1743 revision of the statutes for Heidelberg, reprinted in Stübler, *Heidelberg*, pp. 121–2.

professors joined the faculty. One way was through what Steven Turner has called "horizontal recruitment," the appointment of physicians from outside the ranks of university teachers, to a professorial chair.[66] Although such horizontal recruitment was the most common form of appointment, it was also possible for eighteenth-century professors to come up "vertically" through the ranks. Many students, after taking their degrees and acquiring a bit of polish by traveling, attempted to parley their connections into an appointment as extraordinary professor at a university. Extraordinary appointments carried the right to have one's lectures advertised in each semester's lecture catalogue, and even a small salary in some cases. Most importantly, extraordinary professorships placed the appointee on track to a full professorship.[67]

It was a further mark of the diffuseness of the faculties' role that, no matter what the route to appointment, the standards applied to selection of professors did not attempt to distinguish those who had a special talent for teaching or research. Indeed, nothing qualitatively different was demanded beyond what the applicant had already done in finishing his doctoral degree. The 1737 medical statutes of the University of Göttingen, for example, seemed more interested in fees than in scholarship in specifying that newly created doctors of medicine pay 10 Rthlr (20 for non-Hannoverians) into the faculty treasury for the right to lecture privately and to preside at disputations. After they had presided at three disputations, a payment of an additional 12 Rthlr could permit the doctor "to be dignified with the title of an Assessor of the medical faculty." This title permitted the holder not only to enjoy a rank above that of the private lecturers, but it also freed him from the usual fees for censorship of his publications by the faculty dean. As a final inducement, the statutes promised that purchasers of the title "will be invited by the Dean to the celebratory banquets (*solennia prandia*) of newly promoted doctors"; a painless gesture, it should be noted, because it was the graduate who would be picking up the bill.[68] The Tübingen statutes published in 1752 enjoined the University Senate (comprised of all ordinary professors) from engaging in nepotism or taking bribes (*largitiones*) in selecting new professors, but with respect to academic qualifications they only instructed the Senate to obtain a sample of each candidate's academic writing in making their selection. Only after a candidate had been chosen did the statutes order that he present an inaugural lecture on a

66 R. Steven Turner, "University Reformers and Professorial Scholarship in Germany, 1760-1806," in *The University in Society*, ed. Lawrence Stone, vol. 2 (Princeton, N.J., 1974), pp. 495–531.
67 According to a biographical index I have been compiling of German university medical professors in the eighteenth century, of 193 individuals who occupied a chair as *Ordinarius* between 1750 and 1790, more than 36 percent (70) began as extraordinary professors.
68 See Wilhelm Ebel, *Die Privilegien und ältesten Statuten der Georg-August-Universität zu Göttingen* (Göttingen, 1961), pp. 157–9. The 1743 statutes for Heidelberg directed a candidate to submit a dissertation on the area of medicine that he wanted to lecture on, to be followed by a public disputation over twelve theses, six from the subject to be lectured on. The opponents for this disputation were to consist of two members of the faculty, following which the faculty was to submit a report of the results, along with their votes on whether the candidate should be accepted into the faculty. Stübler, *Heidelberg*, p. 118.

topic designated by the dean of the appropriate faculty, "to find out what skill for teaching he has."[69]

The relatively easy movement of individuals into and out of professorial positions was but one factor among several that blurred the distinctiveness of medical faculties as institutions having a specific function. For it was one of the central facts of life in the medical faculties that although professors received their salaries to give public lectures, they also performed a variety of other tasks. The medical faculty at Göttingen considered these other tasks to be the "principal rights of the faculty," and when the University opened in 1737 they drew up detailed descriptions of those functions in their faculty statutes. One was the professors' right to carry on private practices, an occupation that all too often caused lectures to be interrupted as professors were summoned for consultations, much to the irritation of students and territorial governments. Complaints by the latter often had a disingenuous tinge to them, because many medical professors doubled as personal physicians to local notables, who called them away whenever it suited them.[70] Many medical faculties also were called upon to render written opinions on medical-legal questions, for which they were compensated by the government. Mostly these were routine matters, but on occasion the faculty became embroiled in major controversies. In one particularly notorious case, a formal accusation of witchcraft against a woman in 1749 in the archdiocese of Würzburg included a report in which the university's medical faculty joined with the theological faculty in claiming that witches actually do exist.[71]

In some territories, the faculties exercised broad supervision over the principality's medical system. This combination of functions was especially typical in the ecclesiastical principalities, such as Würzburg, Mainz, and Bamberg. But in Protestant territories too, such as Schleswig-Holstein and the city of Erfurt, the university faculties of Kiel and Erfurt acted as a medical board in examining surgeons, barbers, and midwives, inspecting apothecary shops, and performing other duties that elsewhere fell to local *Physici*. Even in territories where there were central medical boards, the faculties might still enjoy some rights, such as in Württemberg, where a geographical division was made between the responsibilities of the Tübingen faculty and the medical authorities in Stuttgart.[72]

No aspect of the medical faculties' powers and duties aroused more complaint

69 "Electus ad dissertationem publicam, . . . ut pateat, quod artificium docendi calleat, adstringitor . . ." Theodor Eisenlohr, *Sammlung der württembergischen Schul-Geseze*, Bd. 11, Abth. 3, "Universitäts-Gesetze bis zum Jahr 1843" (Tübingen, 1843), p. 418.

70 In his autobiography, Johann Peter Frank complained about one of his professors at Heidelberg, Franz Joseph Oberkamp, that he "paid more attention to his duties as personal physician [to the Count Palatine] than to his professorship, and consequently often had to interrupt his lectures for fourteen days and longer." In "Biography of Dr. Johann Peter Frank . . . written by himself," trans. George Rosen, *Journal of the History of Medicine* 3 (1948): 21.

71 Albert von Kölliker, *Zur Geschichte der medizinischen Facultät an der Universität Würzburg* (Würzburg, 1871), p. 21.

72 Hans-Wolf Thümmel, *Die Tübinger Universitätsverfassung im Zeitalter des Absolutismus* (Tübingen, 1975), pp. 220-1.

than their conduct of examinations. The curious fact that the ceremonies surrounding the students' *Promotionen* in most cases cost a larger sum than the supposedly more important doctoral examinations meant that it made little sense to fail candidates when that entailed losing the respectable rewards to be gleaned from the second half of the process. Besides, even if a faculty wanted to maintain high standards, it availed practically nothing to do so when it was easy enough for candidates to be promoted elsewhere by faculties eager for the business. As a consequence, it was often quite difficult to fail the examinations. Even foreigners remarked upon this, as did one English traveler at the University of Cologne in the 1790s: "to buyers of a certain class, the [exam] has bonus enough to make it pass for a bargain. For, if the fees are heavy, the examinations are light. So that, like a classic done into a vulgar tongue, it is adapted to gentlemen of all capacities!"[73] In a similar vein, Baldinger satirically related how the medical faculty at the "University of ★ ★" never failed any candidate who solemnly vowed that he would not practice in the territory where the university was located.[74] But other commentators found the situation rather less amusing. Ludwig von Hess (1719–84), a writer on administrative policy, pointed out that the state would not dream of allowing a mason or carpenter who was not a member of a guild to build a house, but on the other hand it routinely permits unqualified doctors to practice medicine, a permissiveness "that is so advantageous to mortality. There is no faculty," Hess continued, "in which it is easier to become a doctor than in the medical faculty, and there is none in which it is harder to become learned. . . ."[75]

In the next chapter, we shall examine the ways that territorial governments attempted to alleviate the perceived problems by reforming the universities and medical education. For now, we need to understand what it was about the faculties that created a sense of dissatisfaction after mid-century. Two points appear especially relevant to this question, one having to do with the attitudes of the occupants of professorial positions, and the other concerning what the faculties were expected to be.

There can be no question that a large number of professors held their positions as sinecures. But the term "sinecure" is deceptive, because it has long contained highly negative connotations of indolence and incompetence. By and large, eighteenth-century medical professors were neither of these; yet offices were not completely permeated with an ethos of performance of duty either. It should be recalled that offices in early modern society were given in part as tokens of social recognition. The incomes associated with them represented not so much payment for a job done, but a manifestation of a patron's or sovereign's largesse and favor. Offices represented the ribbons that tied rulers and subjects together in complex networks of patronage and family loyalty. For this reason, petitioners for offices

---

73 Charles Este, *A Journey in the Year 1793 Through Flanders, Brabant, and Germany, to Switzerland* (London, 1795), p. 191.
74 *Neues Magazin für Aerzte* 2 (1780): 573.
75 Ludwig von Hess, *Freymüthige Gedanken über Staatsachen* (Hamburg, 1775), p. 30.

took every occasion to remind a patron of past family ties. "Your Royal Majesty will still remember how my late father served Your Highness long and loyally," wrote one petitioner for a professorial job at Giessen in 1763, "for whose sake Your Highness has most graciously condescended to care for his surviving children, under whose number I find myself."[76] When a position opened up at Tübingen in 1772, Johann Friedrich Gmelin (1748–1804) applied to the university Senate for it by leaning heavily on the memory of his late father, a professor of botany and chemistry. Unfortunately for Johann Friedrich, a powerful advocate – his aunt, Maria Veronica Gmelin (1713–97) – weighed in with a letter to the Senate in support of his cousin, Samuel Gottlieb Gmelin (1743–74). The widow Gmelin too spared no effort to recall her husband's service as a local physician, apothecary and university lecturer in making her pitch.[77]

No doubt Duke Karl Eugen of Württemberg had instances similar to this one in mind when he inveighed against nepotism in the Tübingen statutes of 1752. Yet the same statutes gave the Duke the right to reject candidates of whom he did not approve, which Karl Eugen chose not to exercise in 1772 when confronted by the obvious nepotism of the Gmelins, and he certainly did not scruple at rewarding members of loyal families when it served *his* purposes. Apparently then, both the practices and the complaints emanated from a conflict between two contrasting ideals of bureaucratic service, one based on patterns of personal loyalty, the other on more "objective" criteria of merit and performance. Even Brandenburg-Prussia, supposedly the most "modern" bureaucratic state in eighteenth-century Germany, presented instances of this conflict by making appointments to university posts that were plainly based on family ties.

Even more characteristic than the attitude of professors, however, were some basic ambiguities concerning what the faculties were supposed to *be*. To what extent did the faculties exist to communicate knowledge or to certify it? Governments certainly cared about both, as a constant stream of decrees and admonitions in various territories can testify. Of the two functions, however, it was the examinations that received the weight of attention before 1780. After all, the number of individuals studying medicine at most places was quite small, reflecting the limited range of opportunities that existed for physicians. Even if a government attempted to be rigorous in forcing each professor to hold public lectures every semester, it would prove impossible anyway: as the medical faculty at Frankfurt an der Oder wrote, the students simply were not there. Meanwhile, governments had a keen interest in insuring that newly graduated physicians, who might one day assume elite positions in the medical establishment, display knowledge suitable to their position. Because it touched on the public's welfare, that concern made itself

76 Archiv Universität Gießen, Med K4: *Dozenten der Medizinischen Fakultät*, "Die Wiederbesetzung der professoribus medicinae primariae betreffend," letter from Johann Philipp Berchelmann, dated 16 February 1763.
77 Archiv Universität Tübingen 20/2, 98, nos. 3 & 5.

felt no matter how few physicians there were. In certain respects, therefore, governments seemed to regard medical faculties more as a board of experts than as a collection of teachers. If this was the case, the faculties' other functions, such as preparation of medical-forensic reports and supervision of the health system in some territories, would reinforce this tendency.

One final ambiguity over the faculties' function is evident in the examinations themselves. For although in many territories an academic degree was the sufficient basis to *practice* medicine at mid-century, the exams and the inaugural disputation in essence probed a candidate's ability to perform as a *scholar*. It was entirely characteristic that critics did not attack the contents of the exams, only the faculties' lax standards in administering them. Ludwig von Hess was typical in this respect. After railing at the faculties for unleashing a horde of sanctioned murderers on society, his remedy consisted of compelling professors "under threat of severe penalty" to graduate "no one who has not passed a rigorous (*scharf*) examination, held formal lectures (*lectiones cursorias*), and *pro Gradu* held a disputation."[78] In other words, Hess called for nothing more than a stricter application of the standard requirements. That completing a sequence of academic exams, disputations and lectures might not qualify an individual to practice medicine did not occur to him. Nor should it have done so, for that would have required the perception that medical faculties should perform specialized functions that placed them somewhat apart from both practicing physicians and the administrators of health policy. Hess did not write with such an idea in mind. As we shall see in the next chapter, however, this is precisely the perception that began to take shape during the final third of the eighteenth century.

78 Hess, *Freymüthige Gedanken*, p. 314.

2

Fractures and new alignments

Of necessity, the image of mid-eighteenth century German medicine presented in the preceding chapter was one frozen in time. Yet the constituents of that picture – the intimate connection between medical profession and the universities, and the location of both in the larger society – should be conceived of dynamically, not statically. For all its seeming clarity, as soon as the depth provided by time is added to the picture, the details begin to blur and lose their sharp outline. At no time were there ever institutions such as "the medical profession" or "the universities" for which we can give a precise description. Rather, such institutions are always a more or less discordant blend of meanings and functions, incessantly driven in new directions by unfulfilled expectations (which can themselves be dissonant) and held back by the weight of established practices. If these institutions appear stable at mid-century, it is only in comparison to the changes that would overtake them in the years around 1800.

It is worth remembering this when we consider the forces that acted upon the universities and the medical profession, propelling them into a new relationship. These forces did not act on inert matter. There was no reform "movement" that suddenly arose in the 1700s to resuscitate a group of "outmoded" universities and incompetent physicians. The idea of an eighteenth-century crisis in higher education has roots lying deep in the nineteenth century, and was created at a time when apologists for universities and scientific medicine sought to celebrate their modernity by separating themselves from their ancestors.[1] The decrepit condition of the *ancien-régime* universities, the precarious situation of physicians and the inadequacies of medical knowledge – these were used by historians in Imperial

---

1 James Dennis Cobb attributes the modernism and Prussia-centeredness of many late nineteenth-century university histories to the oppressive influence of Friedrich Althoff, the minister responsible for administering the Prussian universities between 1882 and 1907. Although Cobb may exaggerate Althoff's personal influence on these histories, he surely does not go wrong in attributing their tone to the general political environment and to Prussia's aggressive policies of cultural imperialism. James Dennis Cobb, *The Forgotten Reforms: Non-Prussian Universities 1797–1817* (Ph.D. diss., University of Wisconsin-Madison, 1980), pp. 3–8. For a thorough discussion of Prussia's *Kulturpolitik* in this period, see Suzanne L. Marchand, *Archaeology and Cultural Politics in Germany, 1800–1965: The Decline of Philhellenism* (Ph.D. diss., University of Chicago, 1992).

Germany to celebrate their nation's cultural and economic achievements. We are not bound to accept that story, however, and the time has long since arrived to get a peek behind the shroud it has thrown over the eighteenth century. That there was criticism of the universities and attempts to reform them cannot be questioned. But criticism and reform of education exist in practically every period in which one cares to look. Schools and universities seemingly never correspond exactly to what they are supposed to be, probably because what they are supposed to be is comprised of conflicting elements. Thus there are always calls for reform. What counts for our purposes are the details of the reforms in our particular period and what they can tell us about the perceived social role of higher education and of the professions.

In what follows, three interlocking sets of developments will be discussed that exerted a profound influence on the universities, the structure of the medical profession, and the content of the medical curriculum. The first concerns the attempts to nudge higher education in certain directions by founding new institutions and adding new subjects to the existing curriculum. The thrust of these reforms was to move university curricula toward greater attention to the practical application of knowledge, and their rationale lay in securing bureaucrats for territorial governments. The requirements of bureaucratic supervision – in this case public health – also lay behind the second development, the establishment and strengthening of territorial medical boards, or *collegia medica,* by many states. Finally, concern for public health, especially medical care for the poor, combined with the new utilitarian emphasis of pedagogy in the 1780s and 1790s to create a third innovation, the widespread introduction of clinical courses in the medical faculties of many universities. This development brought for the first time the problem of training students for the practice of medicine inside the universities.

By the end of the century, these changes had made quite urgent the question of the social purpose of higher education and the nature of the learned professions. These problems were intimately related, because the status of the professions derived directly from their place in the universities, and the identity of one could not be altered without affecting the other as well. The vigorous sponsorship of the Enlightenment by territorial governments and the justifications made for expansion of government power on the ideological pillars of reason and utility made the state appear as a disinterested, objective supporter of social progress. The introduction of the new, utilitarian pedagogy was justified by *raison d'état,* in effect an invocation of the Enlightenment itself. Yet this movement engendered a reaction by critics who saw such an educational program as excessively pragmatic and even oppressive. These critics denounced the treatment of students as mere gears in the social mechanism and they began developing a vision of education that stressed personal cultivation of the individual, and not mere training for useful service.

As members of a profession, physicians experienced the quarrel over education as a fracturing of professional identity. The expansion of bureaucratic power under the banner of Enlightenment gave doctors the chance to ally themselves with the forces of progress and reason and to demonstrate the contributions medicine could make to an enlightened society. At the same time, however, emphasis on the utilitarian organization of education and on the practical application of knowledge threatened to diminish the prestige physicians had enjoyed over other healers by virtue of their scholarly credentials. Physicians could choose to stand in the vanguard of progress and Enlightenment, but seemingly only by surrendering one of the very qualities that had constituted them as an elite group.

THE REFORM OF HIGHER EDUCATION

The opening of the eighteenth century marked a new era in more ways than symbolically on a calendar. The previous century had been one in which the political and social tensions sown by the Reformation burst forth in incomparably savage ways, principally in Germany, but also in France and England. The Treaty of Westphalia returned some measure of sanity to Central Europe, and it reduced the occurrence of warfare to a tolerable, if not exactly infrequent level. The restoration of external order permitted the work of cultivating and enforcing proper religious belief to be channeled inside territorial borders, as the eleven Protestant (including three Calvinist) and twelve Catholic universities founded between 1541 and 1669 geared up to produce the foot soldiers of orthodoxy and shout down dissenting doctrines.[2]

By 1700, the pious zeal motivating the Wars of Religion had dampened, helped along no doubt by the bitter and seemingly incessant quarrelling that broke out within individual theology faculties over questions of doctrine. One response to this was the rise in the later seventeenth century of Pietism, a style of religious life that stressed redemption and the cultivation of personal faith over dogmatics and priestly ceremony.[3] Another response was the opening of new universities in Halle (1694) and Göttingen (1734) that sought to downplay one accepted function of higher education, the training of clergymen, in favor of a second, the preparation of effective state functionaries. Indeed as the eighteenth century passed, calls began to be heard, especially in northern Germany, for these two functions to be combined by making the clergy, which traditionally held responsibility for public education, into an arm of the state bureaucracy.[4]

This confrontation with the churches, both Protestant and Catholic, occurred not just at the university level. Although "secularization" has proven to be a rather

2 A useful compilation of university foundations including dates, patrons, and doctrinal orientation is included in William Clark, *From the Medieval Universitas Scholarium to the German Research University: A Sociogenesis of the Germanic Academic* (Ph.D. diss., University of California, Los Angeles, 1986), pp. 604–35.

3 On Pietism, see Mary Fulbrook, *Piety and Politics: Religion and the Rise of Absolutism in England, Württemberg and Prussia* (Cambridge, 1983); and Martin Schmidt, *Der Pietismus als theologische Erscheinung* (Göttingen, 1984).

4 On plans to bureaucratize the clergy in Brandenburg-Prussia and in Hannover and the clergy's resistance to them, see John Stroup, *The Struggle for Identity in the Clerical Estate* (Leiden, 1984).

inexact description of what was going on in the eighteenth century, there can be no mistaking a desire among lay elites in Protestant territories (and perhaps slightly later in Catholic areas as well) to reduce the influence of religious institutions in society. One manifestation of that desire expressed itself clearly in a preoccupation with education of all kinds. Through the new periodical media as well as through agitation for new school curricula and administration, reformers applied the beacons of reason and science to enlighten the public, hector it into abandoning antiquated traditions and superstitions, and teach it civic virtue. Implicitly or explicitly, much of this program amounted to an attack on the clergy, the traditional suppliers of public education.

A second major impulse to educational reform stemmed from the attempts of territorial governments to maximize the wealth they could wring from their economies. A number of reformers stressed that one important means of fostering economic growth was to have a populace educated to be productive and efficient – in short, one inculcated with the values of "industry." A school system designed for this purpose would offer a curriculum tailored to students' future occupations, and convey an ethos of productive labor and entrepreneurial initiative. Equally important in the reformers' minds was the development of new teaching methods to replace what they regarded as the mindless repetition of catechism and Latin exercises of existing schools with a more stimulating method of instruction.[5]

The same values underlay university reforms as well. Because, as the Erfurt Statthalter Karl von Dalberg (1744–1817) wrote, the purpose of a university is "to educate capable instruments (*Werkzeuge*) for the benefit of the State," the problem was how best to accomplish that end.[6] Dalberg, who was charged by the Archbishop of Mainz with submitting proposals for the reform of the University of Erfurt, approached the problem at least partly in terms of methods of instruction. As he saw it, one of the chief principles of education is that if students are to be competent in their occupations, it is not sufficient merely to broaden their knowledge. They must also become proficient at applying it. Accordingly, he urged professors to set their students problems to be solved that will illustrate how theoretical knowledge is put to use.[7]

The movement to bring more practical instruction to university curricula made its way into a wide variety of subjects. In medicine, for example, candidates for M.D. degrees at Göttingen and Erlangen were ordered to conduct anatomical demonstrations to display their facility for carrying out dissections. In making this requirement, officials surely had one eye on the students' future occupations as *Physici*, who had responsibility for conducting forensic medical inquiries.[8] The

5 Manfred Heinemann, *Schule im Vorfeld der Verwaltung* (Göttingen, 1974), pp. 23–5.
6 Wilhelm Stieda, *Erfurter Universitätsreformpläne im 18. Jahrhundert* (Erfurt, 1934), p. 101.
7 Ibid., pp. 105–6.
8 See the decree by Margrave Christian Friedrich of Ansbach-Bayreuth, dated 15 January 1770, ordering anatomy demonstrations at the University of Erlangen. Staatsarchiv Bamberg Rep. C14, Nr. 290: "Hochfürstliche Verordnungen die Friedrichs-Universität betreffend." The government in Hannover ordered the same for Göttingen in 1751, yet in 1763 there were indications the order was not being carried out. In that year, the Privy Council admonished the medical faculty for not

drive for more practical instruction also contributed to the rapid spread of teaching clinics in medicine during the 1780s and 1790s, a development to which we shall return later on.

Nor was medicine the only discipline affected. When new statutes for the University of Greifswald in Swedish Pomerania were issued in 1775, they underscored the university's role in occupational training, not only for government officials and members of professions, but also for "landlords, merchants, seamen, or craftsmen and manufacturers." For this purpose, the statutes ordered that none be appointed as professor but those who are "not only thoroughly learned and proficient in academic lecturing, but also practically experienced" in one area or another.[9] They further specified the type of practical teaching to be given in each of the higher faculties: theology students were to be taught their priestly obligations and how to preach and conduct catechisms; law students were to be taught "judicial as well as extra-judicial practice"; finally medical students were to learn the exercise of their profession through "diligent dissections, surgical operations, and birthings."[10]

The guiding force behind many of these reforms, insofar as they developed out of initiatives by territorial governments, was cameralism. That "baroque science," as Mack Walker so aptly named it,[11] might best be defined as the science of fiscal administration, so long as it is understood that under "fiscal" affairs a cameralist might include an impressive range of topics. The basic principle of cameralism was perhaps nowhere better expressed than by young Crown Prince Friedrich of Prussia, not yet "the Great," but already in 1739 well schooled in his future duties. "The might of a state," he wrote, "does not at all consist in the extent of its lands, nor in the possession of vast wastes or immense deserts, but in the wealth of its inhabitants and in their number. The interest of a prince is thus to populate a country, to make it flourish, not to devastate and destroy it."[12]

> reporting on each candidate's performance in their anatomy demonstrations, as it had been ordered to do. To this the professors replied that the requirement carried with it many problems and that in any case it was their business how candidates were examined in anatomy. Archiv Universität Göttingen 4IVa, Nr. 4: "Verfügungen, daß die medicinische Facultät über die Examina der promovierten Candidaten jährlich zu berichten habe."
>
> 9 Johann Carl Dähnert, *Sammlung gemeiner und besonderer Pommerscher und Rügischer Landes-Urkunden, Gesetze, Privilegien, Verträge, Constitutionen und Ordnungen,* Supplement, Bd. 2 (Stralsund, 1786), p. 112.
>
> 10 Ibid., pp. 113–14. It should be noted that students who intended to become physicians would not actually perform surgical operations and birthings in most places, but as future *Physici* they would be responsible for examining and supervising the surgeons and midwives who would be carrying out those duties.
>
> 11 Mack Walker, *German Home Towns: Community, State, and the General Estate, 1648–1871* (Ithaca, N.Y., 1971), p. 145.
>
> 12 Quoted in Keith Tribe, *Governing Economy: The Reformation of German Economic Discourse 1750–1840* (Cambridge, 1988), p. 19. Tribe's book is an excellent general introduction to cameralism, and my treatment leans on it heavily. See also Marc Raeff, *The Well-Ordered Police State: Social and Institutional Change through Law in the Germanies and Russia, 1600–1800* (New Haven, Conn., 1983), and Walker, *German Home Towns* pp. 145–84. Finally, Charles Ingrao, *The Hessian Mercenary State: Ideas, Institutions, and Reform Under Frederick II, 1760–1785* (Cambridge, 1987), offers a case study of attempts to put cameralist principles into action. See pp. 46–52 for comments on the program's inherent contradictions and limitations.

Make no mistake about it. This was not the stuff of liberal, laissez-faire capitalism centered in free individuals seeking their own ends. Cameralism placed the primary motive power for economic growth in wise intervention by state government. It was nothing if not creation by design. But probably for this very reason the promise of cameralism – contented, wealthy, and well-governed subjects supplying a treasury brimming with tax revenues – proved quite seductive to princes. Thus planners and others seeking the ear of a prince quickly learned to deploy cameralist principles to sell their ideas. Physicians too showed themselves adept at presenting medical policy in terms of the new discourse.

Cameralism made itself directly felt in higher education as a subject for university courses. The first chairs of administrative science and economics were created by the Prussian government at Halle and Frankfurt an der Oder, both in 1727. Three years later, the Landgrave of Hesse-Kassel made a similar appointment at the University of Rinteln. From there, the spread of cameralism stagnated for a time, at least as a subject of regular unversity lectures. Following its successful introduction at the University of Vienna after mid-century and the publication of comprehensive treatises by Justi and Sonnenfels, however, cameralism became a standard offering at most universities in Protestant and Catholic Germany.[13] The appeal of cameralism in university education was neatly summed up by Dalberg in his memorandum on the University of Erfurt. "One can say what one will," he wrote in a section calling for the introduction of *Policeywissenschaften* (administrative sciences) at Erfurt, "those who administer the State or serve it must be familiar with these unalterable principles, otherwise their administration will be painful and miserable bungling (*Pfuschwerk*)."[14] Because princes looked to the universities to produce the future counselors and administrators, the benefits promised by a "science of administration" were attractive indeed.

The second impetus for reform came not so much from cameralism itself as from the kind of bureaucratic and fiscal thinking that nurtured the cameralists. Along with their role in educating "instruments for the State," as Dalberg so charmingly put it, universities also came to be seen as money-making ventures in their own right. If only inhabitants of a territory could be prevented from going elsewhere and foreigners induced to attend the local university, so the thinking went, the territory's economy would be greatly enriched. This viewpoint guided planning for the University of Göttingen during the early 1730s every step of the way. "It is easy to prove," wrote one planner,

that up to now over 100,000 fl have been taken from the principality and wasted, money which through establishment of a local university will not only be retained in the country, but two or three times as much will be drawn in. The calculation of 200,000 fl follows automatically, if one reckons on only 1000 students and 200 fl per student, of whom the majority customarily require much more.[15]

13 Tribe, *Governing Economy*, pp. 42–44, 91–118.
14 Stieda, *Erfurter Universitätsreformpläne*, p. 112.
15 Emil Franz Rössler, *Die Gründung der Universität Göttingen* (repr. ed. of Göttingen, 1855), first memorandum of J. D. Gruber, dated 30 August 1732, p. 1.

In the event, Göttingen was designed with just these considerations in mind, as a sort of academic resort for well-to-do young men. It offered the full range of currently fashionable subjects, it hired a large law faculty because law was the subject that young men on their way up (or already there) most preferred to study, and most importantly, Göttingen paid top dollar for famous scholars. Students who came to the university, therefore, could be assured of making the acquaintance of individuals who had valuable connections for their future careers.[16]

There can be little question that Göttingen succeeded spectacularly. Although no one ever seems to have reckoned whether it actually made money for the Hannoverian government, it certainly stimulated the local economy by drawing hundreds of well-heeled students.[17] Even more importantly, Göttingen's perceived success markedly altered the way that universities conceived of themselves and were conceived of by their territorial governments as revenue sources. One memorandum from the late 1760s, for example, opened by declaring that if only five hundred "foreign" students could be drawn to the University of Erfurt, they would bring at least 100,000 Rthlr yearly to the benefit of the area's economy.[18] Although the next university founded after Göttingen, the University of Erlangen (1743), attempted to serve as a bridge between academically oriented secondary schools (*Gymnasien*) and full universities, it too attempted to present an attractive assortment of subjects for well-to-do students. Among these were instruction in the "gallant studies," which were outside the normal faculty curricula (as they were at Göttingen): French, fencing, riding, and dancing. Emphasizing its position as a bridge institution, Erlangen initially hired five professors in the philosophy faculty, two theologians, two jurists, and only one professor of medicine. The low priority placed on the latter discipline no doubt derived from the overall scarcity of medical students.[19]

16 Charles E. McClelland, *State, Society and University in Germany, 1700–1914* (Cambridge, 1980), pp. 35–41; Notker Hammerstein, "Die Universitätsgründungen im Zeichen der Aufklärung," in *Beiträge zu Problemen deutscher Universitätsgründungen der frühen Neuzeit,* ed. Peter Baumgart and Notker Hammerstein (Nendeln/Lichtenstein, 1978), pp. 263–98.
17 Hans-Jürgen Gerhard, "Göttingens Verfassung, Verwaltung und Wirtschaft in der ersten Hälfte des 18. Jahrhunderts," in *Göttingen im 18. Jahrhundert* (Göttingen, 1987), pp. 7–23.
18 Stadtarchiv Erfurt, 1-1/X, B, XIII, Nr. 39; memorandum labeled "Unterthänigste Vorschlag, über die Mittel zur Wieder-Aufnahme der Erfurtischen Universität." The memo is undated, but it refers to the recent death of the medical professor Mangold, which occurred in July 1767.
19 On Erlangen, see Hammerstein, "Die Universitätsgründungen im Zeichen der Aufklärung," pp. 280–2. Erlangen was not the only school to attempt to fill this niche. The Collegium Carolinum in Kassel (founded 1709) also attempted to bridge the *Gymnasium* and the full university, although it never attempted to obtain imperial patents as a university. A similar institution with the identical name – Collegium Carolinum – was also opened in Braunschweig in 1745. Theodor Hartwig, "Mitteilungen aus der Geschichte des Collegium Carolinum in Cassel," *Zeitschrift des Vereins für hessische Geschichte* 41 (1908): 68–96; Otto Berge, "Beiträge zur Geschichte des Bildungswesens und der Akademien unter Landgraf Friedrich II von Hesse Kassel (1760–1785)," *Hessisches Jahrbuch für Landesgeschichte* 4 (1954): 229–61; Ingrao, *The Hessian Mercenary State,* pp. 31–3, 77–9; and Friedrich Koldewey, *Geschichte des Schulwesens im Herzogtum Braunschweig von den ältesten Zeiten bis zum Regierungsantritt des Herzogs Wilhelm im Jahre 1831* (Wolfenbüttel, 1891), esp. pp. 147–53. These sources emphasize the new schools' orientation toward the "modern" disciplines of natural science, mathematics, and modern history.

Not only did Göttingen change the way universities thought about themselves, it also changed the way they talked about themselves. Göttingen had a boundless capacity for self-promotion, and it advertised itself in the press with all the verve of a market huckster, if with somewhat more refinement. One pamphlet published in 1748 was cleverly constructed in the form of two letters to a "distinguished gentleman" who was thinking of sending his son to Göttingen. The writer of the letters emphasized the city's healthy air and water, wide and brightly lit streets, beautiful surroundings, and reasonable cost of living. Turning then to the university itself, the writer had little to say in his first letter about theology or medicine at Göttingen, not surprisingly, because these subjects were unattractive to wealthy students. In contrast, he devoted considerable effort to the law faculty, including a discussion of the professors' writings and their methods of teaching students the practical business of judicial procedure. The writer also described the philosophical faculty in some detail, and he took care to praise the talents of the riding, fencing, and dancing masters at Göttingen (as well as listing their customary honoraria).[20]

As might be expected, this sort of thing spread to other universities. Very shortly after the Göttingen pamphlet appeared, a similar publication offered a "Trustworthy Report on the Current Situation at the University of Marburg." It too talked about the favorable locale, dedicated professors, and the opportunities for gallant studies at Marburg, and it made a special point of mentioning how young cavaliers could find good society by being welcomed into surrounding aristocratic houses.[21] Puff pieces of this sort appeared to be a particular specialty at Erlangen. One published in 1770 described the trendy new chairs in the philosophical faculty for natural history, "economic and cameral sciences," and applied mathematics.[22] Meanwhile, the University of Erfurt put its best face forward in 1768 by publicly advising prospective students that they would be immune from suits brought by local women for paternity and betrothal. Even the University of Altdorf, not one of the more dynamic institutions during this period, got into the act in 1795.[23]

20 Der gegenwärtige Zustand der Göttingischen Universität in Zweeyen Briefen an einen vornehmen Herrn im Reiche (Göttingen, 1748).
21 Johann Nikolaus Schwendler, Zuverlässiger Bericht von der gegenwärtigen Verfassung der Universität Marburg (n.p., 1748).
22 [Johann Georg Krafft], Schreiben an einem Freund von dem gegenwärtigen Zustande der hochfürstlichen Friedrichs Alexanders Universität zu Erlangen (Ansbach, 1770), p. 22. See also Johann Ernst Wiedeburg, Nachricht von dem gegenwärtigen Zustand der Akademie Erlangen (Erlangen, 1759); and Johann Georg Papst, Gegenwärtiger Zustand der Friedrich Alexander Universität zu Erlangen (Erlangen, 1791).
23 The advertisement for Erfurt is reprinted in Stieda, Erfurter Universitätsreformpläne, pp.79–82. On Altdorf, see Georg Andreas Will, Geschichte and Beschreibung der Nürnbergischen Universität Altdorf (Altdorf, 1795). Although it contains an obvious pitch for parents thinking of sending their sons to Altdorf, Will's book is too long and pedantic to be a successful exemplar of this genre. It should also be noted in passing that this sort of university propaganda eventually engendered its counterpart: a literature consisting of criticisms of individual universities. See, for example, [Carl Friedrich Hochheimer], Göttingen, nach seiner eigentlichen Beschaffenheit zum Nutzen derer die daselbst studieren wollen (Lausanne, 1791). In this case, the writer was by no means an unalloyed critic of Göttingen, although he had unfavorable comments about, among other things, several of the professors, the quality of student life, the wine and beer, and the excessive number of dogs in town.

Most interesting of all is the way that universities applied their learned periodicals to the purposes of advertisement. Although *gelehrte Zeitschriften* had been published previously in towns such as Jena, Hamburg, and Frankfurt am Main, the *Göttingische Zeitungen von gelehrten Sachen,* begun in 1739, became a model for a host of similar publications in which the ends of scholarship dovetailed with university self-promotion. One of them, the *Erlangische Anzeigen,* launched in 1743, the same year that the university opened, published along with its book reviews and "useful" scholarly essays occasional reports of what was going on at the university even when there was not much to talk about. Thus there appeared in 1744 a notice declaring how the number of students was increasing daily, and adding that not a single student had died at Erlangen in the preceding year, owing to the town's healthy location and the university's "good order."[24] The same reform memorandum from the University of Erfurt in the 1760s that talked about how more foreign students would improve the local economy also urged the launching of a learned periodical, "which is the custom at all well-established universities."[25] A few years later, regulations issued for the University of Tübingen in 1771 also urged publication of a learned periodical that would be a collection of articles, notices and reviews of "important and useful books," and a report of scholarly goings-on in Tübingen and the entire duchy of Württemberg.[26] Eventually, learned periodicals were at least attempted during the eighteenth century in Jena (several), Tübingen, Erfurt, Halle, Kiel, Leipzig (several), Mainz, Würzburg, Königsberg, and Rinteln.[27]

The extent to which universities were transformed into market-driven institutions should not be exaggerated. When the University of Mainz was reorganized in 1784, Anselm Franz von Bentzel (1738–86), the university's curator, explicitly denied that raising money from foreign students was his goal. His purpose instead was to create an institution that would train local men for state service.[28] Moreover, while discussion of their economic aspects occupied a major portion of the public and state attention devoted to the universities, few significant structural changes seem to have been implemented. True, the eighteenth-century German universities gradually introduced new subjects into the curriculum, and the impe-

---

24 *Erlangische Anzeigen* Nr. XLVI, 9 November 1744, p. 366.
25 See note 18, above.
26 Theodor Eisenlohr, *Sammlung der württembergischen Schul-Geseze* Bd. 11, Abth. 3, "Universitäts-Gesetze bis zum Jahr 1843" (Tübingen, 1843), p. 494. The merits of learned periodicals for burnishing the reputation of a university were also mentioned in connection with the University of Mainz. See Helmut Mathy, "Das Gutachten des Juristen Franz Joseph Hartleben zur Reform der Mainzer Universität 1783," *Archiv für hessische Geschichte und Altertumskunde,* Neue Folge 30 (1969/70): 241.
27 On these journals, see Joachim Kirchner, *Bibliographie der Zeitschriften des deutschen Sprachgebiets bis 1900,* Bd. 1 (Stuttgart, 1969), pp. 1–28.
28 *Neue Verfassung der verbesserten hohen Schule zu Mainz* (1977 repr. of Mainz, 1784), p. 10. On Bentzel's role in introducing enlightened reforms into Mainz, see Horst-Wilhelm Jung, *Anselm Franz von Bentzel im Dienste der Kurfürsten von Mainz* (Wiesbaden, 1966).

tus behind these introductions undoubtedly arose from a desire to attract students. But taken as a whole, the reforms instituted by governments at various times aimed at correcting abuses or inadequacies in the operation of the universities, rather than completely transforming them into new institutions. What is unmistakable is the redirection of university curricula toward the teaching of practice.

TERRITORIAL GOVERNMENTS AND THE PUBLIC'S HEALTH

The reform of university curricula constituted but one avenue of activity on the part of princely governments as they attempted to extend bureaucratic control over the complex social, political, and economic structures of their territories. University reforms contributed significantly to this larger project, because after all it was the university-trained administrators who devised the policies of enlightened statecraft and attempted to implant them in the routine of governance. Among these graduates, it was obviously the jurists who played the biggest role. In their role as administrators of the school system, ministers too were involved in the reforms, if only in some cases as opponents to removal of control of education from the governing church consistories.

Although it might appear at first glance that physicians stood to the side as onlookers to these developments, there was one area of policy making where they had an opportunity to contribute significantly: public health. Governments wanted to minimize the economic consequences of human and animal epidemics and improve the level of health care available to the population, which in turn would raise its productivity. For their part, physicians were eager to demonstrate that they too could stand in the vanguard of "enlightened" administration. By doing so they hoped to glean some of the prestige, remuneration, and social advancement that government sevice offered, no meager compensations in a land where the middle class had few avenues for upward mobility. Consequently in the 1770s medical writers began publishing works that prompted the various city-states and principalities toward greater vigilance in the area of public health, and promoted themselves as the ideal framers and executors of the new policies. The advocates of *medicinische Policey,* as the program was called, attached their arguments to one of the central principles of eighteenth-century cameralism: the size of a state's population as the cornerstone of its economic and political power. The same arguments that cameralists used to encourage immigration and preservation of some tenure rights for the peasantry were appropriated by physicians to urge the establishment of programs for public health. As one of the major proponents, Christoph Ludwig Hoffmann (1721–1807), expressed it in 1777, "The population is the true means for making a state vigorous and increasing a treasury's revenues without the subjects feeling it."[29] This sort of talk, as Hoffmann well knew, made

---

29 Quoted in Alfons Fischer, *Geschichte des deutschen Gesundheitswesens,* Bd. 2 (Berlin, 1933), p. 46.

princes sit up and take notice, and their interest provided support for the creation of territorial medical boards (*collegia medica*) and other public health structures.

Alongside the support lent public health by the economic motives of cameralism, the creation by the states of a supervisory apparatus for public health intersected with other goals as well.[30] One was the attempt to bring formerly independent institutions under closer bureaucratic supervision, or where that proved impossible, to peel away some of those institutions' functions. Mostly this involved territorial governments and university medical faculties, although in certain respects governments also limited the independence and usurped the position of the town and district physicians. The faculties, it will be recalled, were characterized by a collection of sundry privileges and duties, for which they were rarely answerable directly to higher authorities, and from which the faculty members obtained no small portion of their incomes. It was to create a medical authority more directly responsible to the central government that various territories inaugurated the medical boards.

Unquestionably the principal conflict between territorial governments and medical faculties occurred over admission to medical practice. Governments displayed considerable dissatisfaction with what they saw as the faculties' lax standards in the granting of degrees. Part of the problem arose from the fact that a doctorate of medicine represented a license both to teach *and* to practice medicine, and the actions taken by governments attempted to separate those rights. At no time during the eighteenth century did governments attempt to intervene in the granting of licenses to teach at the university. But it was quite another matter with the license to practice. As early as 1651, the Bavarian Collegium Medicum (organized in 1616) was granted authority to conduct a second examination of prospective physicians, an innovation that took place over the strenuous objections of the medical faculty at Ingolstadt.[31]

The elaborate medical system that evolved in Brandenburg-Prussia between 1685 and 1725 ultimately represented a far greater restriction on the privileges of the territory's four universities. The initial edict of 1685 created a Collegium Medicum in Berlin, consisting of the court physicians resident in the capital, along with the two full medical professors at Frankfurt/Oder. Although Frankfurt lay only some seventy-five kilometers from Berlin, that distance was sufficient to insure that the Collegium would be dominated by its Berlin members, who were dependent on the Elector for their support. One of the Collegium's principal duties was the certification of all existing and future physicians, who were ordered to present themselves to the Collegium either in person or in writing, along with their diplomas and testimonials. The Collegium was also charged with yearly inspection of all apothecary shops in the Hohenzollern lands – a well-nigh

---

30 On cameralism and public health, see George Rosen, "Cameralism and the Concept of Medical Police," in idem, *From Medical Police to Social Medicine* (New York, 1974), pp. 120–41.

31 Alexander von Hoffmeister, *Das Medizinalwesen im Kurfürstentum Bayern,* Neue Münchner Beiträge zur Geschichte der Medizin und Wissenschaften, Bd. 6 (Munich, 1975), p. 25.

impossible task, considering the distances to be covered – and the certification of new apothecaries, midwives, barbers and surgeons.[32]

These requirements for admission to practice underwent a significant modification in 1718. Whereas previously a practitioner simply had to display his qualifications, a new edict issued early in 1718 specified that henceforth no one, "whether he has received a university degree or not," would be permitted to practice before presenting himself in person before the Collegium Medicum, and passing an examination including the "resolution of practical cases (*Casuum Practicorum*)."[33] Although from the description it is clear that the "practical cases" were merely written case histories and therefore answerable using standard textbook procedures, the inclusion of this subject in the exam – along with the introduction of the examination itself – suggests the importance attached by the Prussian government to raising the qualifications of physicians for practice.

The final major piece of the medical system that would prevail in Prussia for most of the eighteenth century was added in 1725, with the issuance of a new general medical code and the opening of the Collegium Medico-Chirurgicum (not to be confused with the Collegium Medicum) in Berlin. The new Collegium was established by Friedrich Wilhelm I, ever mindful of the needs of his army, as a training school for military surgeons. But it also became for Berlin, which did not have a university, a sort of shadow medical faculty. To say that the Collegium Medico-Chirurgicum rivaled the existing Prussian universities would be to cast it into rather shabby company, for it enjoyed the use of the anatomical theater and botanical garden of the Berlin Academy of Sciences and the Court Apothecary's well-equipped chemical laboratory. Six professors were appointed to the Collegium, making it the largest medical faculty in Prussia and one of the largest in Germany. To complement the Collegium's primary task of educating military and civilian surgeons, the edict of 1725 ordered all candidates for medical degrees to complete a course of six lectures in anatomy offered during the winter in Berlin.[34] The Collegium's role was augmented once again in 1781, with the inclusion of a mandatory clinical course for all students wishing to practice medicine in Prussia.[35]

Needless to say, the Collegium and the new requirements for an anatomy course in Berlin were unwelcome developments to the medical faculties. Although a university degree was required to sit for the examinations and the anatomical course, the faculties justifiably felt the new institution made dangerous inroads into their prerogatives and incomes. It now became possible for a student to spend

---

32 Christian Otto Mylius, *Corpus Constitutionum Marchicarum, oder Königl. Preußis. und Churfürstli. Brandenburgische in der Chur- und Marck Brandenburg, auch incorporirten Landen publicirte und ergangene Ordnungen, Edicta, Mandata, Rescripta, etc.*, Teil 5 (Berlin, 1740), pp. 11–13, 17–21.
33 Ibid., p. 205.
34 Ibid., p. 224
35 Wolfram Kaiser et al., "Collegium Clinicum Halense," in *250 Jahre Collegium Clinicum Halense 1717–1967*, Beiträge zur Geschichte der Medizinischen Fakultät der Universität Halle (Halle, 1967), pp. 65–6.

a minimum time at a university digesting the theoretical courses, take his degree, and then travel to Berlin, where he could complete his anatomical training and also receive bedside clinical instruction at the city's large Charité hospital (which was required after 1781). This not only took a significant portion of medical training out of the faculties' hands; it also set up Berlin as an alternate center of patronage, and a far more useful one than provincial towns such as Halle, Duisburg, or Königsberg. Worse still, the creation of the Collegium Medico-Chirurgicum raised the danger of medical degrees from non-Prussian universities being accepted as a basis for practice in Brandenberg-Prussia, so long as the candidate took the anatomy course in Berlin and passed the exams there. In fact this did not happen, and Friedrich the Great even issued a decree in 1751 forbidding Prussian students from attending any non-Prussian university. But this did little to dispell the belief that the traditional medical faculties were being bypassed.[36]

The example set by Bavaria and Prussia, establishing a territorial medical board with authority to regulate admission to internal medicine as well as other branches of healing, was followed by various German principalities during the eighteenth century. The duchy of Braunschweig-Wolfenbüttel published a medical ordinance in 1721 ordering practitioners to present their credentials, without specifying to whom the credentials were to be presented. This oversight was corrected in 1747 with the creation of a Collegium Medicum, before which anyone wishing to practice in the duchy must display his credentials and then submit to an oral examination.[37] Collegia medica with jurisdiction over admission to the healing occupations were also established in the duchies of Jülich and Berg in 1773, in the Palatinate as early as 1775, and in the ecclesiastical principality of Hildesheim in 1782.[38]

This general trend toward creation of medical boards separate from university faculties was not universal. New ordinances published in Mecklenburg-Schwerin in 1751 and Ansbach-Bayreuth in 1770 confirmed the sufficiency of medical degrees from their respective universities, Rostock and Erlangen, for practicing medicine.[39] The ordinance issued for Swedish Pomerania in 1779 took a middling

36 Reinhold Koser, "Friedrich der Große und die preußischen Universitäten," *Forschungen zur Brandenburgischen und Preußischen Geschichte* 17 (1904): 131–2.
37 *Serenissimi Reglement und Verordnung das Collegium Medicum in Braunschweig betreffend* (n.p., 1747), pp. 4–7. See also *Hoch-Fürstliche Braunschweig-Wolfenbüttelsche Medicinal-Ordnung nebst beygefügter Apotheker-Taxa* (Braunschweig, 1721). My thanks to Mary Lindemann for furnishing me with copies of these two ordinances.
38 For Jülich and Berg, see "Churfürstlich-Pfälzische Medizinalordnung für die Herzogthümer Jülich und Berg," *Archiv der medizinischen Polizey und der gemeinnützigen Arzneikunde* 3 (1785): 26–63, esp. pp. 28–31. According to Eberhard Stübler, *Geschichte der medizinischen Fakultät der Universität Heidelberg 1386–1925* (Heidelberg, 1926), p. 130, an order issued in 1775 directed all physicians wishing to practice in the Palatinate to be examined before the Consilium Medicum in Mannheim. For Hildesheim, see *Hochfürstlich-Hildesheimische Medicinal-Ordnung* (Hildesheim, 1782). It should be noted that this list of collegia medica is not meant to be exhaustive.
39 *Herzoglich Mecklenburg-Schwerinsche Medicinal- und Taxordnung vom 20. Juli 1751*, 2nd ed. (Schwerin, 1779). The second edition includes several ordinances published between 1751 and 1775 as

course between the others. It created a *Gesundheits-Collegium*, consisting of the medical professors from the University of Greifswald, the first and second *Physici* from the town of Stralsund, along with the doctor to the army garrison stationed there, the "collective *Physici* in the districts and remaining cities," and finally two members of the Greifswald magistracy trained in jurisprudence. In theory then, the influence of the professors should have been more than balanced by the number of other members. But because the Collegium's seat was put in Greifswald, the senior professor from the faculty was appointed as director, and, most importantly, only the Greifswald members had any claim on the Collegium's income, one might suppose that the other members' engagement with its business was less than passionate. Still, giving medical professors as individuals an influential role in the *Gesundheits-Collegium* was not the same thing as vesting those powers in the faculty.[40]

Certainly the most ambitious and comprehensive of the plans for Collegia Medica devised during the eighteenth century were those created by Christoph Ludwig Hoffmann. Hoffmann's first project, the Münster medical ordinance of 1777, combined three goals. First, like previous ones, it set procedures for examination and approval of healers. Hoffmann's procedures, however, were far more elaborate than any yet devised. Each member of the Collegium was to give the candidate a question to work on, for which the answer could be either known or unknown. Any member who asked a question with an unknown answer must compose a written response to the candidate's answer and prove his response. Hoffmann especially encouraged this kind of question, because any candidate who showed himself unable to create his own answer or to understand the board member's proof would clearly be lacking a fundamental knowledge of logic. "From such a man," he noted, "there is certainly little promise of anything scientific."[41]

Hoffmann's second goal was to create a distribution of practititioners that would insure adequate health care for the entire population. As an explicit goal of

---

supplements to the original. For Ansbach-Bayreuth, see Staatsarchiv Bamberg Rep. C14, Nr. 290, "Hochfürstliche Verordnungen die Friedrichs Universität betreffend," dated 15 January 1770.

40 *Medicinal-Ordnung für Schwedisch Pommern und Rügen* (Stralsund, 1779), reprinted in Dähnert, *Sammlung,* Supplement, Bd. 2, pp. 552–62. The ordinance called for an examination consisting of an anatomical course in Greifswald (apparently following the Prussian example) and the written solution of a clinical problem. The reason for the specification of the Stralsund members is that Stralsund, along with its attached estates, comprised a separate district under the supervision of its three members and two members of the Stralsund magistracy. They had the right to examine healers and presumably to collect the resulting fees.

41 "Von einem solchen Manne hat man sich aber gewiß wenig Wissenschaftliches zu versprechen, . . ." *Unterricht von dem Kollegium der Aerzte in Münster wie der Unterthanen bey allerhand ihm zustoßenden Krankheiten die sichersten Wege und besten Mittel treffen kann seyne verlohrene Gesundheit wieder zu erhalten nebst den Münster Medizinalgesezten entworfen* (Münster, 1777), pp. 126–7. On Hoffmann and Münster, see Paul Druffel, "Das Münstersche Medizinalwesen von 1750–1818," *Zeitschrift für vaterländische Geschichte und Altertumskunde* 65 (1907): 44–128; and Manfred Stürzbecher, "Zur Geschichte der Medizinalgesetzgebung in Fürstentum Münster im 17. und 18. Jahrhundert," *Westfälische Zeitschrift* 114 (1964): 165–99.

medical ordinances, this was quite novel, as was the method devised for attaining it. Hoffmann proposed that physicians, surgeons, and other healers be ranked according to their performance on the examination. Accordingly, he defined six classes of physicians: the lowest class consisted of "Empiricists" who do not know enough semiotics (the interpretation of symptoms in diagnosing a disease) even to look a disease up in a standard reference work; the fifth class, also called "Empiricists," who do understand semiotics but who do not understand the causes of diseases; the fourth class of "capable" physicians, who have an appropriate knowledge of logic, natural philosophy (*Naturlehre*), and the "demonstrative method"; the third class or "very capable" doctors, who add to the preceding class a knowledge of dissection, physiology, pathology, therapeutics, and who know what has been discovered to treat illness; the second class of "excellent" (*fürtreffliche*) doctors, who also know auxiliary sciences such as chemistry, botany, and mineralogy; and finally the "excellent and distinguished" (*fürtreffliche und ausgezeichnete*) doctors, who not only dispose of all medical knowledge, but have also contributed something to it. This final group, Hoffmann added, is "astonishingly rare."[42]

Once assigned their proper class on the basis of their exams, physicians would receive a certificate testifying to their standing. The certificate for the lowest class would list the diseases they were qualified to treat. The certificate for the next class would testify to the physician's ability to treat all illnesses, and the higher categories would designate progressively greater knowledge and accomplishment with their honorific titles: "capable," "very capable," "excellent," and so on. Hoffmann expected the classification to promote a better distribution of healers in the territory, because he placed restrictions on the right of a lower-class healer to settle into an area where a higher class one already resided. This, he claimed, would force healers to spread out, and it would also encourage those on the lower rungs to study and be reexamined as a way of bettering their economic situation. At the same time, Hoffmann called for periodic examination of higher class physicians as well, to insure that they did not slack off in their attempts to improve their knowledge. Through all of this he expected to produce a dramatic melioration in the level of health care.[43]

Hoffmann's plan for Münster attempted to remove the unofficial and unqualified healers who vexed administrators of health policy by simply incorporating them into the official system and assigning them to their proper place on the ladder. Although he eliminated the requirement that physicians hold an M.D., he retained it as a requirement for *Physici* and members of the Collegium, which meant it remained effectively mandatory for those hoping for real social advancement. While appearing to open up opportunities for social and economic advancement through reexamination, in fact the plan did just the opposite. The retention of the M.D. for official positions and especially the definition of higher classes of practitioner on the basis of knowledge that one obtains routinely in

42 *Unterricht*, p. 122.
43 Ibid., pp. 134–51.

university medical study effectively closed off the upper classifications to healers from the lower strata of society who could not afford a university education.

Hoffmann knew full well that merely proclaiming a set of laws would do little to change the health system if the public did not understand the reasons behind it. Therefore his third goal was to educate the public about why they should consult only healers certified by the Collegium Medicum and why physicians who understood the true causes of disease were more capable than those who made a diagnosis and started therapy simply by reading off a patient's symptoms. The centrality of this goal was demonstrated by the title of the volume in which Hoffmann published the new laws: "Instruction from the College of Physicians in Münster How a Subject Can Obtain the Most Secure Way and Best Means to Recover his Lost Health. . . ." Interspersed with sections containing the laws dealing with physicians, surgeons, and other healers, were long didactic portions meant to teach the public about healers and health care. Unfortunately this project was seriously undermined by the way it was presented. The publication contained hundreds of pages and was written in a baroque prose that made it horribly unwieldy, scarcely the sort of thing one would want to use for enlightening the masses.

Whatever its didactic shortcomings, Hoffmann's plan for Münster proved quite successful, if success is measured by its influence on other medical codes. After consultations with Hoffmann, the Margrave of Hesse-Kassel adopted a plan that was virtually identical to the Münster code in 1778.[44] The next summons to Hoffmann came from the Archbishop-Elector of Mainz, who engaged him in 1787 to set up a medical board in the principality.

When Hoffmann arrived in Mainz, he encountered a situation far different from that in Münster and Kassel. In Münster, there had been no medical faculty to deal with in creating a central medical authority, and while Hesse-Kassel possessed two universities, at Marburg and Rinteln, those schools enjoyed relatively little influence at the court in Kassel, where there was already an academic institution, the Collegum Carolinum, with its own medical faculty. As a consequence, Hoffmann's establishment of a medical board in Kassel was supported by the local medical elite, who saw this board as giving them an advantage over the university faculties. Mainz, by contrast, had its own university and a medical faculty that had effectively functioned as the chief medical authority in the principality.

Hoffmann's call to Mainz must be seen too against the background of more than forty years of attempts by successive Electors to introduce administrative,

---

44 *Erneuerte und erweiterte Ordnung für das Collegium Medicum zu Cassel; sammt den Gesetzen, welche das Medicinal- und Sanitätswesen überhaupt, und im ganzen Lande, betreffen* (Kassel, 1778). Hesse-Kassel already had a Collegium Medicum holding broad supervisory powers over medical practitioners. The Collegium, established in 1770 and resident in Kassel, was another example of the erosion of the powers of medical faculties, in this case the faculties at Marburg and Rinteln. See Ingrao, *The Hessian Mercenary State*, p. 111; and Hans Braun, "Hessische Medizinverhältnisse im 18. Jahrhundert," *Hessenland* 17 (1903): 102–4, 126–8, 144–5.

educational, and fiscal reforms into the principality. A special target of the reform efforts was the sumptuous wealth held by the Jesuits and other religious orders in the principality, along with their total domination of the educational system. With the aim of restricting the amount of wealth that could be salted away in religious institutions, a series of laws declared in the early 1770s severely restricted new endowments of monasteries and other religious foundations, created a secular School Commission with broad powers over education, and established a College of Education to provide future teachers with an up-to-date training free of Jesuit influence and methods.[45] The dissolution of the Jesuit order by Pope Clement XIII in 1773 freed up teaching positions at all levels, including the university, and it allowed the Elector to confiscate the Jesuits' former properties.[46] He intended that these be sold and the proceeds used for primary education, but this plan was stalled for some time by aristocratic opposition. Other monastic properties were confiscated in 1781, and their assets became the endowment of the University of Mainz when it was refounded in 1784.[47]

Even before Hoffmann's arrival, the question of whether the medical faculty should continue acting as the chief medical authority in the territory had been the subject of disagreement among the professors themselves. Two memoranda written in 1773 took opposing stances, with one professor calling for the affairs of public health to be separated from teaching positions. Another argued that because there were only a few opportunities for physicians in the territory, there would never be many medical students at Mainz. Therefore it would be wise to permit professors to supplement their incomes through "governmental medical practice (*staatliche Praxin medicam*)."[48]

Almost from the day he began his new duties, Hoffmann ran into trouble. He fell into an acrimonious dispute with one of the medical professors, Karl Strack (1722–1806), over where a new hospital should be located. His high-handed attitude toward the faculty was amply displayed in a memorandum he wrote for the Elector, outlining an appropriate medical curriculum for the university. After

45 T. C. W. Blanning, *Reform and Revolution in Mainz 1743–1803* (Cambridge, 1974), pp. 114–6 and 126–33. See also Jung, *Anselm Franz von Bentzel*, pp. 5–53.

46 The dissolution of the Jesuits was the occasion for significant reforms at other Catholic universities as well, a topic that has been treated recently by Anton Schindling, "Die Julius-Universität im Zeitalter der Aufklärung," in *Vierhundert Jahre Universität Würzburg*, ed. Peter Baumgart (Neustadt an der Aisch, 1982), pp. 77–127, and Winfried Müller, *Universität und Orden* (Berlin, 1986), which provides an excellent portrayal of Ingolstadt between 1773 and 1803. Funds confiscated from the Jesuits after 1773 also contributed to the transformation of an academic secondary school (*Gymnasium*) in Bonn into an academy like the ones in Kassel and Braunschweig in 1777 (see note 18 for more about these schools), and into a full university in 1784. See Max Braubach, *Die erste Bonner Hochschule* (Bonn, 1966), pp. 23–44.

47 On the reform of the University of Mainz, see Blanning, *Reform and Revoltion in Mainz*, pp. 166–72; and Helmut Mathy, *Die Universität Mainz 1477–1977* (Mainz, 1977), pp. 115–53.

48 The two memoranda are cited in Anton Ph. Brück, "Um die Reform der Mainzer juristischen und medizinischen Fakultäten im 18. Jahrhundert," in *Die alte Mainzer Universität. Gedenkschrift anläßlich der Wiedereröffnung der Universität in Mainz als Johannes-Gutenberg-Universität* (Mainz, 1946), p. 63.

describing the courses that should be taught and their rationale in the curriculum, Hoffmann concluded by castigating the medical professors for their "pitifully bad" teaching of natural philosophy and the "still greater improvements" needed in physiology, pathology, materia medica, and the "entirety of practical subjects (*das ganze Praktische*)." Hoffmann also lost a valuable ally in Georg Christian Wedekind (1761–1831), a medical professor and personal physician to the Elector, about whose alleged membership in a secret society Hoffmann helped spread innuendos to the Elector.[49]

Whether for these reasons or others, such as the occupation of Mainz by the French army in October 1792 and the subsequent Jacobin uprising there, Hoffmann never did succeed in establishing a new Collegium Medicum in Mainz. But the conflict over his plan and its eventual failure should not be seen as arising merely from local circumstances and personalities. For embedded in it was a fundamental conflict in the medical profession itself. By long tradition, a medical degree had conferred on its holder the right both to teach at a university and to undertake treatment of internal illnesses. The standards used to judge conferral of those rights were those of physicians themselves, and while it would not be accurate to describe the profession as based upon a seamless joining of bedside practice and university teaching, every doctor of medicine could claim both as the pillars of his identity.

This professional unity began dissolving in the eighteenth century. The interest of governments in promoting public welfare and in leveling and regulating society's institutions was met by the desire on the part of physicians to provide enlightened health care and to design the best possible system for delivering it to the public. Physicians eagerly enlisted in the territorial governments' campaign, which they saw as progressive, but their service cost them a measure of professional independence and unity. To be sure, the distance between physicians in government service and their colleagues elsewhere was not large. Whether rendered for practice or for teaching, approval remained under the control of physicians. But it was no longer the same physicians who provided that approval.

THE INTRODUCTION OF CLINICAL INSTRUCTION

Beyond question, the most conspicuous innovation in medical curricula during the second half of the eighteenth century was the introduction of clinical instruction. Whereas at mid-century only one university in Germany, Halle, offered students such training, by 1800 no fewer than twelve universities (Erlangen, Jena, Marburg, Altdorf, Halle, Kiel, Tübingen, Greifswald, Göttingen, Würzburg, Bamberg, and Leipzig) were offering medical students clinical courses. What is noteworthy about this development is how the founding of these clinics was

---

49 Hermann Terhalle, "Das Projekt eines 'Collegium medicum' in Mainz," in *Medizingeschichte in unserer Zeit,* ed. Hans-Heinz Eulner et al. (Stuttgart, 1971), pp. 291–3.

clustered in a fairly limited period. With the exceptions of Halle (1729), Göttingen (1764), and Würzburg (1769), all were started between 1778 and the end of the century.

In a general way, the creation of these clinics was a response to the reforms already discussed in this chapter. By assuming functions that had formerly belonged to medical faculties, the new territorial medical boards in effect redefined the faculties by subtraction: the faculties ceased being professional "colleges" in the sense of the Faculté de Médecine in Paris or the Royal College of Physicians in London, and became teaching units. The university reforms enacted during the century, especially those designed to utilize the universities' potential for generating income, worked to the same end. Any school that hoped to succeed in this venture had not only to offer an attractive selection of courses, but also to persuade potential customers that they would be taught well. Certainly the economic impact of a renowned medical faculty was minor in comparison to the rewards to be collected from a good law faculty. But it was not negligible, and as universities such as Erlangen, Marburg, and Würzburg learned toward the end of the century, a good medical faculty headed by a widely respected clinical teacher could draw medical students all out of proportion to a university's size.

The medical boards probably prompted the creation of clinics in another way as well, by setting up a second examination. This exam solidified the functional side of the physician's identity, and it avoided the ambiguities between scholarship and practice inherent in the faculties' examinations. Those who passed it were certified as *practitioners,* even if the standards were those used by the faculties themselves: candidates' command of textbook doctrine in the theoretical and practical subjects. The importance attached to the practice of medicine is evident in the condemnation of the medical faculties made by the university reformer Christoph Meiners (1747–1810) at the opening of the nineteenth century: "If experience teaches that the faculties . . . all too often distribute to incompetent people the right to bring unpunished damage upon the life and health . . . of their fellow residents; then one cannot become angry if the government subjects those doctors promoted by one of the territorial universities to a second, stringent examination."[50] The faculties did respond to Meiners' criticism; indeed, they had already begun doing so when he published it in 1802. More than any other course, clinical training embodied that portion of a physician's identity connected to healing.

Although these conditions provided an environment favorable to the spread of clinics, evidence for their role in the creation of specific clinics is lacking. In part this is because the initiative for clinical instruction seems not to have come from the states in most cases. Instead, nearly every clinic was the project of an individual professor. The motivations behind the establishment of these clinics are unknown,

50 Christoph Meiners, *Ueber die Verfassung und Verwaltung deutscher Universitäten,* Bd. 2 (Göttingen, 1802), p. 360.

but whatever their personal reasons, professors' public justifications emphasized one common theme: clinics' contribution to public welfare, particularly among the poorer strata of society.[51] The merits of clinics in educating future medical practitioners, by contrast, received at best a secondary emphasis. Thus when the Altdorf professor Christian Gottlieb Hofmann (1743–97) published an announcement of his clinic in the *Journal von und für Deutschland* in 1786, he called it an "institute for poor patients (*Anstalt für arme Kranke*)," and he related how contributions collected from benefactors represented the fulfillment of every upright person's duty to aid his or her neighbor.[52]

The application of teaching clinics as a medium of poor relief was one more development in a long tradition of state and municipal sponsorship of medical care to the poor. The office of town physician, or *Physicus,* included medical care for the poor as one of its primary responsibilities, and it was easy for a professor who also held a post as *Physicus,* such as Christian Gottlieb Hofmann, to apply his practice among the poor to the purpose of giving students first-hand experience with healing. Poor patients were especially suitable for this, because as welfare recipients they were in no position to object to being gawked at and discussed by a group of strangers. Wealthier patients would not have suffered the indignity of such treatment, and simply would have found themselves another doctor.

A change that began in the 1770s in the orientation of public health policies also prompted the establishment of clinics. Up to that time, medical codes had concerned themselves mainly with regulating the activities and credentials of healers, be they physicians, surgeons, midwives, or apothecaries. This form of policy saw its culmination in the medical codes written by Christoph Ludwig Hoffmann. In the 1770s, however, a new type of policy began to appear, one based not on regulating practitioners but on controlling the environments and activities of citizens in order to preserve them from injury and illness. Public health policy began to intrude upon the affairs of everyday life.

The principal example of this new attitude toward public health was Johann Peter Frank's (1745–1821) epochal *System einer vollständigen medizinischen Polizey* (System of complete medical police). Calling his work a "system" was no empty boast; as it unwound through its first four volumes between 1779 and 1790, Frank's treatise pointed to an astonishing range of topics where government could act to improve the health of its subjects. Regulation of marriage, care of pregnant women and newborns, encouragement of mothers to nurse their own infants, establishment of orphanages, education, regulation of food, drink, and housing, prevention of accidents; he had suggestions for all these and more.[53] While

---

51 The role of university clinics in providing poor relief is discussed by Dieter Jetter, "Die ersten Universitätskliniken westdeutscher Staaten," *Deutsche medizinische Wochenschrift* 87 (5 October 1962): 2037–42.

52 Christian Gottlieb Hofmann, "Ankündigung einer Anstalt für arme Kranke zu Altdorf im Nürnbergischen," *Journal von und für Deutschland* 3, no. 1 (1786): 96–100.

53 Johann Peter Frank, *System einer vollständigen medicinischen Polizey.* 6 Bde., 3rd ed. (Vienna, 1786–1817).

nowhere was Frank's *System* adopted in its entirety – which given its immense scope is not surprising – it did lead to a heightened awareness of the possibilities for an active role for the state in improving public health. Clinics were justified by their founders in just these terms. Frank himself, who was hired by Göttingen in 1784, published an announcement of a clinic he intended to operate, in which the aims of the clinic were linked to public welfare. "How lucky is the society," he proclaimed,

whose leaders do not merely depend upon the sympathy of the better citizens and doctors, but who allot some aid to the needy father who has taken ill, [and] to all truly indigent down-at-the-heel (*baufälligen*) people; and who testify thereby to the influence that the well-being of the last link has on the great chain, through which citizen is linked to citizen, and in which [chain] no part can suffer without a corrosive rust affecting the others![54]

Although the link to public welfare may have provided an essential boost to the rapid spread of clinics during the 1780s and 1790s, clinical instruction was by no means unknown before then. The fountainhead of modern clinical teaching has been traditionally regarded by generations of historians as Boerhaave's *collegium medico-practicum*, a small, twelve-bed section of the St. Caecilia hospital in Leiden.[55] A second influential source of clinical teaching was Johann Juncker's clinic at Halle, which began in 1717, only three years after Boerhaave was appointed director of the Leiden clinic. Juncker was staff doctor in the enormous philanthropic institution in Halle known as the *Waisenhaus*, (although it included far more than an orphanage) run by the noted Pietist theologian and pedagogue, August Hermann Francke (1663–1727). Almost from the moment of his appointment, Juncker determined to use the *Waisenhaus* hospital and the money Francke made available for treatment of needy walk-in patients for the practical education of medical students. The course was developed entirely out of Juncker's personal initiative; it had no formal connection to the university, aside from being listed in its catalogue. Indeed, not until 1729 would it be officially attached to the university with Juncker's appointment to a professorial chair.[56]

---

54 Johann Peter Frank, *Ankündigung des klinischen Instituts zu Göttingen* (Göttingen, 1784), p. 6.
55 Guenter Risse summarizes current thinking about Boerhaave's clinical teaching in "Clinical Instruction in Hospitals: The Boerhaavian Tradition in Leyden, Edinburgh, Vienna, and Paris," *Clio Medica* 21 (1987/88): 1–19, esp. pp. 1–5. Boerhaave's significance for the introduction of clinical instruction has been questioned in recent years from a number of directions, first by Jetter in "Die ersten Universitätskliniken westdeutscher Staaten," who called attention to the link between clinical instruction and urban poor relief. Michel Foucault contrasted the "structured nosological field" manifested in Boerhaave's clinic to a more authentic training in bedside practice that developed later in *The Birth of the Clinic*, trans. A. M. Sheridan Smith (New York, 1975), p. 59. More recently, Beukers' examination of the number of patients admitted to the clinic during the 1720s and early 1730s – that is, during the period of Boerhaave's greatest activity and widest influence – has cast doubt on how much clinical instruction Boerhaave actually offered during that period. See Harm Beukers, "Clinical Teaching in Leiden from Its Beginning Until the End of the Eighteenth Century," *Clio Medica* 21 (1987/88): 139–53, esp. pp. 146–8.
56 The story of Juncker's clinic in Halle has been developed in a number of excellent articles by Wolfram Kaiser. See in particular his "In memoriam Johann Juncker (1679–1759)," in *Johann Juncker (1679–1759) und seine Zeit (I)*, ed. Wolfram Kaiser und Hans Hübner (Halle, 1979), pp. 7–28,

By including consultations with ambulatory patients as part of his clinical program, Juncker offered students a far wider opportunity for learning practice than was possible in Boerhaave's clinic, or in Juncker's own stationary clinic. As Juncker himself wrote, through this arrangement "the students have the great advantage that they become old practitioners in their youthful years; for they send 12,000 patients on their way with help in one year, which is a number that even many an old practitioner cannot point to."[57] This quote indicates a second and decisive difference beyond mere numbers between Boerhaave's and Juncker's clinics: Juncker allowed more advanced students to take partial responsibility for treating patients. In Juncker's hands, the clinic became not merely a set of animated engravings to illustrate the doctrines of pathology and therapeutics, but the first occasion for a student to collect his own practical experience.

Juncker's initiative did not rapidly spread to other universities. One of his students, Johann Wilhelm Baumer (1719–88), opened a clinic for consultation with ambulatory patients at Erfurt in 1755. At first, Baumer's clinic was funded privately – whether from Baumer's own resources, student fees, or donations is not clear. By 1758, however, the clinic's popularity with patients and students had induced the government in Mainz to order that patients be given medication free of charge. Despite this encouraging start, the clinic did not become integrated into the university's structure, and it closed when Baumer moved to Giessen in 1764.[58]

A more lasting institution developed at Göttingen, even though no clinical courses were taught for nearly twenty years after the university opened. This is surprising in light of the fact that Paul Gottlieb von Werlhof (1699–1767), who wrote a memorandum on how to set up the medical faculty in 1733 before the university opened, specifically called for the inclusion of clinical teaching in the curriculum. Such training, he argued, was what made Paris, Leiden, and Strasbourg popular with medical students. Closer to home, Werlhof also pointed to the success of Juncker's clinic, saying that it explained why Halle, which was otherwise "badly staffed," continued to flourish.[59]

Be that as it may, apparently no Göttingen professors taught any clinical courses before the 1750s. But starting in 1755 no fewer than three professors – Johann Gottfried Brendel (1712–58), Rudolph Augustin Vogel (1724–74), and Johann Georg Roederer (1726–63) – began offering them. What these "clinics" actually

for a concise discussion of the clinic, its place in Francke's institution, and Juncker's methods; and Kaiser et al., "Collegium clinicum Halense," pp. 9–66, for a more extensive treatment. For Kaiser's most recent work on this subject, see "Theorie und Praxis in der Boerhaave-Ära und in nachboerhaavianischen Ausbildungssystemen an deutschen Hochschulen des 18. Jahrhunderts," *Clio Medica* 21 (1987/88): 71–94.

57 Quoted in Kaiser, "Theorie und Praxis," p. 77.

58 Baldur Schyra, "Die Bedeutung Johann Wilhelm Baumers (1719–1788) und Christoph Andreas Mangolds (1719–1767) für die Geschichte der Medizin und der Medizinischen Fakultät in Erfurt. Mit einer Einleitung von Dr. phil. Horst Rudolf Abe," *Beiträge zur Geschichte der Universität Erfurt (1392–1816)* 5 (1959): 27–52.

59 Werlhof's memorandum is published in Rössler, *Die Gründung der Universität Göttingen*, pp. 301–2.

were is uncertain. They were not official university institutes, for no funds were as yet allotted to this purpose. Vogel's course, at least, seems to have allowed students to take some responsibility for visiting bed-ridden patients in their homes and keeping journals of cases, but nothing is known of the others. They may have been stationary clinics consisting of a few beds set in a corner of the professor's house, an ambulatory clinic for consultation with poor patients, or nothing more than the old practice of taking students along when the teacher made regular calls on patients. Finally, none of these clinics, not even Vogel's, were offered on a regular basis, if listings in the university's lecture catalogues are any indication.[60]

Göttingen finally established a university clinic in 1773, when Ernst Gottfried Baldinger was appointed professor of practical medicine. Immediately upon his arrival, Baldinger busied himself with setting up the clinic, for which he requested a subvention of 200 Rthlr from the government to cover the cost of medications. Baldinger further stipulated that each student pay one and a half Rthlr to attend the clinic, which too was applied to the cost of medications. In structure, Baldinger's clinic was an ambulatory clinic or dispensary; it had no beds. It appears to have been run out of his home, with consultations on Mondays, Wednesdays, and Fridays from one to two o'clock. Patients too ill to come to the consultation were visited in their homes.

In spite of its promising beginnings and "official" status, all did not go smoothly for Baldinger's clinic. During the next decade he twice attempted to receive funds for installation of a stationary clinic to supplement the existing dispensary; both times he was refused. Disappointing too was the level of student participation. One reason for this was a competing private clinic run by Johann Friedrich Stromeyer (1750–1830), who as town *Physicus* enjoyed access to the city hospital, where Baldinger had neither official status nor access. Baldinger's situation at Göttingen was also poisoned by quarrels with his colleagues on the medical faculty. Embittered by the competition and fighting, Baldinger left Göttingen in 1782 for Hesse-Kassel, where he later opened a successful clinic at the University of Marburg. However, the dispensary at Göttingen remained after his departure, and in 1784 it was joined by a new stationary clinic. There also continued to be an assortment of private clinics run by professors and private lecturers.

By the time Baldinger left Göttingen for Kassel, other official clinics (that is, those supported at least in part by state funds) had begun appearing in different parts of Germany. The spread of clinical teaching, however, did encounter opposition from city governments and town physicians. Control of admission to local hospitals often lay with municipal authorities, who had their own agendas for the institutions. The town *Physici*, whose responsibilities included caring for the poor and who sometimes controlled the town hospital as well, not unreasonably saw the new clinics as a threat to their offices and their livelihoods. At Halle, Johann

60 This and the following discussion of Göttingen is drawn from Renate Kumsteller, *Die Anfänge der medizinischen Poliklinik zu Göttingen* (Göttingen, 1958), pp. 15–21, 27, 37–41.

Juncker had not faced this problem, because he directed his own hospital. But other professors did not find it so easy. Before Juncker began his clinic, another Halle professor, Friedrich Hoffmann, found the doors of the city hospital closed to him when he sought to conduct clinical demonstrations there for his students. Baldinger's plans for expansion of the university clinic at Göttingen were frustrated by the city government, which pointed out that it already provided adequate medical care through the *Stadtphysicus*. The city also complained about the influx of indigents from the surrounding region, who arrived in the city seeking aid from Baldinger and his students.[61]

Similar opposition was encountered by Friedrich Wendt when he started an extremely successful clinic in Erlangen in 1778. Like Baldinger's clinic at Göttingen, Wendt's began as a private endeavor, but it soon received support from the territorial government. It was also supported by donations from wealthy benefactors and by student fees.[62] And like Baldinger's, Wendt's clinic quickly ran afoul of the local *Physicus*, a certain Fleischmann, who produced a long series of charges against Wendt and his clinic in 1782, including neglect of patients, refusal of treatment to seriously ill patients, and misappropriation of local poor-relief funds. After Fleischmann's initial complaints were sharply rejected by the government with a decree directing that Wendt's clinic take full responsibility for medical care for the poor in Erlangen, the *Physicus* renewed his campaign with a colorful portrayal of his professional devotion and the clinic's transgressions:

Since the beginning of this century our *Physici* have been bound by a personal oath to succor the poor with word and deed, by day and night, without pay; . . . To this same oath I have pledged myself for 15 years. . . . Never did we count up the number of recovered cases at the end of the year in order to be noticed. It was reward enough to have served the true subjects of our princely Highness. With this diligence to service we looked upon the blossoming of the princely clinical institute, recognized it as a true blessing that many hands could work toward the well-being of humanity, persuaded many of our patients that they should enter the clinic, and never did it enter our minds to give offense to the clinic. Certainly we needed great magnanimity as we saw this worthy institute soon depart from its circle, remaining not with the poor but instead taking responsibility for rich and poor without distinction, authorizing every medical student to practice in the city, and we quietly looked on as still inexperienced youths took on patients and . . . dispatched them into the next world, and as our practice was taken from our hands; . . .

Fleischmann went on to describe the fear that Wendt's clinic inspired in his patients, with one being overcome by convulsions at the mere suggestion that she go there for treatment, and another saying he would rather die than be handled by Wendt's students.[63]

61 Kaiser et al., "Collegium clinicum Halense," p. 25; Kumsteller, *Die Anfänge der medizinischen Poliklinik*, p. 26.
62 See the balance sheets included at the end of Friedrich Wendt, *Nachricht von der gegenwärtigen Einrichtung und dem Fortgang des Instituti Clinici* (Erlangen, 1780).
63 Archiv Universität Erlangen, Teil I, Pos. ii, Nr. 8: "Der Stadt Physici Hr. D. Flesichmanns Vorstellung wegen der Instituti Clinic betr.," letter from Fleischmann dated 22 August 1782.

Fleischmann's complaints only gained him the increasing disfavor of the territorial government, which stood squarely on Wendt's side. Yet we should not be too quick to conclude from this that clinics represented growing state power and modernity while Fleischmann and other town doctors were relics of the feudal and corporatist past. Certainly the incidents in Erlangen and Göttingen embodied a more general struggle between territorial and municipal governments for political control, a struggle in which public health and poor relief were one arena. But at the same time, clinics such as Wendt's depended heavily on networks of local, personal patronage for monetary support. Consequently they added several strands to that dense web of dependence and favor that bound early modern societies together. While such networks often operated implicitly and informally, at times they revealed themselves in unexpectedly open ways. Christoph Gottlieb Hofmann's announcement of his new clinic in Altdorf in 1786, for example, stated forthrightly that benefactors not only would be receiving reports on the clinic's operation, they would also have the right to recommend patients for admission.[64]

Therefore in contrast to the struggle between Christoph Ludwig Hoffmann and the medical faculty in Mainz, Fleischmann's opposition to Wendt's clinic presents a more subtle pattern of cleavage and conflicting responsibility between physicians in official positions. On the one hand, the clinic obviously enjoyed strong support from the territorial government of Ansbach-Bayreuth, and in this way it manifested the standard opposition between states and municipalities. On the other hand, it was also a part of the university's medical faculty, a group that in Mainz and elsewhere had formed an obstacle to the extension of central authority. It should be recalled too that the faculty in Erlangen operated relatively independently and enjoyed a good share of control over the principality's medical system.[65] Thus the government's support of the Erlangen clinic cannot be read off as yet another case of the state's bureaucracy extending its tentacles ever deeper into the social structure.

It is at the local level that the fractures in the profession emerged most clearly. By giving medical care to the poor and by cultivating the support of well-placed benefactors, Wendt's clinic presented the *Physicus* with a competing source of authority and influence at the local level. If his situation was like that of most of his fellow *Physici*, Fleischmann probably received a pittance for his salary. The less tangible fruits of his office, therefore, were most likely Fleischmann's principal reward, and an observer would be hardhearted indeed not to see how deeply injured he felt by Wendt and his students.

---

64 Hofmann, "Ankündigung einer Anstalt für arme Kranke zu Altdorf," p. 97. The role of medical institutions as a vehicle of patronage at the local level has been discussed for English voluntary hospitals in John Woodward, *To Do the Sick No Harm: A Study of the British Voluntary Hospital System to 1875* (London, 1974).
65 See the discussion in the section "Territorial Governments and the Public's Health" in this chapter.

In some ways, the values of the Enlightenment were deeply threatening to physicians. Their identity and claims to status, as we have seen, rested largely on elements other than their function as healers. It is not that physicians did not heal people, but what distanced them from the myriad other healers in society was their learnedness. Learnedness, however, was precisely that quality in danger of being emptied of its significance by a set of values based on utility and function. Consequently physicians faced an uncomfortable dilemma. They could oppose an ideology adopted by leading reformers both inside and outside of government, and pass up a chance to attach themselves to the progressive state. Or they could sign on to the movement and put at risk the very elements of their professional identity on which they had traditionally staked their status.

Put this way, the choice between the alternatives appears more conscious than it probably was. Most physicians rallied enthusiastically around the Enlightenment because it represented progress and efficiency. But the tensions that resulted from their association with the new ideology were never too far from the surface of their rhetoric. Just as a rational, enlightened social order based on "merit" and expert knowledge threatened to subvert the traditional estates of birth and strip the aristocracy of its claim to social preeminence, so too did the emphasis on useful knowledge and its application in work undermine one of the professions' key sources of status.

Nowhere were these dangers more clearly displayed than in the rising status of surgeons. For centuries, surgery had been learned and exercised through guilds, a tradition that provided a ready target for medical reformers during the eighteenth century. They attacked the guilds' monopolistic practices, and charged them with hindering the discovery of new methods and perpetuating the crudest kind of surgical technique and training. Above all, the reform of surgery was conceived of as a pedagogical problem. Christoph Ludwig Hoffmann echoed a commonly sounded theme when he caricatured the three-year apprenticeship in surgery as a period when novices are not required "to do much more than brush their masters' shoes, watch their children, and work in their gardens."[66]

In an attempt to raise the standards of surgical training and to break the control of guilds over surgery, surgical academies were erected in several principalities, including Brandenburg-Prussia, Braunschweig-Wolfenbüttel, Saxony, Hesse-Kassel, and Württemberg. These schools offered surgeons not only an introduction to the manual craft of surgery, but also a comprehensive survey of the theoretical subjects. In effect, the graduates of surgical academies possessed knowledge and skills virtually identical to the physicians who graduated from universities. All they lacked were the legal privileges attendant with an M.D.

Even those remaining distinctions seemed to be disappearing. Calls began to be

---

66 Quoted in *Deutsches Museum*, Bd. I (1778), p. 37.

heard for elimination of the legal distinctions between the kinds of healing that physicians (internal illnesses) and surgeons (wounds, breaks, extractions, removal of swellings) could undertake. Hoffmann's medical ordinance for Münster dismantled most practical barriers between the two groups, a step that received enthusiastic approval from one commentator.[67] Toward the end of the century, the Academy of Useful Sciences in Erfurt sponsored a prize essay competition on the question of whether surgery and medicine should be united. Five of the six entries answered in the affirmative. The winning entry was the only one to take a negative position. Significantly, however, the winner's argument drew not upon any of the traditional sources of physicians' higher status, but on the time and expense necessary to become expert in both medical and surgical practices. In this case, functional and utilitarian considerations were turned into a defense of the legal separation of physicians and surgeons.[68]

Along with raising persistent questions about the separation of medicine from surgery, the new surgical academies also symbolized a feasible alternative to the university education. This was true especially in Brandenburg-Prussia, where the Collegium Medico-Chirurgicum in Berlin demonstrated how a flourishing medical faculty could exist independently of a university. By the end of the century, the universities' standing with the Prussian government was at its nadir. In 1798, Julius von Massow (1750–1816), who represented the most extreme wing of utilitarian pedagogical reformers, was appointed Interior Minister, which included responsibility for the universities. Massow made no secret of his lack of sympathy for the universities. Calling them a "monstrous agglomeration (*Zusammenwuchs*) of several schools," he advocated their dissolution and replacement by individual schools offering specialized, occupationally oriented education. In his eyes, the model for such a school was the Collegium Medico-Chirurgicum. Although Massow's plans never came to fruition, they reflected how much both the universities and the learned professions stood to lose from the new emphasis on utilitarian education.[69]

As if the disfavor of government ministers and the increased status of surgeons were not damaging enough already, physicians toward the end of the century began to feel besieged by ever-growing numbers of medical students.[70] In part, the feeling was fully justified. It does appear – although hard evidence is difficult to come by – that medical enrollments were increasing at a number of universities

67 "Ueber die Münsterschen Medicinalgeseze," *Deutsches Museum*, Bd. 3 (1778), pp. 167–78.
68 Karl Schubert, *Die Kampf um die Gleichberechtigung der Chirurgie und der inneren Medizin um die Wende des 18. zum 19. Jahrhunderts* (med. Diss., Düsseldorf, 1938).
69 Max Lenz, *Geschichte der königlichen Friedrich-Wilhelms-Universität zu Berlin*, Bd. 1 (Halle, 1910), pp. 36–43, quoted on p. 37.
70 Friedrich Hildebrandt, "Ein Wort über die zunehmende Menge der Mediciner auf unsern Academieen," *Der Reichs-Anzeiger*, nr. 75 (29 March 1797), pp. 797–9; J. H. G. Heusinger, "Ein Wort über die zunehmende Menge der Mediziner auf unsern Universitäten," *Allgemeines Jahrbuch der Universitäten, Gymnasien, Lyceen, und anderer gelehrten Bildungsanstalten in und ausser Teutschland* 1 (1798): 32–7; Christian Gottfried Gruner, "Deutsches Medicinalwesen am Ende des achtzehnten Jahrhunderts," *Almanach für Aerzte und Nichtärzte* (1790), p. 242.

during the last three decades of the century. Medical enrollments, in fact, represent a major exception to a general decline in the number of university students between 1750 and 1800.[71] But it is unlikely that the moderate increases in enrollment would have substantially increased the level of competition too. Competition had always been a part of professional life. What made it intolerable was where physicians thought the competition was coming from.

The medical press during the 1780s and 1790s spilled over with the complaints of physicians who detected an unprecedented rush by surgeons to enroll in medical faculties and take an M.D. by the shortest route possible. The lamentations had a repetitive cast to them: not satisfied with the better training and status they had enjoyed, impudent surgeons sought to climb above their station through buying a degree from a disreputable faculty, and then using that degree as a lever to gain entrance into respectable society. As the Jena professor, Christian Gottfried Gruner (1744–1815), put it in 1790,

If every reckless individual, every depraved cobbler can become a physician and adorn himself with a doctoral degree, can usurp thereby dignity (*Rang*) from another deserving man, and be permitted to blunder around with human life; when every useless barber can practice [medicine] as soon as he has money and be protected against every justified complaint; then the title of physician will become a despicable one, and the exercise of the art (*Kunst*) will sink down to the most wretched handicraft (*Handwerk*).[72]

Gruner's grumbling provides a vivid reminder that, for all its beguiling hints of modernity, the Enlightenment often remains alien territory to the modern traveler. We take for granted that the eighteenth century introduced the notion of reason as the foundation for the evaluation of "objective" qualifications, and that for the first time careers were opened to "talent" instead of birth. From the modern perspective of "merit," Gruner's complaint appears oddly askew. As long as a student, no matter what his background or previous occupation, has taken the prescribed courses and passed the required exams, why should he not prove just as capable a physician as the next person? Yet that was precisely the point at issue. Being a physician involved not merely acquiring a set of intellectual tools for a

---

71 Eulenberg reported that the total number of German university students declined from approximately 4,350 in 1750 to a plateau in the 1760s and 1770s, when there was an average of 3,600 students, and finally 2,930 in 1800. Although his data for individual universities are far from complete, increasing medical enrollments are evident at Duisburg, Erfurt, Freiburg, Göttingen, Jena, Würzburg, and Tübingen from 1770 to 1800. Halle also showed an increase in the period 1770–1800, but that represents a partial recovery from a period of decline that had begun in the 1730s. Although Heidelberg and Erlangen did not show a clear increase between 1770 and 1800, both universities' medical enrollments during those years well exceeded anything they had had previously. See Franz Eulenberg, "Die Frequenz der deutschen Universitäten von ihrer Gründung bis zur Gegenwart," *Abhandlungen der philologisch-historischen Klasse der königlichen sächsischen Gesellschaft der Wissenschaften* 24, no. 2 (1906): 132, 309–16. It appears too that the medical faculty at Kiel saw at least a modest increase in enrollment during this period. Heinrich Schipperges, "Geschichte der medizinischen Fakultät," in *Geschichte der Christian-Albrechts-Universität Kiel* Bd. 4, Teil 1 (Kiel, 1967), pp. 85–90.
72 Gruner, "Deutsches Medicinalwesen am Ende des achtzehnten Jahrhunderts," p. 242.

job; it required character and personal dignity. Schooling was not merely a set of doctrines and techniques to be communicated; it was the opportunity to become cultured, to develop one's understanding and judgment.

The complaints by Gruner and others against what they saw as surgeons' grasping after higher status was a particular instance of a more general phenomenon toward the end of the century. In the press and in scores of decrees issued by territorial governments, there is evident an anxiety over what contemporaries thought was an unseemly degree of social climbing by the lower classes through the taking of university degrees. Poor students, who may possess the intellect to complete a university degree but who lacked the bearing and background to move comfortably in society, were thought to be overwhelming the universities in the hope of bettering their station.[73]

It was in complaints such as these that the contradiction between the egalitarian and the elitist strains in Enlightenment ideology came most clearly into focus. As Anthony La Vopa has pointed out recently, the majority of German pedagogical reformers were committed to the notion that governance was best left to a small, well-educated vanguard. Schooling for the general population demanded reform not so much to create a level playing field for all members of society as to train students for their proper station in life. Although such a system left the door open for poor students of exceptional talent to make their way into the elite – and not a few reformers had done just that – the experience of negotiating the ladder of education, patronage and deference effaced whatever identification they might have had with their poorer brethren. They articulated what La Vopa described as a "neocorporatist" conception of merit as something that inhered in individuals, but under the modulating influences of birth, wealth, and education.[74]

Physicians shared this attitude, and it became a foundation for defense of their professional status. Even those reformers who most ardently promoted reform, such as Christoph Ludwig Hoffmann, set strict limits to how far they would erase the professional distinctions between physicians and other types of healers. Hoffmann's plans may have allowed both physicians and surgeons an open field with respect to practice, but the qualifications on which they were to be judged were those of academic medicine. More significantly still, he wrote into the laws for Münster and Hesse-Kassel that only holders of the M.D. would be appointed to positions as *Physicus* and to the all-important seats on territorial medical boards.

The emphasis on character by which Gruner and others defended the privileged status of the learned professions represented a subtle but significant transformation from the former appeal to learnedness. The old foundation had been eroded

73 See, for example, "Mittel und Vorschläge, die Menge derer zurückzuhalten, die sich jetzt aus den niederen Ständen, ohne natürlichen Beruf zum Studiren auf Universitäten, und in die Stände der Gelehrten einzudrängen," *Deutsches Magazin* 13 (1797): 80–94. The seminal work on this subject is Anthony J. La Vopa, *Grace, Talent, and Merit: Poor Students, Clerical Careers, and Professional Ideology in Eighteenth-Century Germany* (Cambridge, 1988). See esp. chap. 1 for the standard contemporary depiction of poor students.

74 Ibid., pp. 197–215.

considerably by the Enlightenment rhetoric of utility, and by developments within the profession itself. The creation of medical boards, the opening of teaching clinics, the very standards by which physicians were judging themselves all pointed to a profession that was beginning to see itself as serving a particular *function* in society. In such a profession, learnedness no longer held the same value it had previously, and there was some question whether it had any value at all. In its place, therefore, physicians began adopting the argument advanced by other university apologists, that a proper university education – not one through which a student raced merely to complete the requirements for a job – conferred a unique form of character development, almost a form of spiritual transcendence. They referred to this cultivation of personal character with nearly mystical reverence as *Bildung*.

Bildung is one of the great totems of German historical scholarship, and it is virtually impossible to approach the subject with anything resembling detachment. But separated as we are from the eighteenth-century origins of *Bildung* by mountains of nineteenth-century (not to mention twentieth-century) rhetoric, it is all too easy to forget that the ideology of *Bildung* originally took root in the rather modest justifications advanced by mid-eighteenth century philologists for the study of ancient languages, especially Greek. They defended the teaching of Greek not, as the humanists had done, in order to inculcate a capacity for imitating the ancients, but instead to awaken students' taste, judgment and imagination through contact with Greek literature.[75]

Bildung presented an attractive alternative to what some critics saw as an excessively pragmatic approach to education. In assigning training for useful occupation as the only desideratum for education, reformers had ignored the role that education could play in formation of the individual. The *Sturm und Drang* literary movement of the 1770s, depicting the pathos of individual genius and freedom stifled by the oppressive organization of society, gave voice to a kind of alienation that the ideology of *Bildung* later captured. The emphasis placed by *Bildung* on individual character and freedom also gave poorer students an escape from the neocorporatist view of merit and education that had dismissed them as social climbers. Claiming possession of *Bildung* offered those students a means of rendering ambition socially acceptable.[76]

Historians have often presented the ideology of *Bildung* as the source of the philosophical faculty's claims to prestige against the position of the three "higher" faculties, and as the basis of the growth of the philosophical faculties in the nineteenth century. Kant's defense of the philosophical faculty as the only one that

75 Friedrich Paulsen, *Geschichte des gelehrten Unterrichts auf den deutschen Schulen und Universitäten*, Bd. 2, 2nd ed. (Leipzig, 1897), pp. 9–46. The most important recent treatment of this concept is Rudolf Vierhaus, "Bildung," in *Geschichtliche Grundbegriffe: Historisches Lexikon zur politisch-sozialen Sprache in Deutschland*, ed. Otto Brunner, Werner Conze, and Reinhart Koselleck, Bd. 1 (Stuttgart, 1972), pp. 508–51. See also Lenore O'Boyle, "Klassische Bildung und soziale Struktur in Deutschland zwischen 1800 und 1848," *Historische Zeitschrift* 207 (1968): 584–608.

76 This latter quality is emphasized in La Vopa, *Grace, Talent, and Merit*, pp. 249–86.

cares exclusively for "the interests of scholarship (*Wissenschaft*)" as opposed to the more pragmatic functions of the higher faculties, is well known.[77] What has often been overlooked, however, is how broad the appeal of *Bildung* actually was. Not only did it become the slogan of an educated flotsam of disaffected young men; it also penetrated the most elite cultural circles, and it was adopted by members of the higher professions. In place of the now-discarded *Gelehrsamkeit*, *Bildung* became a new bulwark for maintaining professional status. In many ways, it acted in a virtually identical fashion, by tying the professional identity of physicians to their university education. Only now that education formed the foundation of physicians' corporate prestige not because of the erudition it conferred, but instead because of the depth of character and quality of insight it developed in the student.

But if the new ideology of *Bildung* helped define and justify physicians' place at the pinnacle of the medical world, it left unanswered nagging questions about just who physicians were. Claims about *Bildung* of doctors did not eliminate other, more utilitarian conceptions of education and the professions. Far from displacing those values, it actually merged with ideas of function and utility through the medium of the traditional Lutheran virtues of "calling" and duty. Therefore physicians were faced at the end of the eighteenth century with several competing ideals of professional identity: they could describe their profession as relatively divorced from particular social functions and present themselves as a group of spiritually cultivated individuals pursuing knowledge of nature; or they could emphasize the contributions made by physicians toward social progress and relief of suffering, justifying this work either in the secularized language of Enlightenment or in more religious terms of calling; or they could combine elements of both views. Whatever the choices made by individual physicians, the fracturing of professional identity into several competing identities left physicians with considerable room to disagree over the relationship between theory and practice in medicine. That disagreement became distinctly pointed when physicians began pondering the content and purposes of medical knowledge and how it should be taught to students.

77 "Der Streit der Facultäten," in *Kants gesammelte Schriften*, Bd. 7 (Berlin, 1907), pp. 18–19.

3

Physicians and writers: Medical theory and the emergence of the public sphere

The previous chapter described how the eighteenth-century medical profession was shaped by (and in turn gave form to) reformist impulses that were proclaimed under the banners of Enlightenment, social welfare, and the pragmatic uses of knowledge. The responses formulated by physicians to those impulses, as that chapter suggested, were a complex amalgam of defensive and offensive postures. At the most general level, those responses were structured by two issues. The first issue, hinted at by the discussion of *Bildung,* consisted of how someone conceived of the profession's relationship to the state. Did medicine exist to promote the state's enlightened ends (for example, by means of public health), or should physicians stake their identity on a more individual and personal level, for example in terms of their selfless service to patients, or their claim to cultivation of personal freedom through *Bildung?* The second issue concerned physicians' sense of the relationship between theory and practice in medicine. Should theory be cultivated with an eye toward its application at the bedside, or could medical theory rightly lay claim to being a profound inquiry into the mysteries of organic nature? How in fact did bedside practice represent an "application" of a physician's theoretical knowledge?

Two points must be made to clarify these issues. First, in some ways their presentation as choices between alternatives is deceptive, because they did not necessarily represent mutually contradictory stances. It was possible, for example, for one person to believe *both* that medicine was a profound inquiry into nature *and* that its theoretical discoveries could inform therapeutics. Nevertheless, we can also identify disputes at the end of the century that turned precisely on the issues as framed above. Second, as the reader may have suspected already, the two issues were not entirely independent of each other. Physicians who identified the profession with enlightenment and the promotion of social welfare also tended to be those who discounted the value of pursuing medical theory for its own sake. Yet the correspondence of stances was far from being invariable.

Thus at the turn of the century German physicians entered into a complex and highly fragmented debate over the nature of their profession, medical knowledge, and medical education. This chapter and the two following will attempt to sort out prominent themes from this cacophony of overlapping debates. Here the emphasis will be on the elaboration of medical theory (taken here to mean physiology) during the eighteenth century and through the first decade of the nineteenth. The development of physiology will be examined from two frames of reference, one of them internal to medicine and the second an external frame that sets medical writing in the larger literary culture. Internally, the most conspicuous feature of theory in this period was the tendency for physiology (that portion of medicine most intimately tied to natural philosophy) to evolve in a direction separate from other branches of medicine and define its own problem domain: the study of vital forces. By the 1790s this research program had developed to a point at which some critics began to call for a reform of physiology that would encourage its reintegration with bedside practice. But such calls turned out to be futile, for almost as soon as they had been articulated there arose new opportunities to take medical theory in directions quite alien to bedside practice. Inspired by the doctrines of Friedrich Schelling's *Naturphilosophie,* and by the dream of incorporating medical theory into a unified science of nature, many younger writers of the late 1790s pictured their scholarship not in the service of bedside practice, but instead as an inquiry into the most profound truths of living nature.

To understand why *Naturphilosophie* proved so attractive to these physicians, however, we need to move to the second frame of reference, which lies outside the professional and scholarly context of medicine. For debates about the future course of medical theory existed not in some hermetically sealed professional space, but instead amongst a public composed of physicians and non-physicians alike. Recalling a point made previously in the introduction, a distinctive feature of this new public sphere is the emergence of "criticism," a type of cultural exchange embodied in a host of new review periodicals such as *Allgemeine deutsche Bibliothek* and the *Allgemeine Literatur-Zeitung.* So prominent did criticism become in the new cultural awareness that even Immanuel Kant, planted virtually on the marches of civilization in Königsberg, could observe in the preface to the first edition of the *Critique of Pure Reason* (1781):

Our age is, in especial degree, the age of criticism, and to criticism must everything submit. Religion through its sanctity, and law-giving through its majesty, may seek to exempt themselves from it. But they then awaken just suspicion, and cannot claim the sincere respect which reason accords only to that which has been able to sustain the test of free and open examination.[1]

This developing public sphere was important not just as a forum for establishing cultural and intellectual values, but also for allowing individual writers to create themselves as public figures.[2] For if criticism itself often wore the mask of anonymity as an incantation to the universality of judgments of taste, the objects

---

1 Immanuel Kant, *Critique of Pure Reason,* trans. Norman Kemp Smith (New York, 1965), p. 9.
2 Hans-Jürgen Haferkorn, "Der freie Schriftsteller. Eine literatursoziologische Studie über seine Entstehung und Lage in Deutschland zwischen 1750 und 1800." *Archiv für Geschichte des Buchwesens* 5 (1964): 523–711; and Rudolf Vierhaus, "Der aufgeklärte Schriftsteller. Zur sozialen Charakteristik

of criticism nonetheless consisted of very visible authors and their works. Even if one could not earn a sufficient living from writing, one could still achieve a measure of success through public notoriety. Because medical writing participated in that larger arena formed by the public sphere, physician–writers confronted possibilities and pursued goals not available to earlier generations. Of course in becoming writers for the public these physicians did not necessarily lose contact with their professional identities and cease being doctors. But the chance to appear before the public allowed them, as we shall see in the case of *Naturphilosophie*, to conceive of that identity in new ways.

THE DEVELOPMENT OF MEDICAL THEORY IN THE EIGHTEENTH CENTURY

Decades before the emergence of anything that could be called a "public sphere" in central Europe, medical theory had begun to evolve in a direction that would open a considerable gap between physiology and the remaining areas of medical writing in both theory and practice. The traditional role assigned to physiology had been as a bridge between medical theory proper and the larger domain of natural philosophy. Physiology embodied medicine's claim to be a learned *scientia*, and it existed primarily – and, before the seventeenth century, exclusively – to be taught.[3] During the seventeenth century, however, the introduction of new methods of studying nature through experiment in the work of scholars such as William Harvey opened new venues for the subject, although experimentation had by no means displaced the traditional pedagogical forms of physiological scholarship.

The seventeenth century also saw the final overthrow of Aristotelian natural philosophy in favor of one of several corpuscular and mechanical theories.[4] These changes resonated in physiology too, just as one would expect of the subject that

einer selbsternannten Elite," in *Über den Prozess der Aufklärung in Deutschland im 18. Jahrhundert*, ed. Hans Erich Bödeker and Ulrich Herrmann (Göttingen, 1987), pp. 53–65. On the development of the book trade over the course of the eighteenth century, see Rudolf Jentzsch, *Der deutsch-lateinische Büchermarkt nach den Leipziger Ostermeß-Katalogen von 1740, 1770 und 1800 in seiner Gliederung und Wandlung*, Beiträge zur Kultur- und Universalgeschichte, Heft 20 (Leipzig, 1912). Jentzsch's data clearly display a decrease in devotional and professional literature (of which much of the latter was published in Latin in 1740) and a corresponding increase in novels, as well as in subjects such as agriculture, history and geography, and natural sciences.
3 On the teaching of medical theory in the Renaissance, see Nancy G. Siraisi, *Avicenna in Renaissance Italy* (Princeton, N.J., 1987). Siraisi describes the transmission via editions and commentaries of Book I of Avicenna's *Canon*, which contained an overview of Galenic physiological doctrine. See esp. pp. 9–11 for general comments on the teaching of physiology in Renaissance Italy.
4 The best recent general history of biology is *Geschichte der Biologie*, ed. Ilse Jahn et al. (Jena, 1982). Also useful are Thomas S. Hall, *Ideas of Life and Matter*, 2 vols. (Chicago, 1969); and Karl E. Rothschuh, *Physiologie, der Wandel ihrer Konzepte, Probleme und Methoden vom 16. bis 19. Jahrhundert* (Freiburg, 1968). The latter was translated as *History of Physiologie*, trans. and ed. with a new English bibliography by Guenter B. Risse (Huntington, N.Y., 1972). For discussions of physiology in a more strictly medical context, see Lester S. King, *The Medical World of the Eighteenth Century* (repr. ed. Huntington, N.Y., 1971); and idem, *The Philosophy of Medicine: The Early Eighteenth Century* (Cambridge, Mass., 1978). Still valuable too are the chapters on physiology and pathology in the *Handbuch der Geschichte der Medizin*, ed. Max Neuburger and Julius Pagel, 3 Bde. (Jena, 1902–1905).

linked medicine and natural philosophy. Among other places, the triumph of the mechanical philosophy is evident in the writings of the influential Leiden medical teacher, Hermann Boerhaave. For Boerhaave, physiology still served an undisputedly propaedeutic function for the rest of medicine. As illustrated by his introductory textbook, the *Institutiones medicae,* first published in 1708, the universe of medical knowledge was divided among five areas: physiology, pathology, semiotics (the interpretation of symptoms), hygiene (the rules for preserving health), and therapy. By no means was Boerhaave the first to make such a division. Similar introductory surveys had been a staple of seventeenth-century medical teaching, for example as presented in Daniel Sennert's *Institutionum medicinae libri V* (1632), which was itself a direct descendent of the commentaries made on Book I of Avicenna's *Canon* during the Renaissance.[5]

Although Boerhaave's partitioning of medical subjects was rooted in long-standing tradition, the doctrines he presented within that structure were based on the most up-to-date brand of natural philosophy, which meant of course the mechanical philosophy. In 1703, when he was still only a reader in medicine (if already by then a popular one) at Leiden, he held an oration entitled "On the usefulness of the mechanical method in medicine." Boerhaave described mechanics as "a marvelous science, almost superhuman as to its results which exceed all expectations! For its most subtle and complicated discoveries are based on principles which are sure, yet very few in number and generally known."[6] Only in medicine, Boerhaave continued with more than a little exaggeration, is mechanics despised and its results ignored. Yet there is no legitimate reason for physicians not to adopt the principles of mechanics in formulating medical theory. "The senses testify and reason pronounces," he asserted, "that the human body is in no way different from the rest . . . except that it is composed of several different mechanisms which are set in motion by the liquids which flow through them."[7]

Although Boerhaave regarded mechanics as applicable to virtually all of the most important physiological phenomena, such as the motion of the skeletal muscles and the action of the circulatory system, no less evident to him was its usefulness for bedside practice. In these instances it aided the practitioner by furnishing a ready explanation for his therapeutic interventions: "Are we not a thousand times obliged, in treating our patients, to thicken what is fluid, to loosen what is congested, to move on what has stagnated, to restrain what is loose, to dilute what is too thick, to condense what is too light?" In stark contrast to this everyday experience, Boerhaave set the improbable "principles" of the iatrochemists. Only rarely, he noted sardonically, are we "compelled to attend to the conflict between salts, the flames of sulfur, or to the hidden spirit of mercury."[8]

5 Siraisi, *Avicenna in Renaissance Italy,* p. 101.
6 *Boerhaave's Orations,* trans. with an introduction by E. Kegel-Brinkgreve and A. M. Luyendijk-Elshout (Leiden, 1983), pp. 85–120, quoted on p. 95.
7 Ibid., p. 96.
8 Ibid., p. 106.

For Boerhaave, a proper theory of physiology would provide the framework for pathology as well. Beginning at the most fundamental level, the basic fibers comprising the body's solid fabric, he described how these fibers can suffer from excessive hardness or softness, rigidity or looseness, or even dissolution. Boerhaave insisted that all such physical attributes depended not on the chemical properties of the constituent particles, but on their physical coherence.[9] Moving from the level of individual fibers to organs, Boerhaave defined organic diseases as infirmi- ties of the body's solid parts which affect their ability to perform vital functions. Such functional defects could arise from any of four causes: (1) damage or alteration to the organ's internal or external surfaces, which change its ability to interact with fluids that surround and penetrate it; (2) excess or deficiency in the number of organs, such as having only one kidney instead of two; (3) dispropor- tionate size; and (4) defects in the location of the organ and its connection to other bodily tissues. In this way, Boerhaave discussed tumors as examples of the third category of infirmity, that of immoderate size.[10]

Even infirmities of the body's humors, which for the ancients had given rise to a bountiful variety of qualitative differentiae, could be rendered by Boerhaave in mechanical terms: "A particle of a humor goes wrong with respect to its shape in the first instance, when in receding from its spherical form it acquires acute angularity; hence in applying its entire motion to a small portion [of itself] it becomes sharp (*acris*);. . ."[11] We should take care to avoid portraying Boerhaave as a rigidly dogmatic mechanist. He did, for example, concede the presence of a fermentation in digestion that was not simply the mechanical separation of nutri- tive particles. Moreover, as time went on and he immersed himself more in chemistry – he added that subject to his collection of professorial chairs at Leiden in 1718 – his view of the body became more nuanced. Yet it is no exaggeration to say that over his career Boerhaave largely held to doctrines that allied him most closely with iatromechanists such as Borelli, Bellini, and the Cartesians.[12]

Boerhaave's adoption of the mechanical philosophy was not meant to dislocate physiology from the rest of medicine; clearly, he intended just the opposite. There can be no doubt that he believed mechanical principles would both link medicine

9 Hermann Boerhaave, *Praelectiones academicae, in proprias institutiones rei medicae*, vol. 5 (Leiden, 1758), p. 15.
10 Ibid., pp. 21–2. Interestingly, Boerhaave's partitioning of pathological conditions bore a pronounced similarity to the categories of 16th-century Galenists, which suggests that the novelties bestowed on medicine by the mechanical philosophy were in some respects less than claimed by its apologists. See Ingo Wilhelm Müller, *Iatromechanische Theorie und ärztliche Praxis im Vergleich zur galenistische Medizin* (Stuttgart, 1991), p. 77.
11 "Peccat particula humoris sua figura tum inprimis, quando a natura sphaerica recedens angulosam acutam induit; hinc motum suum integrum parvae parti applicans acris fit; . . ." Ibid., p. 43.
12 For useful summaries of Boerhaave's mechanical viewpoint, see G. A. Lindeboom, "Hermann Boerhaave," in *Dictionary of Scientific Biography*, vol. 2, ed. Charles Coulston Gillispie (New York, 1981), pp. 224–7; and King, *The Philosophy of Medicine*, pp. 121–4. On early eighteenth-century iatromechanism, see Müller, *Iatromechanische Theorie und ärztliche Praxis*, which provides a thorough examination of the *Medicinae rationalis systematicae* of the Halle professor Friedrich Hoffmann.

to the latest developments in natural philosophy and render intelligible the physician's experience at the bedside. For all of Boerhaave's optimism, however, the doctrine did constrain the physician in significant ways, constraints that had not existed in the Galenic-Aristotelian theory. According to Boerhaave's pathology, diseases exist as disruptions in the function of particular organs, for example a blockage in the intestines or the accumulation of blood in a given part of the body. By specifying disease in this manner, Boerhaave adopted what Temkin has called a "physiological" view of disease.[13] On this principle the symptoms of the disease, the outward signs discernible to the doctor or the patient, are to be interpreted as direct manifestations of the internal condition. And indeed certain symptoms lend themselves to a causal explanation based on mechanical principles. Visible swellings (non-tumorous ones, anyway) are easily comprehended as accumulations of fluid in a part of the body. Constipation does point immediately to some kind of intestinal blockage.

But other routine aspects of the doctor's experience with illness contravene this model. Many diseases present themselves as distinctive and characteristic collections of symptoms indicative of some entity, some "X" which gives rise to them, which could not straightaway be rooted via mechanistic explanations in a single physiological disorder.[14] Furthermore, many symptoms commonly attended to by physicians, such as color, smell, dampness, or texture, were not amenable to mechanical explanations. Because mechanical philosophers drew a distinction between the primary qualities of matter itself (such as impenetrability, size, and shape) and the secondary qualities of sensation (such as color and smell), they could not explain the origin of particular secondary qualities in matter. That is, they were unable to account for the fact that a given configuration of particles produces the sensation "red" as opposed to "yellow" or any other color, or why it produces a color and not a particular taste, for that matter.[15]

---

13 Owsei Temkin, "The Scientific Approach to Disease: Specific Entity and Individual Sickness," in idem, *The Double Face of Janus* (Baltimore, 1977), pp. 441–55.

14 This "ontological" view, whose most prominent early modern advocate was Thomas Sydenham (1624–89), treated diseases as the products of some kind of morbific entity. Therefore it is possible to think of different people as suffering from the "same" disease, even when its actual manifestation is somewhat modified between one person and another. The ontological model of disease held certain advantages over the physiological model, most notably in explaining the occurrence of epidemics. On the conflict between the mechanists and followers of Sydenham at the very end of the 17th century, see Andrew Cunningham, "Sydenham versus Newton: The Edinburgh Fever Dispute of the 1690s between Andrew Brown and Archibald Pitcairne," in *Theories of Fever from Antiquity to the Enlightenment.* Medical History, Suppl. 1, ed. W. F. Bynum and V. Nutton (London, 1981), pp. 71–98. See also Kenneth Dewhurst, *Dr. Thomas Sydenham (1624–1689): His Life and Original Writings* (Berkeley and Los Angeles, 1966), pp. 60–7. Dewhurst, however, downplays the significance of this aspect of Sydenham's thought.

15 Peter Alexander has argued that the traditional distinction between primary qualities as "objective" and secondary qualities as "subjective" rests on a fundamental misinterpretation of Locke's *Essay Concerning Human Understanding.* According to Alexander, *both* primary and secondary qualities for Locke resided in matter itself and differed in the ideas they give rise to in the mind, with secondary qualities being those that create in us ideas of color, taste, and so forth. Yet even if secondary

For physicians of earlier generations, who did not adhere to mechanical doctrines, the connection between pathological doctrine and symptoms of a given disease, however speculative it might have seemed to later critics, had been less difficult to maintain. This was because, following Aristotelian natural philosophy, these writers had accepted various qualities such as smell and color as properties of objects and not as sensations produced by matter. The yellowish tinge of the skin observable in jaundice, for example, was said to arise from the excess of yellow bile (which by its nature is yellow) that characterizes the disease. Because the liver removed yellow bile from the blood, the color of the skin pointed directly to an underlying impairment of the liver's function. Galen's medical theory, depending as it did on humors consisting of varying amounts of warmth, cold, wetness and dryness, was readily applicable to the symptomatic manifestations of illness. In describing the various humoral imbalances (*dyskrasias*) that affect the liver, for example, Galen wrote the following:

In regard to the liver, . . . the various hot dyskrasias digest and burn those humors which the liver contained before, and also those which were brought up from the mesenteric veins. On the other hand, in a cold dyskrasia the humors already present in this organ are rendered thick, sluggish and difficult to move, while the [humors] brought up [by emesis] become phlegmatic, crude and half-digested. This also applies to the two other dyskrasias: the dry dyskrasia produces humors drier and thicker, and the moist dyskrasia, which produces thinner and more watery humors.[16]

To be sure, Boerhaave's mechanical pathology could lay claim to explaining thick and viscous or thin and watery humors at least as well as Galen's dry and wet *dyskrasias*. However, in contrast to the rich lexicon that a Galenic physician could bring to the description of symptoms, only a comparatively scanty assortment of descriptive terms could be pulled out of the mechanist's medical bag. Not that this stopped mechanical physicians from deploying the same descriptive terms as their colleagues. But the dependence of mechanical natural philosophy on the motions of qualitatively undifferentiated particles lent those symptomatic descriptions a meager theoretical substrate.[17] Thus the adoption of the mechanical philosophy by Boerhaave and other medical teachers opened a rift between physiology on one side and those portions of medical theory related more closely to practice and

qualities thereby lost their subjective character, what remained unresolved was the relationship between primary qualities, which were of significance for natural philosophy, and particular secondary qualities such as smells, tastes, and colors, which were important for medical semiotics. See Peter Alexander, *Ideas, Qualities and Corpuscles: Locke and Boyle on the External World* (Cambridge, 1985), chaps. 5, 6, 8. For a somewhat different interpretation, see Arnold I. Davidson and Norbert Hornstein, "The Primary/Secondary Quality Distinction: Berkeley, Locke, and the Foundations of Corpuscularian Science," *Dialogue* 23 (1984): 281–303.

16 Galen, *On the Affected Parts*, trans. Rudolph E. Siegel (Basel, 1976), p. 160.
17 In this regard, Lester King has noted how pathological concepts became increasingly abstract and divorced from bedside experience during the 17th and 18th centuries. This process, I would argue, was promoted by the adoption of the mechanical philosophy. See King, *The Philosophy of Medicine*, pp. 189–195.

dependent upon the interpretation of symptoms on the other. As we shall see, this rift grew wider over the course of the eighteenth century.

Boerhaave is important for our story in still another way. As one of Europe's most sought-after teachers, he played a major role as Newton's earliest and most influential advocate on the continent.[18] Paradoxically, Boerhaave championed Newton without ever applying the key Newtonian concept of "force" to his medical theory. Just what Boerhaave saw in Newton is something of a puzzle. Lindeboom, his most recent biographer, argued that he drew his "empirical tendency" from Newton, which at best places Boerhaave in the large crowd of natural philosophers who found the fashion of Newton's glory very much to their liking and showed this by embracing a faintly Newtonian empiricism.[19] In any case, and for whatever reasons he chose to present himself as standing at Newton's side, Boerhaave was, in the apt phrase of LeeAnn Hansen Le Roy, an "incomplete Newtonian."[20]

The same cannot be said of Boerhaave's students, of whom the most prominent, Albrecht von Haller, placed forces at the foundation of his natural philosophy. In contrast to Boerhaave, for whom physiological theory consisted of an *explanation* of phenomena articulated in terms of hydraulics and motions of particles, Haller used forces as a *description* of the phenomenal world. No attempt was made by Haller to account for the underlying causes of phenomena. Instead, he and his contemporaries used "force" as a way of asserting the lawlike behavior of phenomena without going through the tiresome business of actually justifying such an assertion. So compelling was Newton's concept of gravity that it made such justifications appear unnecessary to the majority of eighteenth-century natural philosophers, at least before Kant stepped into the discussion. Thus according to Haller, physiology's task consisted of describing the forces

through which the forms of things received by the senses are presented to the soul; through which the muscles, which are governed by the commands of the mind, in turn have strength; the forces through which food is changed into such different kinds of juices; and through which, finally, from these liquids both our bodies are preserved and the loss of human generations is replaced by new offspring.[21]

Leaving aside the messy question of how the mind can interact with the material world, what is noteworthy about this statement is the way that Haller consistently enumerated forces as categories of phenomena: as sensations, muscular action, digestion, and so forth. This concept of force became for Haller an entire program

18 G. A. Lindeboom, *Herman Boerhaave: The Man and His Work* (London, 1968), p. 100.
19 Ibid., p. 268.
20 LeeAnn Hansen Le Roy, *Johann Christian Reil and "Naturphilosophie" in Physiology* (Ph.D. diss., University of California, Los Angeles, 1985), p. 21.
21 Quoted in Shirley A. Roe, "Anatomia animata: The Newtonian Physiology of Albrecht von Haller," in *Transformation and Tradition in the Sciences: Essays in Honor of I. Bernard Cohen*, ed. Everett Mendelsohn (Cambridge, 1984), pp. 273–300, quoted on p. 276.

of experimental research, in which he attempted to locate forces such as sensibility and irritability in particular parts of the body.[22]

Haller's formulation of irritability as a vital force distinct from sensibility and the soul rapidly became entangled in larger conflicts over the properties of matter.[23] However, that did not hinder his program from striking a responsive chord with many natural philosophers, whatever their metaphysical inclinations. Whereas Haller himself had circumspectly attempted to limit the number of forces to two, so as to grant them maximum generality (and make them analogous to the Newtonian forces of attraction and repulsion), subsequent writers on physiology eagerly began multiplying their number. Johann Friedrich Blumenbach (1752–1840), who like Haller taught at Göttingen, identified no fewer than five of them. In addition to Haller's sensibility and irritability, Blumenbach's catalogue of vital forces included contractility, the property of non-muscular cellular tissue to shorten itself; the generative force (*Bildungstrieb* or *nisus formativus*), which accounted for the majority of phenomena associated with generation and reproduction; and finally the "particular life" (*besonderes Leben* or *vita propria*) of each organ whose functions cannot easily be accounted for in terms of irritability or some other recognized force. The "particular life" represented a category of forces, thereby opening the door to the description of many new vital forces. Along with adding several new forces to the organic inventory, Blumenbach also conceptualized vital forces in a way different from Haller. Haller had attempted as far as possible to define sensibility and irritability operationally: irritability, for example, was the property of tissue to contract upon stimulation. Using these forces more or less heuristically as descriptions of experimentally produced phenomena allowed Haller to sidestep the question of their ontological status. However, as James Larson has argued, Blumenbach, together with Carl Friedrich Kielmeyer (1765–1844) and other late eighteenth-century scholars, was far more willing to grant vital forces some kind of material existence.[24]

22 On Haller's doctrine of sensibility and irritability and on his general philosophy of science, see Roe, "Anatomia animata"; Le Roy, *Johann Christian Reil and "Naturphilosophie,"* chap. 1; and Richard Toellner, *Albrecht von Haller: Über die Einheit im Denken des letzten Universalgelehrten,* Sudhoffs Archiv Beiheft 10 (Wiesbaden, 1971), esp. pp. 89–118. For a helpful description of the intellectual climate when Haller's doctrine was announced in 1752, see G. Rudolph, "Hallers Lehre von der Irritabilität und Sensibilität," in *Von Boerhaave bis Berger: Die Entwicklung der kontinentalen Physiologie im 18. und 19. Jahrhundert mit besonderer Berücksichtigung der Neurophysiologie,* ed. K. E. Rothschuh (Stuttgart, 1964), pp. 14–34.

23 One major arena in which these issues were joined was in connection with embryogenesis, as described in Shirley A. Roe, *Matter, Life and Generation: Eighteenth-Century Embryology and the Haller-Wolff Debate* (Cambridge, 1981), pp. 32–6ff. See also R. K. French, *Robert Whytt, the Soul, and Medicine* (London, 1969).

24 My interpretation agrees most closely with that of James L. Larson, "Vital Forces: Regulative Principles or Constitutive Agents?" *Isis* 70 (1979): 235–49. For a somewhat different view of Blumenbach and vital forces, see Timothy Lenoir, "Kant, Blumenbach, and Vital Materialism in Germany," *Isis* 71 (1980): 77–108; and idem, *The Strategy of Life: Teleology and Mechanics in Nineteenth-Century German Biology* (Dordrecht, 1982).

While writers such as Haller and Blumenbach were engaged in their "Newton-ian" project of defining physiology as a survey of vital forces, academic writing on pathology was proceeding along a divergent path, indeed several divergent paths. The first represented for the most part a continuation of the treatment given pathology by Boerhaave. The *Institutiones pathologiae medicinalis* (1758), by the Leiden professor Hieronymous David Gaub (1705–80), became one of the more widely used pathology textbooks. Gaub defined illness as any condition of the human body whereby it is unable to perform its normal functions.[25] Like Boer-haave, Gaub hung his notion of disease on his conception of physiology. Accord-ingly, he spent a considerable portion of the book cataloguing the changes to which the body's solid and fluid parts are susceptible. Dislocations of joints no less than chemical corruptions of fluids and laxity of the fibers found their place in this scheme. Gaub presented other traditional topics from pathology as well, including an overview of the various categories of causes of disease: remote versus proximal, internal versus external, and predispositions versus occasional causes. As part of his discussion of the occasional causes (i.e., those that trigger disease by acting on a body made susceptible by one or more predispositions), Gaub reviewed the ancient doctrine of the six non-naturals which affect the body: air, food and drink, motion and rest, excretion and retention, sleep and wakefulness, and emotions.[26]

The textbook published in 1754 by the Leipzig professor Christian Gottlieb Ludwig (1709–73) handled its subject somewhat differently. Instead of approaching pathology primarily as a survey of the body's possible pathological changes, Ludwig sought to guide readers from the "outside in," from the symptoms to the internal conditions underlying them. Ludwig too sketched the varieties of pathological change that overcome the body's solid and fluid parts, but his princi-pal interests lay with etiology, the causes of disease, and with semiotics, the interpretation of symptoms. Thus while Ludwig's overall notion of disease resem-bled Gaub's – Ludwig too identified disease as changes in the body's solid or fluid parts and not as a specific entity – his presentation of pathology was less natural philosophy than practical handbook.[27]

This same treatment of pathology with an eye toward practice permeated what was probably the century's most prominent treatise on pathology, *De sedibus et causis morborum* (On the seats and causes of diseases, 1761), by Giovanni Battista Morgagni (1682–1771). Morgagni took as his task the correlation of particular

---

25 "Status ille corporis humani viventis, quo sit, ut actiones, homini prorpiae, non possint apposite ad leges sanitatis exerceri, *Morbus* dicitur." *Institutiones pathologiae medicinalis* (Leiden, 1758), 34.

26 On the history of the doctrine of the non-naturals, see L. J. Rather, "The 'Six Things Non-Natural,'" *Clio Medica* 3 (1968): 333–47. For a general discussion of the theory of disease causation in early modern medicine, see King, *The Philosophy of Medicine*, pp. 209–32. Among King's topics is a helpful review of Boerhaave's thought on causation.

27 Christian Gottlieb Ludwig, *Institutiones pathologiae praelectionibus academicis accommodatae* (Leipzig, 1754).

symptoms with their underlying anatomical changes, and in the five dedications and preface with which he opened the treatise he clearly laid out his desire to provide a tool for medical practice. He expressed the hope that his work would be presented to medical students to guide their future practice, claiming that "it is far more advantageous to show them by medical anatomy the causes of those diseases which they will frequently encounter in their medical practice than of those few which they possibly will never meet."[28] To this end, he organized his treatise first by the major portions of the body ("Disorders of the Head," "Disorders of the Thorax") and then within each division by individual symptoms or groups of symptoms ("suffocation and cough," "spitting of blood," "pain in the Breast, Sides, and Back"). Morgagni spoke too at great length of the desirability of compiling indexes of pathological anatomy, with which practitioners could rapidly locate information about the anatomical basis of particular symptoms.[29]

As the subject that bridged the theoretical and practical portions of medicine, pathology expressed the fullness of medicine's complex relationship to natural philosophy and to bedside practice. Gaub, Ludwig, and Morgagni would have found considerable agreement among themselves concerning the causes and nature of disease. Where they differed, or more precisely, where they chose to place different emphases, was on the question of pathology's role in medical learning. At mid-century, when their major works appeared, the profession was flexible enough to comprehend without much dissension a broad vision of medical theory and practice. However, developments during the second half of the century made the relationship between theory and practice increasingly contentious. Whereas Gaub in 1758 could present his version of a pathology closely linked to physiological theory and have it adopted as a standard textbook, by the late 1790s the Brunonians' attempt to do the same thing created an uproar.

The reasons for this are complicated, and will be developed as we go along. But one element of the explanation – the tendency of physiology to develop its own complex of problems based on Newtonian forces – has already been alluded to. The description of vital forces as part of a more comprehensive inquiry into the nature of life tended to draw physiology away from its moorings in medicine. As they had always done, writers on physiology attended closely to the currents of philosophical doctrine and adjusted their own direction accordingly. But over the course of the eighteenth century, physiology increasingly developed its own research agenda, one defined by the search for vital forces and their correlation with anatomical structure. Not surprisingly, this trend found its reflection in medical textbooks. After Boerhaave, it became uncommon for physiology to

28 Giovanni Battista Morgagni, *The Seats and Causes of Diseases Investigated by Anatomy*, vol. 1, trans. Benjamin Alexander, repr. ed. with an introduction and translation of five letters by Paul Klemperer (New York, 1960), quoted from the dedication to Johann Friedrich Schreiber.
29 Ibid., author's preface, pp. xxix–xxxi.

appear as one topic in an *institutiones medicae,* becoming instead the subject of its own separate *institutiones physiologiae.*[30]

CRITICISM AND THE REFORM OF MEDICAL SCIENCE IN THE 1790S

As he surveyed the medical scene from his editorial perch in 1794, Christian Gottfried Gruner, professor of medicine at Jena and editor of the *Almanach für Aerzte und Nichtärzte,* could see only a bleak landscape of decay and ruin. His profession had forfeited its erstwhile dignity and sobriety to an unruly mob of arriviste surgeons and squabbling sectarians. "The ruling spirit of the age," Gruner declared, "which is interested in idolatry, in enlightenment and superstition, in revolution and recasting of all things, in the overthrow of the previous world order and estates; which hates everything old and seeks through the new to dazzle and mislead, has also seized the heads of physicians."[31] He denounced the tendency of writers in auxiliary sciences such as physiology to spin theories empty of practical content; he savaged followers of fashionable "foreign" theories, such as William Cullen's neuropathology; and he pronounced anathema on anyone who would deviate in the slightest from the cautious empirical path to knowledge marked out by the ancients.

To be sure, Gruner rarely had a kind word for medical novelties of any stripe. His was the most conservative wing of the medical establishment, a group that apprehended a period of political revolution and growing medical pluralism with considerable alarm. But his voice was by no means the only one sounding these themes. Ernst Gottfried Baldinger, professor in Marburg and an indefatigable medical journalist, satirized the spirit of the age in his *Neues Magazin für Aerzte* and *Medicinisches Journal,* although he avoided Gruner's histrionics. Perhaps most characteristic of this era of controversy was the *Journal der Erfindungen, Theorien, und Widersprüche in der Natur- und Arzneywissenschaft* (Journal of discoveries, theories, and controversies in natural philosophy and medicine), launched in 1792 by the Erfurt professor August Friedrich Hecker (1763–1811). Like Gruner, Hecker railed against the prevailing tendency to construct medical systems and seek novelty, which generates controversy among adherents of different systems. The effects of this are particularly harmful for students, in whom, Hecker wrote, "we

---

30 Johann Samuel Ersch, *Literatur der Medizin seit der Mitte des 18. Jahrhunderts bis auf die neueste Zeit mit Registern* (Leipzig, 1822). See cols. 73–8 for a list of textbooks and systematic treatises on physiology. It should be noted that a variant of the *institutiones medicae* persisted into the nineteenth century as introductory surveys, such as Karl Friedrich Burdach's *Propädeutik zum Studium der gesammten Heilkunst* (Leipzig, 1800). But such texts no longer were vehicles for a serious treatment of physiological theory, as Boerhaave's *Institutiones* or Haller's *Elementa physiologiae* had been. On the separation of physiological writing from medical pedagogy, see Thomas H. Broman, "J. C. Reil and the 'Journalization' of Physiology," in *The Literary Structure of Scientific Argument,* ed. Peter Dear (Philadelphia, 1991), pp. 13–42.

31 *Almanach für Aerzte und Nichtärzte* (1794), p. 85.

always perceive the greatest inclination for reform, new theories, speculations, systems and so forth; *but their mania for system* (Systemsucht) *is our ruin!*"[32]

What is noteworthy about such complaints is not their content, but their medium, for the periodicals in which Gruner and Hecker so ardently censured the latest trends were in fact their very embodiment. The last quarter of the eighteenth century witnessed an explosion in the number of periodicals, a funda-mental reorientation of the publishing business that also encouraged new forms of social organization of reading, such as lending libraries and reading societies.[33] Medicine too succumbed to the new taste for periodical reading, as some seventy new titles were launched in the 1790s alone.[34] These publications served a variety of ends. Some were expressly didactic and aimed at the general public; they participated in the great project of spreading Enlightenment. Others were in-tended primarily for medical practitioners and contained case histories and other material for a professional readership.

Most distinctive were those periodicals, such as Gruner's and Hecker's, that used journalism to engage in debates over the nature of the medical profession and the proper basis of medical knowledge. Moreover, although the participants in the debates may have been almost exclusively physicians, the audience for them consisted of that much broader, vaguely defined "public." As a consequence, the standards of argument conformed to the universally accessible canons of "reason," rather than being accessible only to a privileged clique of specialists. Medical journalists sought to appropriate the new periodical medium to establish the proper boundaries of medical theory and practice, and establish themselves as the arbiters of those boundaries. Hecker's *Journal der Erfindungen* was most explicit in this respect. Citing the number of theories and systems in circulation, Hecker gave his journal the task of criticizing new ones as they appeared. Paradoxically, it proved impossible to impose closure on debates in this way. The only product of public criticism was the generation of ever more criticism and periodicals.

Yet periodicals could be used more than just reactively; they could also be applied positively to building the critical foundations for a theoretical position.

32 *Journal der Erfindungen Theorien, und Widersprüche in der Natur- und Arzneywissenschaft*, Stück 1 (1792), p. 17. The emphasis was Hecker's. One can gather Hecker's attitude toward novelty from the epigraph with which he opened the first issue: "Truth is not the daughter of respectability (*Ansehens*), but of time."

33 Much good work has been done on the sociology of literature in Germany. With particular reference to reading societies, see Klaus Gerteis, "Bildung und Revolution: die deutschen Lese-gesellschaften am Ende des 18. Jahrhunderts," *Archiv für Kulturgeschichte* 53 (1971): 127–39; Marlies Prüsener, "Lesegesellschaften im achtzehnten Jahrhundert: ein Beitrag zur Lesergeschichte," *Archiv für Geschichte des Buchwesens* 13 (1972): 369–574; Barney M. Milstein, *Eight Eighteenth Century Reading Societies: A Sociological Contribution to the History of German Literature* (Berne, 1972); Rolf Engelsing, *Der Bürger als Leser: Lesergeschichte in Deutschland 1500–1800* (Stuttgart, 1974), pp. 216–258; and Otto Dann, "Die Lesegesellschaften des 18. Jahrhunderts und der gesellschaftliche Auf-bruch des deutschen Bürgertums," in *Buch und Leser*, ed. Herbert G. Göpfert (Hamburg, 1977), pp. 160–93.

34 Joachim Kirchner, *Das deutsche Zeitschriftenwesen: seine Geschichte und seine Probleme* (Wiesbaden, 1958), p. 116.

This is exactly what we see in the *Archiv für die Physiologie,* which began in 1795 under the editorship of the Halle professor Johann Christian Reil (1759–1813). Reil believed the proper foundation for a science of medicine was physiology which, as he saw it, required a thoroughgoing critique of its aims and methods. "There lacks an appropriate, prescribed plan," he wrote, "and also a knowledge of the rules by which we must investigate physiology."[35] Reil made it the task of the *Archiv* to supply those rules and restore physiology to its proper place as the cornerstone of medical theory.

Like Baldinger and Hecker, this critic and reformer began life as the son of a Lutheran pastor.[36] For young men such as Reil, medicine offered an opportunity to receive a university education without the bleak prospect of spending years as a tutor, schoolmaster, or curate while waiting for a parsonage. Although the medical profession may have appeared less overcrowded than the clergy, it too demanded patronage for making a successful career, and Reil found his patron at Halle in the person of Johann Friedrich Goldhagen (1742–88), professor and town *Physicus.*[37] For a short while following his graduation, Reil returned to his home town (in East Frisia) and took up medical practice, but his chance to return to Halle was not long in coming, for in 1787 he received an appointment as a private lecturer and then extraordinary professor at the university. The very next year Goldhagen, in a display of exemplary considerateness toward his protegé, died, leaving the way open for Reil to assume his chair and his place as *Physicus.*[38] But along with Hecker and Baldinger, Reil was not content to mark professional success simply by settling down into a well-connected position at a prestigious university. He sought to make his presence felt in the public arena as a writer, critic, and editor.

What is striking about Reil's treatment of medical theory is the extent to which he redefined physiology's traditional concerns in terms of more fundamental questions about the general possibility of scientific knowledge. This is not to say that earlier writers had naively supposed that empirical evidence produces indubitable knowledge of nature's universal order. But in the wake of Kant's critical philosophy Reil placed the subjective conditions of knowledge at the center of his discussion, thus linking medical theory to a broader public discussion about the role of subjective consciousness in understanding and shaping the world.[39] In a

---

35 *Archiv für die Physiologie* 1, no. 1 (1795): 4.

36 Many years ago, Hans Gerth identified the prominent role played by sons of clergymen in the cultural and political movements of the 1790s, which he attributed to the value placed on education in clerical families and the simultaneous lack of social mobility for sons of the lower clergy. See Gerth, *Bürgerliche Intelligenz um 1800: Zur Soziologie des deutschen Frühliberalismus* (repr. Göttingen, 1976), pp. 29–31; and Anthony J. La Vopa, *Grace, Talent, and Merit: Poor Students, Clerical Careers, and Professional Ideology in Eighteenth-Century Germany* (Cambridge, 1988), pp. 266–78.

37 For a discussion of how patronage shaped the experience of poor students in the 18th century, see La Vopa, *Grace, Talent, and Merit,* pp. 83–110.

38 For biographical details, see Max Neuburger, *Johann Christian Reil* (Stuttgart, 1913), p. 12; and Hans-Heinz Eulner, "Johann Christian Reil, Leben und Werke," *Nova Acta Leopoldina,* Neue Folge 22 (1960): 7–50.

39 On the reformulation of physiology as an epistemological problem, see Brigitte Lohff, *Die Suche nach der Wissenschaftlichkeit der Physiologie in der Zeit der Romantik* (Stuttgart, 1990), pp. 35–46.

series of essays in the *Archiv's* first three volumes, Reil argued that the phenomena accessible to the senses arise from the properties of the matter at the origin of those phenomena, especially from the form and mixture of matter. If the phenomena undergo a change, so too must there have been an alteration in the form and mixture of the matter. "That we do not find in inanimate Nature the same phenomena as in animate Nature," he concluded, "depends on the particular properties of organic matter, which [matter] is not found in inanimate Nature."[40] Reil rejected as pointless the common notion of a non-material *Lebenskraft* imparting life to matter:

The peculiar nature of the matter, of which animal bodies consist, contains the preeminent basis of their peculiar animal phenomena. *Lebenskraft*, which we regard as the cause of these appearances and bring to organic matter, is not something separate from the same; rather the matter itself, as such, is the cause of these appearances. . . . We do not need, therefore, any *Lebenskraft* as an elementary force to explain [the phenomena of organic Nature]; we use this word merely to designate the manifestation of the physical, chemical, and mechanical forces of organic matter.[41]

But wherein exactly do the differences in matter lie? The key to this problem is provided by the method of analysis. Through analysis of the complex phenomena of the organic world, Reil reasoned, we follow out the chains of cause and effect, until we come up against that "general cause" of phenomena, the form and mixture of matter. However, the analysis does not end here. It continues until we finally reach elements of which all matter is composed. "Among these elements," Reil wrote, "we distinguish nothing further than a different nature of each, by means of which their combination produces not mere increases of mass, but rather substances of a unique sort."[42] Thus according to Reil physiology could be founded upon objective knowledge furnished by chemistry.

That Reil set himself the task of bringing chemical enlightenment to physiology was ambitious enough, but what he presented as the methodological compass of physiology was meant to orient a unified science of medicine as well. "Illness is a deviation from the healthy mixture and form of the body and its parts," he wrote, "which becomes visible to us through anomalies in the body's phenomena."[43] Reil attacked the belief that illness is the product of an abnormal stimulus acting on organs that are otherwise healthy, arguing instead that every illness resulted

40 Johann Christian Reil, "Von der Lebenskraft," *Archiv für die Physiologie* 1, no. 1 (1795): 14. See also Le Roy, *Johann Christian Reil and "Naturphilosophie,"* pp. 106–35. Le Roy's dissertation presents an exceedingly thorough and reliable interpretation of Reil's thought, and my reading of Reil finds many points of contact with it. The major difference between our interpretations is that whereas Le Roy sets Reil in a philosophical context defined by the work of Kant and Schelling, my own interpretation emphasizes Reil's place within the medical profession.
41 Johann Christian Reil, "Veränderte Mischung und Form der thierischen Materie, als Krankheit oder nächste Ursache der Krankheitszufälle betrachtet," *Archiv für die Physiologie* 3 (1799): 424.
42 "Von der Lebenskraft," pp. 16–17.
43 Johann Christian Reil, "Ueber die nächste Ursache der Krankheiten," *Archiv für die Physiologie* 2 (1797): 212.

from an abnormal form and mixture of a particular organ.[44] Although he did not deny that pathology's traditional assortment of causes was useful in describing the instances of disease, he maintained that these causes worked only mediately through changes in the form and mixture of organs. Pathology and physiology thus were inextricably united by their mutual dependence on knowledge of the chemical properties of matter. As a consequence, the essential understanding of illness rested on knowledge of the composition of the healthy and diseased organ, and Reil bemoaned the backwardness of physiology for impeding attainment of that knowledge. The primitive state of physiology, Reil complained, leaves the physician to grope almost blindly for the relation between the causes of disease and its symptoms.[45]

In his effort to provide the broadest scientific foundation for medicine, Reil extended his systematic grasp to therapeutics. He supported the traditional and much-maligned division of his profession, between surgery and internal medicine, on the grounds that they pursue different courses in the treatment of illness. Surgery uses "physical and mechanical forces" to alter the form of matter, while the medicaments of internal medicine change the body's mixture through "chemical forces."[46] Although the precise mode of action of medicaments remained a mystery, Reil confidently believed in the potential for chemical explanations of their effects.

Reil's reformulation of medicine as an empirical Kantian science placed it squarely before a public – and not just a medical public – that was in a position to follow and appreciate its development in general, if not in all its details. Other writers pitched in as well, such as Johann Heinrich Varnhagen (1770–1805), whose *Versuch einer Kritik der wichtigsten physiologischen Grundbegriffe* (1796) presented a criticism of medical theory similarly founded on Kantian principles.[47] The outstanding example of this literature is *Physiologie philosophisch bearbeitet*, published in 1798 by Carl Christian Erhard Schmid (1761–1812). Schmid's work is all the more remarkable for having been enthusiastically received by medical reviewers despite the fact that the author was not a doctor at all: Schmid was a professor of theology at the University of Jena.[48]

That a theologian could write a work on physiology and have it accepted by physicians as a major contribution testifies to how inclusive the public sphere was

---

44 Johann Christian Reil, *Ueber die Erkenntniß und Cur der Fieber*, Bd. 1, "Allgemeine Fieberlehre," 3rd ed. (Halle 1820), pp. 12–13, 16–17; and "Ueber die nächste Ursache der Krankheiten," pp. 214–18 and 225–6.
45 "Ueber die nächste Ursache der Krankheiten," p. 213.
46 *Ueber die Erkenntniß und Cur der Fieber*, Bd. 1, pp. 23–4.
47 Lohff, *Die Suche nach der Wissenschaftlichkeit*, p. 44.
48 Schmid was already by that time well-known as a leading exponent of Kantian philosophy. For an example of the welcome Schmid's book enjoyed in the medical press, see the *Medicinisch-chirurgische Zeitung*, 15 August 1799, pp. 243–8. It was favorably reviewed in more general literary periodicals as well, such as the *Allgemeine Literatur-Zeitung*, 12 September–14 September 1799, nos. 292–94. In the latter review, the critic leaves little doubt that Schmid has made a major contribution to shaping a science of medicine.

in the 1790s. It also illustrates how different subgroups within that "public" shared a common language for science, taken in its broader German sense of *Wissenschaft* rather than its narrow English connotations. By his own admission, Schmid's knowledge of physiology was derivative, garnered through attending various medical lectures at Jena.[49] His intention was not to add to the store of physiological facts in any way; his book made use of information that was well known among physiologists. But no special expertise or familiarity with the content of physiology was needed to discuss the general principles according to which any subject, including physiology, is a *Wissenschaft*.

The biggest drawback facing medicine, Schmid wrote in the introduction to his treatise, is its lack of an adequate theoretical foundation for practice. Far from attaining anything remotely resembling this, medicine actually was

for the most part nothing more than a quasi-systematic collection (*systemartiges geordnetes Aggregat*) of individual observations and more or less useful rules of thumb (*Kunstregeln*) derived from them, for which we still do not possess scientific proof from the highest and most general principles. The reality [of these rules] rests exclusively on their usefulness in practice, not on theoretically valid grounds, and therefore they have absolutely no scientific value, but rather merely technical worth.[50]

As an example of such rules of thumb, Schmid cited medical specifics. Specifics were medicaments known to be effective against particular diseases, but without the knowledge of how they work. Schmid conceded that as practitioners, physicians might have every reason to be confident in such treatments. "But so long as medicine has and must have specifics, so long is it . . . a merely empirical art."[51] Beyond their failure to stand proof as scientific knowledge, Schmid continued, specifics can actually hinder the transformation of medicine into a science. The existence of the seemingly firm rules provided by specifics tempts physicians to test theories by their conformity with practice, which reverses the process by which they ought to be testing their knowledge. He urged physicians not to give in to this temptation and instead to derive their theories from first principles, if they want to claim possession "of a medical theory that deserved the name of a science."[52]

This of course states the gulf separating academic *Wissenschaft* from practical exigency rather nicely, for the practitioner might well remain content knowing that the reality of his rules depended on their usefulness in practice. For practitioners, it was only fitting that medical theories be made to pass the test of the bedside. If the physician's identity depended to any significant extent on his role as a healer – and it manifestly did, according to many writers – then standards of knowledge such as those Schmid was proposing might seem less than compel-

49 Carl Christin Erhard Schmid, *Physiologie philosophisch bearbeitet,* Bd. 1 (Jena 1798), p. xxxi(n).
50 Ibid., pp. vii–viii.
51 Ibid., p. x.
52 Ibid., pp. x–xi.

ling. And indeed some physicians did reject them, as we shall see in the next chapter.

By bringing discussions of medical theory into the public sphere, the writings of Reil and Schmid and others attempted to reform physiology through criticism. Reil certainly knew that critical prolegomena such as the one presented in "Von der Lebenskraft" would not themselves suffice for construction of a new medical *Wissenschaft*, and for that reason the *Archiv für die Physiologie* prominently featured empirical studies alongside critical essays. But if criticism alone was not sufficient, it was unquestionably necessary, as Reil noted when he launched the journal. Through criticism physiology might at last be set on secure foundations, and in turn provide the theoretical grounding for a reformed medical therapeutics.

THE APOTHEOSIS OF *WISSENSCHAFT*

The cautious path toward a medical *Wissenschaft* advocated by Reil and Schmid, the path of public criticism and empirical investigation, proved not to be the most prominent one taken by German physicians in the two decades following the inauguration of the *Archiv.* Instead, in direct opposition to their intentions, medical writing in Germany became increasingly doctrinal and systematic. One prominent example of this trend is Brunonianism, a controversial medical system that is the subject of Chapter 5. A second example is the system of philosophical idealism known as *Naturphilosophie*, first articulated by Friedrich Wilhelm Schelling (1775–1854) and developed by a host of writers beginning around 1800. In its metaphysical and epistemological stances, indeed in its very language, *Naturphilosophie* represented an emphatic rejection of the Kantianism that guided Reil and Schmid.

As an historical phenomenon, *Naturphilosophie* presents two distinct problems that have made it difficult to interpret. First, the content of *Naturphilosophie* is formidably otherworldly. Especially for scholars trained in the traditions of Anglo-American empiricism, it can seem virtually unintelligible, based as it is on a notion of the "transcendental" that is not part of their standard philosophical approach. Even those who have taken *Naturphilosophie* seriously have tended to do so in one of two ways. One group of scholars, by focusing on certain key concepts in *Naturphilosophie*, such as polarity, has argued for the fruitfulness of some of its doctrines for the later development of science. Such a position has not required that *Naturphilosophie* itself be taken seriously as natural science; rather, the story allows it to be the parent of unintended consequences.[53] A second group has

53 The idea that *Naturphilosophie* opened up fruitful paths for later science is suggested by, among many others, Thomas S. Kuhn, "Energy Conservation as an Example of Simultaneous Discovery," in *Critical Problems in the History of Science,* ed. Marshall Clagett (Madison, Wis., 1959), pp. 321–56, esp. pp. 338–9; R. C. Stauffer, "Speculation and Experiment in the Background of Oersted's Discovery of Electromagnetism," *Isis* 48 (1957): 33–50; Everett Mendelsohn, "The Biological Sciences in the Nineteenth Century: Some Problems and Sources," *History of Science* 3 (1964): 39–59; L. Pearce Williams, "The Physical Sciences During the First Half of the Nineteenth Century," *History of Science* 1 (1962): 1–15; and H. A. M. Snelders, "Oersted's Discovery of Electromagne-

assimilated *Naturphilosophie* to the broader history of transcendental idealism in German philosophy and philosophy of science, allowing for a serious examination of its doctrines.[54]

What these two interpretive approaches share is a tendency to accept *Naturphilosophie* as a speculative form of knowledge, instead of an empirical science. The distinction between "speculation" and "empiricism" has long proven useful for polemical purposes in the history of science, and it has been an especially attractive weapon against *Naturphilosophie*.[55] A second point of agreement between them concerns the perceived necessity of penetrating beyond the language deployed by writers of *Naturphilosophie* to the doctrines beneath it. Even as sympathetic a commentator as William Coleman pronounced *Naturphilosophie* "inherently obscure," while assessments considerably less charitable are typically deployed to provide a ready source of comic relief amidst the sober business of relating histories of science and medicine.[56] It is precisely here, however, in the handling of the language of *Naturphilosophie*, that I believe historians have gone most seriously astray. For all its maddening, metaphorical inscrutability, the language is not something to be "decoded" and thereby swept aside. Quite to the contrary, as we shall see shortly, the *Naturphilosophen* redefined the role of language in the scientific enterprise, which led them to use it in distinctive ways. Once this essential point is grasped, the denigration of *Naturphilosophie* as a merely speculative exercise can be shown to be utterly inappropriate to what it actually set out to do.

An elucidation of the linguistic project of *Naturphilosophie*, important as it is, only takes us part way toward understanding it. For we immediately encounter

tism," in *Romanticism and the Sciences*, ed. Andrew Cunningham and Nicholas Jardine (Cambridge, 1990), pp. 228–40. The varying assessments of *Naturphilosophie*'s contribution to Robert Mayer's ideas on the conservation of energy are summarized in Kenneth L. Caneva, *Robert Mayer and the Conservation of Energy* (Princeton, N.J., 1993), pp. 275–80.

54 Andrew Bowie, *Schelling and Modern European Philosophy* (London, 1993), provides an excellent introduction to Schelling's thought and emphasizes its continuing relevance to contemporary philosophy. See also Manfred Frank, *Eine Einführung in Schellings Philosophie* (Frankfurt, 1985); Joseph L. Esposito, *Schelling's Idealism and Philosophy of Nature*, (Lewisburg, Pa., 1977); and the introduction by Robert Stern in Friedrich Wilhelm Joseph Schelling, *Ideas for a Philosophy of Nature*, trans. Errol E. Harris and Peter Heath (Cambridge, 1988), pp. ix–xxiii.

55 See for example Timothy Shanahan, "Kant, *Naturphilosophie*, and Oersted's Discovery of Electromagnetism: A Reassessment," *Studies in the History and Philosophy of Science* 20 (1989): 287–305. Thankfully, recent scholarship has begun to transcend this simple-minded distinction. See Nicholas Jardine, *The Scenes of Inquiry* (Oxford, 1991), pp. 33–55; and Caneva, *Robert Mayer and the Conservation of Energy*, pp. 275–319, who wavers a bit on the speculation/empiricism issue (compare pp. 280 and 285), but whose presentation of the central doctrines of *Naturphilosophie* generally downplays such distinctions. Finally, Lohff, *Die Suche nach der Wissenschaftlichkeit*, pp. 169–202, describes the complex semantic field that characterized the concepts *Empirie* and *Spekulation* in the early nineteenth century.

56 William Coleman, *Biology in the Nineteenth Century* (Cambridge, 1977), p. 49. In an early article, Timothy Lenoir described *Naturphilosophie* as a "strange and nearly impenetrable offshoot of the Romantic Movement." Timothy Lenoir, "Generational Factors in the Origin of *Romantische Naturphilosophie*," *Journal of the History of Biology* 11 (1978): 57–100, quoted on 57. Similar sentiments are expressed in Hall, *Ideas of Life and Matter*, vol. 2, p. 174. See also John Reddick, "The Shattered Whole: Georg Büchner and Naturphilosophie," in Cunningham and Jardine, *Romanticism and the Sciences*, pp. 322–40; and Rothschuh, *Physiologie*, pp. 191–203.

the problem of explaining why it proved so appealing, especially to physicians, who comprised the majority of Schelling's early followers.[57] What does it say about the professional situation of medicine in the 1790s that *Naturphilosophie* became for physicians a dominant mode of theorizing about nature? The absence of an adequate answer to this question has forced historians to make helpless gestures toward the "spirit of the age," or "Romantic influences" as a way of explaining the phenomenon. But as I will argue below, there are at hand better explanatory tools, ones that take account of the structure of professional and cultural life in 1800.

Before turning to the "why" of *Naturphilosophie*, however, let us begin with the "what." What did it all mean? At a technical philosophical level, *Naturphilosophie* offered a solution to problems raised by Kant's treatment of epistemology. As is well known, Kant's critical philosophy displaced the object from the center of knowledge and replaced it with the subject. A priori synthetic knowledge of the world is possible, Kant argued, not because our cognitive faculties conform to the objects of experience. Rather it is the objects of possible experience that must conform to our faculties of intuition, as a general condition for the possibility of knowledge. Therefore in this sense it becomes knowledge *for us,* and not knowledge of things in themselves.

The critical philosophy bequeathed two problems that bear upon our story. First, the hardened duality between subject and object appeared unsatisfactory to many, for it left unexplained matters such as why nature exhibits law-like behavior. Although one might suppose some sort of regularity among the objects themselves, Kant's system could provide no rigorous and final justification for such a supposition. Second, the mind described by Kant was a satchel full of diverse faculties and categories, but lacking a crucial trait of empirical mind: self-consciousness.[58]

These two legacies furnished the starting point for Johann Gottlieb Fichte's (1762–1814) philosophical system. The basis for a transcendental bridge between subject and object would be for Fichte the self, elevated to self-consciousness. In his system, the self has two drives that constitute its essence. On the one hand, the self is regulated by an active, expansive drive to extend itself into infinity. As pure activity, the self is unbounded and limitless. On the other hand, Fichte attributed to the self the power of theoretical reason, by which the self reflects on itself. At that moment of reflection, the self sets limits to itself and achieves self-consciousness. It sees itself as some*thing:* "A self that posits itself as self-positing, or

57 For a more detailed discussion of the participation of physicians in *Naturphilosophie*, see Ernst Hirschfeld, "Romantische Medizin. Zu einer künftigen Geschichte der naturphilosophischen Ära," *Kyklos* 3 (1930): 1–89; and Thomas Broman, "University Reform in Medical Thought at the End of the Eighteenth Century," in *Science in Germany: The Intersection of Institutional and Intellectual Issues,* ed. Kathryn M. Olesko, *Osiris,* 2nd ser., 5 (1989): 36–53.

58 Self-consciousness does make an appearance in the *Critique of Pure Reason,* but only as the by-product of the synthesis of representations by the understanding. It plays no part in the creation of knowledge.

a subject, is impossible without an object brought forth in the manner described (the determination of the self, its reflection upon itself as a determining [being] is only possible under the condition that it bounds itself by means of an opposite)."[59] Thus the possibility of knowledge is given in the moment when the self constitutes itself as an object of reflection.

Now, the positing of the self as an object of reflection seemed to the young Friedrich Schelling a sufficient answer to the question of what kind of identity is possible between an object and our representations of it. Such an identity, he wrote, can only arise in the case of "a being that contemplated itself" (*sich selbst anschaute*).[60] But it soon became apparent that such identities foundered on what became a central problem for the circle of young intellectuals that gathered around Friedrich Schlegel (1772–1829) and August Wilhelm Schlegel (1767–1845) in Jena, a circle that included Schelling. Reflection by the self is possible only because the object of reflection is a *representation* of the self, rather than the self itself. Were it the latter, then there would be no knowledge, because the putative object would be completely indistinguishable from the subject. Consequently self-consciousness, and by extension all knowledge, is based on representations that manifest the self or subject to itself, but in a formal way, through devices such as language, images, or symbols. Such devices obviously are not and cannot be the same thing as the subject itself; indeed, this difference constitutes the possibility of knowledge. But if the act of representation makes knowledge possible, it also reenacts the gap between representation and the objects of representation, the very gap that Kant had pointed to.[61]

From the standpoint of transcendental philosophy, the problem of representation could be sidestepped by positing an original entity, usually referred to as the Absolute, which exists prior to any act of representation. As Schelling formulated it in his *Ideen zu einer Philosophie der Natur* (Ideas for a philosophy of nature) in 1797, subject and object are not merely joined in the Absolute, they are literally one. In its essential act of knowing, the Absolute gives itself a form, which means that it apprehends itself as an object: that being whose essence is knowing. Schelling described this as a moment (*Einheit*) in the Absolute where its being as subject is entirely subsumed by objectivity. Correspondingly, there is a second moment where the object – the Absolute as a being that knows – is comprehended in another act of knowing. At that moment, the Absolute as object is entirely subsumed by subjectivity. Finally, along with these two moments of absolute

59 Johann Gottlieb Fichte, *Gesammtausgabe*, ed. Reinhard Lauth und Hans Jacob, Bd. 1, Teil 2 (Stuttgart, 1965), p. 361. My translation is changed slightly from Johann Gottlieb Fichte, *Science of Knowledge*, trans. Peter Heath and John Lachs (Cambridge, 1982), p. 195.

60 Friedrich Wilhelm Joseph Schelling, "Abhandlungen zur Erläuterung des Idealismus der Wissenschaftslehre," in *Sämmtliche Werke*, Bd. 1 (Stuttgart, 1856), pp. 365–6.

61 My discussion of the problem of representation in German idealism is deeply indebted to the insights of Azade Seyhahn in "Labours of Theory: The Quest for Representation in Early German Romanticism," *Seminar* 25 (1989): 187–204; and idem, *Representation and its Discontents: The Critical Legacy of German Romanticism* (Berkeley and Los Angeles, 1992), esp. pp. 23–56.

Subject and absolute Object (or, as Schelling sometimes refers to them, absolute being and absolute form), there is a third moment in the Absolute that is the unity of the other two.[62]

These first two moments of the Absolute as Subject and Object constitute the fundamental conformations of the Absolute into the Ideal World (or Spirit) and Nature. Because, Schelling argued, Nature and Spirit themselves each have "a point of absoluteness where the two opposites flow together,"[63] they also contain three moments of objectivity, subjectivity, and the union of the two. In Nature, the moment of objectivity is represented in its essence by the general structure of the universe (*allgemeine Weltbau*), and in its particular form by the given distribution of planets, stars, and other bodies (*die Körperreihe*). The subjective moment – which Schelling observed is subordinate to the objective, "ruling" moment in Nature – is given by universal mechanics (*allgemeine Mechanismus*), the essence of which is light, and whose particular form is corporeal bodies in their dynamic interactions. Finally, the moment of unity is given by the organism, which is "the perfect image of the Absolute in and for Nature."[64]

But if from the standpoint of transcendental philosophy organic nature could be understood as a dialectical moment in the ceaseless activity of the Absolute, from the perspective of empirical science one is placed squarely before the question of how to "interpret" nature for its meaning, or in other words for what it tells us about the Absolute. For it leaves us again confronted with the problem of how to penetrate beyond representations (nature as an "image") to things in themselves. Although members of the Jena Circle recognized that no definitive purchase could be gained on reality beyond any representation, they did hope and expect that alternative modes of representation would yield different insights on that ultimate reality. In calling for a multiplicity of representations, they particularly wanted to deny the privileged position of philosophy in dealing with these questions. For too long, they believed, philosophy had been blind to the representational quality of its own discourse, treating language as if it were a transparent window onto ideas. "Philosophy still proceeds too much in a straight line;" proclaimed one of the fragments in the journal *Athenaeum,* the house organ of the Jena group, "it is not yet cyclical enough."[65] Philosophy, in other words, needed to turn back on itself by expanding its own critical base. It needed to make the ironical gesture of seeing a representation of itself in the objects it handles.

The literary forms most favored by the Romantics were those that emphasized irony, allusion, metaphor, and other tropes manifesting the indirect path between language and object. Poetry obviously had a central role to play here, owing to the metaphorical imagery of verse as well as the fact that poetry only presents its

---

62 Friedrich Wilhelm Joseph Schelling, "Ideen zu einer Philosophie der Natur," in *Sämmtliche Werke,* Bd. 2, pp. 63–4.

63 Ibid., p. 66.

64 Ibid., p. 68.

65 *Athenaeum* 1 (1798): 189.

object evocatively, without attempting to exhaust the object in description. The importance of poetry for the Romantics points to another aspect of representations that is useful for our purposes, and that is the *aesthetic* role of representations such as poetic imagery in mediating between subject and object. Sensory representations provide material to the imagination, which freely combines and recombines them, and even has the power to think beyond the given manifold of sensory representation.[66] "Poetry, which only implies the infinite," wrote Friedrich Schlegel, "does not yield determinate concepts but only intuitions. The infinite is an endless abundance, a chaos of ideas which poetry strives to represent and bring together in a beautiful whole."[67]

The relationship between *Naturphilosophie* and the literary theory of early Jena Romanticism is not a completely straightforward one. Although an adequate exploration of their relationship must be deferred for another opportunity, it might be remarked here that the complexity of their connection stems from, and can be illustrated by, the ambivalence of Schelling's own position. Schelling was a member of the Jena group, yet it appears that he never fit in comfortably. The reasons were in part personal, but they were also intellectual: Schelling was, after all, a philosopher, and he sought to establish himself on the terrain of academic philosophy. He might push the boundaries of that discipline in new directions and appropriate the literary theory of the Jena group, but his project, like Fichte's, remained the completion of the critical philosophy. The same is true for the scholars who took up Schelling's *Naturphilosophie*. Their approach was deeply informed by the literary theory of Jena Romanticism, but the theory was put to work in developing a hermeneutics of nature.[68]

Thus much of *Naturphilosophie,* though by no means all of it, can be understood as an attempt to treat empirical phenomena as representations of the Absolute in nature. As a practical matter, many writers routinely displayed natural phenomena as a series of analogous relationships indicative of the deep structure of the Absolute. The journalist and physician Joseph Görres (1776–1848), for example, attempted to explain the relationship between the body's several organ systems by making an extended play on the opposition between interiority and exteriority. He began with the circulatory and digestive vessels. The muscular arteries, he claimed, are dense structures: they turn in on themselves, presenting the smallest possible surface to the workings of external nature. However, arteries also contain numerous nerves in their interior, so in closing themselves to the outside they open themselves all the more to influences from inside the organism. Görres then pointed out how the veins and lymphatic vessels present a contrastingly large external surface, and are correspondingly unreceptive to the interior influences of

---

66 That is what happens when the imagination confronts the sublime, a confrontation that provides a glimpse of what lies beyond representation. Kant had already broached this function of the sublime in the *Kritik der Urtheilskraft.* See *Kants Gesammelte Schriften,* Bd. 5 (Berlin, 1908), pp. 254–5.
67 Quoted in Seyhahn, *Representation and its Discontents,* p. 33.
68 See Bowie's comments on the hermeneutical aspect of Schelling's philosophy in Bowie, *Schelling and Modern European Philosophy,* pp. 30–44.

nerves. This same structural opposition between interiority and exteriority was then reiterated for the organs of movement and the sensory organs. Görres summarized these relationships as follows: "In the relationship of the arteries to the lymphatic vessels, and of the organs of movement to the sensory organs, of the organism's external hemisphere to its internal, and of both to the organism's sun, the brain, lies the play (*Spiel*) of life."[69]

It merits emphasizing here that analogy was used by Görres not in a heuristic manner, as a working guide for further investigation. Rather he appeared to use his analogies to point the reader toward more fundamental truths. Those analogies work, they *relate* something about the world because the concepts of interiority and exteriority allow the reader's imagination to apprehend the Absolute – even if only fragmentarily and imperfectly – as represented in those same analogies. Other writers of *Naturphilosophie,* such as Lorenz Oken (1779–1851), would develop entire systems of nature out of an elaborate language of analogy and metaphor.[70]

In two ways, therefore, the *Naturphilosophen* took a position that distinguished them from Kant's critical philosophy. First, they attributed to the subject an active role in the creation of knowledge. For them, it was not merely that knowledge ineluctably had a subjective component, as had been true for Kant. Rather the *Naturphilosophen* pointed to the subject's active cognitive and aesthetic apprehension of the world as essential to the creation of knowledge. In effect, the mind and the world produce each other continually. As Schelling put it, "The system of nature is at the same time the system of our mind."[71] Second, and even more characteristically, the *Naturphilosophen* denied that language could act as a transparent window onto its objects. In place of what they believed was the discredited language of philosophy and other academic *Wissenschaften,* the *Naturphilosophen* substituted a language of allusion and metaphor, a language they believed more authentically replicated the nature of our knowledge and the creative work we do in obtaining it.

PHYSICIANS IN THE AVANT-GARDE

If the intellectual program of *Naturphilosophie* embodied such an emphatic rejection of traditional academic discourse and the kinds of natural philosophy it had fostered, why should it have proven so attractive for physicians, who after all

---

69 Joseph Görres, "Prinzipien einer neuen Begründung der Gesetze des Lebens durch Dualism und Polarität," *Allgemeine medicinische Annalen* (1802), cols. 241–79, 561–81, quoted in col. 247.

70 For an interesting interpretation of Oken and *Naturphilosophie* that differs from the one offered here, see Nicholas Jardine, "The Significance of Schelling's 'Epoch of a Wholly New Natural History': An Essay on the Realization of Questions," in *Metaphysics and Philosophy of Science in the Seventeenth and Eighteenth Centuries: Essays in Honour of Gerd Buchdal,* ed. R. S. Woolhouse (Dordrecht, 1988), pp. 327–50. Jardine's discussion is both insightful and important, but its invocation of a "disciplinary context" for natural history at the end of the eighteenth century (see p. 340ff.) raises the question of just how such a disciplinary context was constituted at the time.

71 Schelling, "Ideen," p. 39.

derived their professional identity from their link to the universities? Posing the question this way already hints at a partial answer: that the profession itself had begun to fragment in ways that made the universities and the scholarship they produce an object of contention. As we saw in the previous chapter, even before the appearance of *Naturphilosophie* physicians had become uncomfortable with the utilitarian conception of knowledge that underpinned much of the eighteenth-century reform movement in areas such as medicine and public health. The ideology of *Bildung* was embraced by physicians as a way of replacing mere learnedness with university-sponsored spiritual cultivation as a mark of social distinction.

The emphatic anti-utilitarianism so characteristic of the *Bildungsideologie* was echoed from lecture hall to lecture hall. Friedrich Schiller (1759–1805) played on the common theme of the scholar's freedom from external coercion in his inaugural lecture as professor of history at Jena in 1789. He did this by contrasting a true scholar to the despicable "Bread-Scholar" (*Brodgelehrter*), who designs his education solely around what will suit him for an office of some kind, and who "dedicates all his diligence to the demands that come from the future lord of his destiny."[72] Fichte and Schelling would similarly echo these themes, Fichte in his *Über die Bestimmung des Gelehrten* (On the vocation of the scholar, 1794) and Schelling in *Vorlesungen über die Methode des academischen Studiums* (Lectures on the method of academic study, 1803).[73]

Thus *Naturphilosophie* took shape in a cultural environment grown familiar with the idea of education and knowledge as ultimate ends in themselves, and we should not overlook that the writings of the medical *Naturphilosophen* manifested a desire to cultivate medical theory (and display themselves as cultivated medical theorizers) in a realm liberated from the shackles of practical exigency. But as important as that was, it does not quite exhaust the phenomenon. There was something so aggressive and defiantly outrageous in the doctrines of *Naturphilosophie* that something else is needed to explain its undeniable edge. That edge came from the association of *Naturphilosophie* with the great agitation that swirled around the Jena Romantics, a group that Philippe Lacoue-Labarthe and Jean-Luc Nancy have labeled the first avant-garde in history.[74] Calling the Jena group an avant-garde was a doubly felicitous insight, because it captured both the necessarily prior existence of the public sphere and the Jena group's self-conscious and deliberately provocative distancing of itself from mere bourgeois culture as constituted in and by that public sphere. What is interesting too about avant-garde

72 Friedrich Schiller, *Was heißt und zu welchem Ende studiert man Universalgeschichte?* 2nd repr. ed. of 1789 (Jena, 1984), p. 3.

73 Schiller, Fichte, and Schelling were but three among many scholars who flattered themselves in this way, and we will return to this aspect of the *Bildungsideologie* in Chapter 6. For a nice overview of the scholar's self-appointed role in Romantic culture, see Theodore Ziolkowski, *German Romanticism and its Institutions* (Princeton, 1990), pp. 237–52.

74 Philippe Lacoue-Labarthe and Jean-Luc Nancy, *The Literary Absolute*, trans. Philip Barnard and Cheryl Lester (Albany, N.Y., 1988) p. 8.

movements is that they don't *really* seek to liberate themselves from the public, because that would be self-defeating. Thus when the Jena Romantics wanted to proclaim their independence from the general taste in things, they did so by starting the *Athenäum,* a periodical. Their declaration of independence from the "public" simultaneously disclosed their profound attachment to it. Through their own writings and reviews, and through reviews of their work in other journals, the members of the Jena group became public figures.

Schelling himself became a figure of considerable notoriety. He began his career as a lecturer at Jena while only twenty-two years old, and immediately created a sensation. Henrich Steffens (1773–1845), a Danish mineralogist, traveled to Jena to hear Schelling lecture in 1798, and, as he recalled in his autobiography, was not disappointed:

Schelling stepped up to the podium. He had a youthful appearance . . . and he had in his manner something determined, even defiant. . . . [His] forehead was high, his face was energetically composed, his nose projected somewhat forward, and in his large, clear eyes lay a spiritually commanding power. . . . He spoke on the idea of a *Naturphilosophie,* on the necessity of grasping Nature in its unity, and on the light that would be thrown over all objects if one dared to consider [Nature] from the standpoint of unity of reason. He swept me away completely. . . .[75]

The very same day, Steffens hurried over to Schelling's home to make his acquaintance.

The conversation was indescribably rich. I knew his writings, and I shared his viewpoints, if not all of them, and I anticipated from his undertaking, as he did himself, a great transformation, and not only in natural science. I could not prolong the visit, as the young professor was occupied with his lectures. But the few moments were so rich that they extended in my memory to hours.[76]

Much has been made about the role of personal contact with Schelling in prompting others to take up his ideas.[77] But if personal charisma is a significant factor in the social dynamics of *Naturphilosophie,* surely Schelling's public notoriety was one as well. Steffens chose to travel to Jena because of Schelling's reputation as a writer. Schelling's notoriety also gave Steffens his own entry into the public sphere. One of Steffens' earliest literary efforts was a review of Schelling's writings that ran in the *Zeitschrift für spekulative Physik,* a journal that Schelling himself edited.[78] Nor was it an accident that Steffens' review contributed to a literary feud that was then blazing between Schelling and the *Allgemeine Literatur-Zeitung* in

---

75 Henrich Steffens, *Was ich erlebte,* Bd. 4 (Breslau, 1841), pp. 75–6.

76 Ibid., p. 77.

77 Hirschfeld, "Romantische Medizin," pp. 43–5; Karl E. Rothschuh, "Ansteckende Ideen in der Wissenschaftsgeschichte, gezeigt an der Entstehung und Ausbreitung der romantischen Physiologie," in idem, *Physiologie in Werden* (Stuttgart, 1969), pp. 45–58.

78 Henrich Steffens, "Recension der neuern naturphilosophischen Schriften des Herausgebers," *Zeitschrift für spekulative Physik* 1, no. 1 (1800): 1–48; 1, no. 2 (1800): 88–121.

Jena. By hitching his wagon to Schelling's, Steffens could take a stand, acquire a presence, and become a public figure.

As Steffens' example suggests, publicity itself became a crucial rite of passage for the young men who reached adulthood in the 1790s. Almost half a century ago, Henri Brunschwig presented a collective portrait of this generation, a portrait as acute as it was unsympathetic. None of them, he wrote,

> have any very definite notion of the sort of occupation likely to suit them; official, soldier, merchant, it is all one to them; they will do anything to satisfy their hunger for fame; the sole exception is that they will have nothing whatever to do with the occupation to which they seemed destined from birth. Wackenroder has a horror of law and legal procedure, Schleiermacher will not hear of trade, Kleist resigns from the army.[79]

In short, these were men who felt themselves alienated from the mundane world of affairs.[80] They were educated in universities as their fathers had been, yet they aspired not to settle down into professional life but to leave their mark on the world. It is entirely characteristic that Steffens and and members of the Jena Romantics such as Caroline Schlegel and Ludwig Tieck admired Napoleon as a titan of world history.[81]

Like many others who have also taken up this theme, Brunschwig used what he called a "crisis of the young" to describe the origins of what he believed was the pathologically apolitical condition of the German educated middle classes. Writing as he did in 1947, in the immediate aftermath of World War II, Brunschwig's concerns are understandable. Yet we need not share his motivations, nor even his diagnosis that the German middle class *was* pathological, to agree with him nonetheless that the avant-garde of Romanticism expressed the self-consciousness of a generation that sought to carve out a new niche for itself in deliberate rejection of existing knowledge. The same applies to *Naturphilosophie* as a criticism of prevalent scientific knowledge. For the crowd of physicians who took it up, *Naturphilosophie* was not a subject of strictly medical concern, although as Schelling himself recognized, physicians were in a position to make major contributions to the project by virtue of their education in matters concerning organic nature.[82] It was by contrast precisely the comparative absence of narrowly professional concerns in *Naturphilosophie* that made it a subject of public discourse. *Naturphilosophen* wrote a good deal about health and illness as part of their more general treatments of nature. Those writings, however, consisted more routinely of examinations of the meaning of life, disease, and death than of specific medical

---

79 Henri Brunschwig, *Enlightenment and Romanticism in Eighteenth-Century Prussia*, trans. Frank Jellinek (Chicago, 1974), pp. 138–63, quoted on p. 147.

80 This sense of alienation was reinforced by the perceived surplus of educated men vying for positions in medicine and other professions. See the discussion in Chapter 2, "Responses to utilitarian reform."

81 Brunschwig, *The Prussian Enlightenment*, pp. 174–8.

82 "Medical science is the crown and glory (*die Krone und Blüthe*) of all natural sciences," Schelling wrote in 1805, "as is the organism in general – and the human organism in particular – the crown and glory of the world." *Jahrbücher der Medicin als Wissenschaft* I (1805): vi.

guides to diagnosis and therapy.[83] This is not to say that every piece of writing about *Naturphilosophie* was intended for consumption in the public sphere, nor that every individual who took up these problems wanted to create himself as a public figure. But certainly there was enough of the trendy and avant-garde in *Naturphilosophie* to entice physicians to write about natural philosophy in ways that did not depend on any strictly professional context.

CONCLUSION

At the opening of the eighteenth century, the theoretical portions of the medical curriculum, namely physiology and pathology, provided a foundation in natural philosophy on which could then be built the topics in medical practice such as semiotics, therapeutics, and hygiene. As has been repeatedly emphasized, their function was not so much to regulate the physician's therapeutic efforts as it was to provide a framework for interpreting the phenomena of health and illness. To be sure, physiology did not exist only to fill its propaedeutic function in medical education. Scholars in 1700 were no less interested in formulating general theories of organic nature than they would be in 1800. But one can, I think, reasonably claim that physiology was more closely bound to the rest of medical knowledge at the opening of the century than would be the case at the end of the century.

As this chapter has argued, two developments contributed to this situation. First, the adoption of the mechanical philosophy by physicians early in the century ruptured whatever links had existed between theory and practice in the former Galenic-Aristotelian medical system. Whereas medical theory adapted to the new trends in natural philosophy, medical practice (or more precisely, the theory of medical practice) retained much of the same conceptual toolkit it had used for centuries. Furthermore, the entire complex of questions concerning the existence and characteristics of vital forces – questions raised by the spread of Newtonian natural philosophy – presented physicians with a set of problems for empirical research and scholarly writing. Although it allowed physicians to engage fundamental questions in natural philosophy, this research program moved physiology in directions that loosened its ties to the rest of medicine. Such was the state of affairs that a Reil could appear in 1795, calling for the reconstruction of physiology to bring it back to its position as the foundation of a unified medical science. In a far more radical way, the Brunonians would issue the same call to action, as we will see later on.

But if there was a certain dynamic within medical writing that moved physiology into its own domain, important changes in elite literary culture played a part as well. The creation of the public sphere was distinguished not only by the emergence of a new discourse – the discourse of literary and cultural criticism –

83 A good survey of the medical systems developed by some of the more prominent *Naturphilosophen* is presented in Hans-Uwe Lammel, *Nosologische und therapeutische Konzeptionen in der romantischen Medizin* (Husum, 1990).

but also by the creation of a new persona, the writer, *and* by the appearance of a new medium of communication, the periodical. Together they presented opportunities for physicians to remake themselves as writers and editors, and thereby to claim command over the powerful currents of public opinion. Then again, the public sphere engendered its own dialectical offspring, an avant-garde of young intellectuals who made use of the public sphere while parading their disdain for the common taste in things. Led by Schelling, a coterie of physicians and others eagerly attached themselves to the avant-garde by constructing a theory of nature that strove to break through a science based on mere appearance to grasp an ultimate reality lying tantalizingly beyond the sensible. To the extent that physicians participated in such a program, they too were taken away from more narrowly professional concerns.

Thus by 1800 "medical theory" had become "theories," a welter of systems and proposals for systems and interpretations of nature published by physician-writers seeking to make a name for themselves. The proliferation of such writings suggests that the aspirations held by young scholars for their careers had changed to a considerable degree from the opening or even the middle of the eighteenth century. Some two decades ago, Steven Turner pointed out that whereas in the middle of the eighteenth century a scholar's most important frames of reference were collegial and local, by the middle of the nineteenth century they had come to center on non-localized disciplinary associations.[84] As the preceding chapters have argued, making a career in the mid-eighteenth century certainly depended on being received favorably into one's immediate surroundings, whether a young man aspired to a seat on a university medical faculty or a position as town *Physicus*. And, as we shall see in Chapter 6, by the second decade of the nineteenth century disciplinary identity among various medical specialties had certainly become far stronger than had been the case in the previous century.

With respect to this transformation, what is intriguing about *Naturphilosophie* in this respect is the possibility that it played some kind of mediating role between these conditions. By coming before the public sphere as writers, *Naturphilosophen* learned to perform for audiences beyond their immediate locality. The standards by which they were judged were not those of their neighbors and local patrons, but those formulated in the bright glare of delocalized public criticism. On the other hand, it was from this same public sphere and its implicit appeal to a "Reason" accessible to all that territories of disciplinary and professional specialization would soon begin to be carved out.

---

84 R. Steven Turner, "University Reformers and Professional Scholarship in Germany, 1760-1806," in *The University and Society*, ed. Lawrence Stone, vol. 2 (Princeton, N.J., 1974), pp. 495–531.

4

The art of healing

If *Naturphilosophie* promised to transform medicine into a true *Wissenschaft*, it was a decidedly odd brand of medical science that would emerge from the metamorphosis. For *Naturphilosophie* treated medicine in a way that was virtually oblivious to the practical concerns and social milieu that physicians confronted in their everyday working lives. That was part of its attraction: its siren call was the unity of knowledge through a transcendental poetics of life, with Schelling and his followers playing the role of bards who would sing its truths. But to physicians who did not seek to pursue a larger vision of *Wissenschaft*, and who identified more with medicine as healing than with the avant-garde of Jena Romanticism, the pretensions of the *Naturphilosophen* were not merely by degrees silly or outrageous, they were also fundamentally inimical to the true nature of medicine and medical science. Partly in response to the *Naturphilosophen*, but partly too as their own contribution to shaping public consciousness about the profession, these physicians gave voice to a different version of medicine, one emphasizing its healing mission.

This chapter will explore that alternative vision for medicine, as seen through the writings of physicians who in no way sympathized or identified with the aims of the *Naturphilosophen*. The picture that emerges from these sources consists of three intimately connected elements: first, a justification of the dignity and social worth of the profession; second, an epistemology of medical practice; and finally, a program of medical education. That ideology, epistemology, and education should form the core of this vision should hardly be surprising, since we have seen in previous chapters how by the end of the century physicians were at pains to defend both the social utility of their profession and its status as a learned discipline. By way of preliminary orientation, let us make a brief survey of each element.

The first element, ideology, presented medicine as a profession of service to one's fellows and of sacrifice for the betterment of humanity. As such it was an occupation that one took up in response to a vocation, a term resonant with echoes of a divine calling to the ministry, as portrayed in Lutheran theology. Given this understanding, physicians commonly linked medicine with the ministry, arguing from the one side that physicians like clergymen should work for the physical and moral perfection of their neighbors. Underscoring the links from the other side as well, physicians urged that clergymen in rural areas be given basic medical training that would allow them to provide qualified care in areas underserved by regular practitioners.

Although some physicians described the medical vocation as a divine calling, most writers described it in a more secularized language. The call came not from God, but from Reason, and it urged them to become evangelists not of Christianity, but instead of Enlightenment, Reason's religion. Here too, physicians shared something with clergymen, for in both Protestant and Catholic Germany the Church was largely responsible for education, especially at the primary level. As teachers, both physicians and ministers held the responsibility of directing their audiences toward proper moral and physical conduct. However, physicians lacked an institutional base comparable to the Church's for conducting its "catechism of health," so they did it by means of the press. Through periodicals and through monographs, in almanacs and in a host of other publications directed at the public, physicians attempted to teach their readers the rules for proper living. In effect they appropriated a tradition of medical writings on dietetics and hygiene that stretched back to Hippocrates and shaped it anew for the reading public of their own day.

The second element of this picture was epistemological, and consisted of a theory of medical practice. In opposition to the then-current proliferation of medical theories and "systems" of practice, a number of writers argued that the rules of medical practice could never be derived in any straightforward way from first principles in the manner of a deductive science. Their writings on practice underscored the complexity of medical knowledge and the careful accumulation of experience as the only trustworthy basis of medicine. They used terms such as "talent" and "genius" to describe the practitioner's abilities, and they likened the doctor's therapeutic ministrations to an art, not merely in order to designate therapy as belonging to human artifice but still more to invoke the artistic creativity and intuitive understanding that successful medical practice demanded. In their presentation of the subject, practice aimed not at formulating universals in the manner of other sciences, but at comprehending particulars: the patient and his or her physical condition, individual cases of illness, and hygienic prescriptions for health all displayed this particularizing thrust. In distinct contrast to the emerging clinical sensibility in Paris and elsewhere in Europe, this form of medical knowledge claimed to place the individual patient as much as possible at the center of the doctor's attention.[1]

1 Oft criticized but still unsurpassed is Erwin H. Ackerknecht, *Medicine at the Paris Hospital* (Baltimore, 1967). Significant corrections to Ackerknecht's thesis were presented by Toby Gelfand, *Professionalizing Modern Medicine* (Westport, Conn., 1980); and by Othmar Keel, "The Politics of Health and the Institutionalisation of Clinical Practices in Europe in the Second Half of the Eighteenth Century," in *William Hunter and the Eighteenth Century Medical World*, ed. W. F. Bynum and Roy Porter, (Cambridge, 1985), pp. 207–56. Keel argued that what Ackerknecht and others believed were the

Medical education comprised the third element of this picture. The structure and content of education was a matter of supreme moment for many writers, because a young man's socialization into the profession and the shaping of his attitudes toward it took place through that education. Thus the design of university curricula for medical education became a key arena of contest between alternative visions of medicine. The issue that most concerned the writers discussed in this chapter was the structure of the student's clinical training. As far as possible, they believed, the clinic should introduce the student both to his social role as healer and to the epistemology of medical practice informing that role. To many, though by no means all, writers this meant that the ideal clinic was the dispensary or polyclinic, and not the hospital. In the polyclinic, the student would come to know patients in their real-life circumstances and learn to appreciate how disease and therapy are embedded in a dense web of social and environmental influences. In contrast to the highly unnatural setting of the hospital, where patients were seen only in isolation from the rest of their lives, the polyclinic would teach the student how to deal with patients as he would encounter them in his practice – as surrounded by family, occupation, and his larger social and physical environments.

THE VOCATION OF THE DOCTOR

If anyone exemplifies the ideology of medicine as a vocation to professional service, that person is surely Christoph Wilhelm Hufeland (1762–1836). Professor in Jena and later personal physician to the Prussian royal family and professor in Berlin, founder and editor for some forty years of the extremely successful *Journal der practischen Heilkunde,* Hufeland was an extraordinarily influential spokesman for the dignity of the medical profession. Unlike Johann Christian Reil, his contemporary and rival, who grew up the son of a minister in a remote provincial town, Hufeland was born into an elite medical family. Both his father and his grandfather were personal physicians to the ducal house of Saxe-Weimar. Thus Hufeland's experience with medicine from his earliest days centered on its practice in society: giving comfort to the suffering and bereaved, removing pain, and dedicating one's life to the well-being of others. To these little tokens of professional virtue, Hufeland's family of course could add the social status it derived from its connection to the ducal family, and its location in a town that with Goethe, Wieland, and Herder in residence boasted of a cultural vitality that few locales could match. Hufeland's family lived a life that many physicians must have only dreamed of, with the honor – not to mention the more material pleasures – of being kept on retainer by the local notables, and enjoying the company of people who accorded them the respect owing them as *Gelehrter.* In contrast to Reil, then, for whom

unique clinical perspective and facilities of the Paris hospitals were in fact also present in London, Vienna, and elsewhere at the end of the eighteenth century. But Keel did not challenge Acker-knecht's idea that the dominant (and ultimately progressive) clinical concept was a hospital-based one.

medicine was a ticket to the university and social advancement, for Hufeland medicine manifested itself in the dignity of medical practice.

Hufeland's image of medicine featured personal sacrifice and response to duty, themes which figured prominently in his posthumously published autobiography. As a youth he was handed over to a severe tutor whose grim brand of Lutheran orthodoxy emptied the young boy of whatever blitheness of spirit he might have once had, smothering it with a sense of self-abnegation and duty that became the guideposts for his life. Years later Hufeland would recall his tutor's influence as the decisive one in his life, and he justified a boyhood virtually devoid of social companionship as awakening him to the virtues of contemplation and "scholarly pursuits."[2] In 1780, Hufeland began his medical studies at the University of Jena, which lay within Saxe-Weimar, and, finding the tenor of student life at Jena a shade too riotous, transferred to the University of Göttingen, where he received his degree in the summer of 1783. But at a point when well-to-do graduates typically treated themselves to a grand tour, duty again imposed itself in the form of his father's growing blindness, which forced Hufeland to return to Weimar and begin sharing the burdens of practice. "The years when other youths travel or still enjoy life," he recalled wistfully and self-righteously in his autobiography, "passed for me in work, sorrow, and exertion that often could hardly be overcome."[3]

Hufeland's initial ventures in practice were bitterly disappointing. Shortly after arriving home in Weimar, he was called in his father's place to care for the duke's infant daughter, who promptly died. Some time later, when the duke's mother fell ill, Hufeland was called in at first, but the duke then summoned one of the most prominent professors from Jena to take over the case, and under whose care she recovered. Hufeland's failure in these two cases prevented him from being appointed to his father's position of *Leibarzt* (personal physician). Instead, he remained at the less prestigious and lucrative position of *Hofmedicus* (court physician). So painful was the memory of this incident fifty years later that Hufeland reported in his autobiography how his father's hopes for his future had been ruined. "The sorrow over these dashed hopes," he added, "undoubtedly contributed greatly to my father's early death."[4] Be that as it may, the elder Hufeland lingered for another four years, his blindness growing complete, until finally in 1787 Hufeland found himself alone, with the sole responsibility of providing for his two unmarried sisters. During the next six years, he toiled away at his practice, slowly establishing himself in Weimar. He gave every appearance of being well along the road toward becoming a respected private practitioner whose literary reputation would at best be a modest one.[5] However, Hufeland's career took an unexpected turn in 1793, when a paper he read before a local gathering caught

2 Christoph Wilhelm Hufeland, *Hufeland Leibarzt und Volkserzieher. Selbstbiographie von Christoph Wilhelm Hufeland*, ed. Walter von Brunn (Stuttgart, 1937), p. 33.
3 Ibid., p. 59.
4 Ibid., p. 76.
5 In 1789, Hufeland published *Bemerkungen über die natürlichen und künstlichen Blattern zu Weimar, 1788* (Leipzig, 1789), a small monograph describing his experiences with smallpox inoculation.

the favorable attention of Duke Karl August of Saxe-Weimar, who ordered that Hufeland be appointed to the medical faculty of the University of Jena.

Acceptance of duty also colored the experiences of Ernst Ludwig Heim (1747–1834), who like Hufeland became a prominent figure in the Prussian medical establishment. In Heim's case, however, the acceptance of vocation came with a more redemptive twist. Heim was born into the household of a Lutheran pastor, a severe man who saw to his children's education himself. In contravention of his given name, young Ernst appears to have been a rather carefree lad, much to his father's disappointment, who thought his son too flighty and lacking in the *gravitas* necessary for the clergy. Medicine seemed a more appropriate profession for someone like Ernst. "You are most suited to becoming a charlatan," his father is reported to have said, "You can put anything you want over on people (*du kannst den Leuten Alles weismachen, was du willst*)."[6] At Halle, where he was a student, Heim was diligent enough, but he also fell in among a crowd whose style of living was too extravagant for a clergyman's son, and he began running up debts. Moreover, on one occasion Heim was caught with a packet of tobacco in his possession, which was apparently against the rules, for the academic court sentenced him to a fine of 20–30 *Reichsthaler* or a spell in the student jail. Heim, mortified by the turn of events, appealed to his brother for money, who suggested that incarceration for a week or two would do him no permanent harm.[7] But eventually his family came through with enough money to allow Heim to scrape by, and that incident, coupled with the appearance of a virtuous new friend, seems to have set Heim's life on a new course. For soon we read of him devoting his spare time to giving free medical care to poor people in outlying villages and running up debts again, this time for medicaments given free of charge to his needier patients.[8]

It should be noted that not every physician's life was portrayed as a response to a vocation. Another common story described a medical career as growing from a youthful interest in science.[9] Yet when discussion turned to the practice of medicine, the themes of dedication, sacrifice, and service to one's patients usually came to the fore.[10] Such values brought medicine into proximity with the clergy, which may be surprising, because we are habituated to thinking of the eighteenth-century clergy as suffering from widespread disdain. Spirited attacks mounted on

6 Georg Wilhelm Kessler (ed.), *Der alte Heim. Leben und Wirken Ernst Ludwig Heims* 2nd ed. (Leipzig, 1846), p. 13. Whether Heim's father actually uttered such encouragements is beside the point. What is more important is the way this episode sets up Heim's subsequent achievements as a story of meeting (and exceeding) fatherly expectations.

7 Ibid., pp. 22–5.

8 Ibid., p. 76.

9 See, for example, Johann Peter Frank, *Seine Selbstbiographie*, ed. Erna Lesky, Hubers Klassiker der Medizin und Naturwissenschaften, Bd. 12 (Bern, 1969).

10 See Wilhelm Gottfried Ploucquet, *Der Arzt, oder über die Ausbildung, die Studien, Pflichten, Sitten, und die Klugheit des Arztes* (Tübingen, 1797), pp. 3–8. Among many other examples in this vein see also Christian Gottfried Gruner, *Gedanken von der Arzneiwissenschaft und den Aerzten* (Breslau, 1772), pp. 5–14.

religious superstition and clerical abuses by Voltaire, d'Holbach, Hume, Gibbon, and a score of others have persuaded us that the clergy was everywhere in decline. But it was not so. For in spite of the abuse heaped upon religion and Christian churches both Protestant and Catholic, the fact remains that clerical careers – like medical careers – remained one of the few paths available for social advancement, especially in Germany, where the commercial middle class remained small. As bourgeois occupations enjoying a measure of social prestige, medicine and the clergy were far more closely joined to each other than to the more aristocratically inclined profession of law.

Such links were often made quite explicitly. In one of his early writings the Jena professor Christian Gottfried Gruner called the doctor a "priest of nature," and compared the physician's attempt to alleviate suffering to those of a "compassionate divinity" *(mithleidigen Gottheit)*.[11] Hufeland believed the practitioner's life to be a religious vocation, to which only the blessed few are called. "Only a pure, moral person can be a doctor in the true sense of the word," he wrote near the end of his life, "for only he feels a higher purpose to his existence in his breast, which elevates him above life itself, and over all joy and hardship."[12] Curing physical ailments comprised but one portion of the physician's total mission. Even in the absence of any specific illness, Hufeland believed the physician was called upon to improve the lives of his patients. He wrote on one occasion:

The true purpose of medicine is the physical perfection of man and preservation and restoration of health in the individual as well as in the entirety of mankind. Medicine is therefore one of the most sublime, wide-ranging, and humane *Wissenschaften,* just as eternally inseparable from humanity as is moral teaching *(die Moral),* to which medicine directly connects. The latter has the moral, and the former has the physical perfection of humankind as its final goal. Both work toward a single goal.[13]

Another writer argued that in filling the basic human needs for comfort and happiness, the physician must attend both to a patient's physical situation and to his or her moral and psychological situation.[14]

On the other side of the equation, physicians and public health planners acknowledged that clergymen often dabbled in various kinds of medical practice. Samuel-Auguste Tissot (1728–97), perhaps the eighteenth century's leading writer on popular medicine, wrote one of his most famous works, *Avis au peuple sur sa santé* (1761), with the recognition that rural clergy would comprise a significant portion of his readership. Prompted perhaps by Tissot's work, plans were discussed

11 Gruner, *Gedanken,* p. 5.
12 Christoph Wilhelm Hufeland, *Enchiridion Medicum, oder Anleitung zur medizinischen Praxis* (Berlin, 1836), p. 709.
13 Christoph Wilhelm Hufeland, "Ein Wort über den Angriff der razionellen Medicin im N.T. Merkur. August 1795," *Der neue teutsche Merkur* 1, no. 9 (1795): 147–8.
14 C. E. Fischer, "Ueber die moralische Wirksamkeit des Arztes," *Journal der praktischen Heilkunde* 28 (1809): 56–107. See also the discussion of the importance of religious feelings for doctors in the *Allgemeine medicinische Annalen* (1810), cols. 557–64.

in various German states to transform rural clergy into part-time medical practitioners. Indeed, some critics of the Lutheran clergy urged that ministers be
trained as medical practitioners as a way of increasing the clergy's "utility." Johann
Peter Frank advocated something like this in his *Academische Rede über Priester-
Aerzte* (1803), although he did not tie it to any specific criticism of the clergy.
Hufeland too favored the idea, saying it would constitute a better use of the rural
ministry's abundant free time than its usual pursuits of farming or natural history.[15]

The alliance between physicians and the clergy certainly had its limits, and we
should not exaggerate its intimacy. Several things worked to put distance between
them. In the first place, when rural clergymen engaged in healing, they did
become a source of potential competition for physicians. Any enthusiasm felt by
physicians for extending medical care over the countryside had to be tempered
with concern for lost income. Moreover, in spite of their shared status as members
of a learned profession, it was not always advantageous for physicians to highlight
their association with the clergy. Especially as the eighteenth century drew to a
close, the medical profession came increasingly to rest its dignity on the progress
of scientific knowledge, a badge of honor the clergy could not share. One medical
writer bumped up against these limits when he suggested that physicians would
enjoy more respect if they were ceremoniously received into a town, in the
manner that clergymen are installed in their parishes. This prompted the sarcastic
observation from one reviewer that such an installation would accomplish little,
because the ministry stood in comparatively low repute.[16]

These frictions aside, a good deal of writing about medicine was of a tenor that
placed it in close proximity to the clergy as a profession of service and sacrifice.
Whether the calling to become a physician came as a vocation from God or from
the inner urgings of Reason ultimately made little difference. He who responded
to it could claim to be doing work of great significance, work that shouldered
responsibility for bettering the world in some small measure. Thus the idea of
medicine as a vocation meshed seamlessly with Enlightenment ideas of improvement and social uplift. Against what they considered the hubris of the *Naturphilosophen*, defenders of the medical vocation offered a seemingly more self-denying
vision of trial and devotion. And although it could not compete with *Naturphilosophie* for place of honor in the avant-garde, it was a vision with its own kind of
resonance in bourgeois German society.

---

15 Samuel Auguste Tissot, *Avis au peuple sur sa santé* 2nd ed. vol. 1 (Paris, 1763), pp. xliii–xliv.
   Christoph Wilhelm Hufeland, "Medizinische Praxis der Landgeistlichen," *Journal der practischen
   Heilkunde* 29, no. 5 (1809): 1–10. On plans to use the ministry for medical practice, see John
   Stroup, *The Struggle for Identity in the Clerical Estate* (Leiden, 1984), pp. 104–5; and Robert Heller,
   " 'Priest-Doctors' as a Rural Health Service in the Age of Enlightenment," *Medical History* 20
   (1976): 361–83.
16 The suggestion for a ceremonious installation was made in Johann Karl Ackermann, *Ueber das
   Medicinalwesen in Deutschland* (Zeitz, 1794), pp. 7–16. It was harshly criticized in the *Medicinish-
   chirurgische Zeitung*, 21 August 1794, pp. 258–64.

SPREADING THE GOSPEL OF ENLIGHTENMENT

If medicine was a kind of vocation and the doctor functioned, as Gruner put it, as a "priest of Nature," then the analogy with the clergy reached its completion in the evangelizing mission of spreading medical enlightenment. Probably the activity that most closely joined physicians and ministers was their role as teachers to their patients and congregations. In teaching, ministers and doctors had an opportunity to work creatively, not only acting defensively against sin and disease, but also positively, admonishing and instructing people toward their own moral and physical perfection. The centrality of this didactic activity should come as no surprise. The Hippocratic writers, after all, had made avoidance of illness through proper rules of living a cornerstone of their medical practice, and medical writers ever since had offered themselves as advisors on maintaining health.[17]

Although the aim (and even much of the content) of this literature was not particularly novel in the eighteenth century, the media in which it appeared were. It did not take long for physicians to recognize that periodicals, the numbers of which were growing rapidly in Germany throughout the century, were an ideal device for spreading medical enlightenment, and numerous journals were launched toward this end. The most famous such effort was Johann Georg Unzer's *Der Arzt, eine medicinische Wochenschrift*. Unzer's journal, which appeared from 1759–64 and in reprints thereafter, modeled itself on moral weeklies published earlier in the century, which in turn drew their inspiration from the *Tatler* and the *Spectator*, two successful English weeklies.[18] In other cases, physicians made use of the scholarly periodicals published in many university towns to present essays on medical matters.[19]

Popular medical essays appeared in the general periodical press as well. One of Hufeland's earliest efforts in this direction was an essay written in 1792 for the *Journal des Luxus und der Moden*, a women's fashion journal, on the proper rules for infant care. Hufeland praised recent advances in this area, which had restored the "rights of Nature and of childhood" to their proper place of respect. Raising

17 On the role of physicians as learned advisors, see Harold J. Cook, "Good Advice and Little Medicine: The Professional Authority of Early Modern English Physicians," *Journal of British Studies* 33 (1994): 1–31; and idem, "The New Philosophy and Medicine in Seventeenth-Century England," in *Reappraisals of the Scientific Revolution*, ed. David C. Lindberg and Robert S. Westman (Cambridge, 1990), pp. 397–436.

18 Wolfgang Martens, *Die Botschaft der Tugend* (Stuttgart, 1968). A comprehensive survey of medical periodicals for the public is in Erdmuth Dreißigacker, *Populärmedizinische Zeitschriften des 18. Jahrhunderts zur hygienischen Volksaufklärung* (med. Diss., Marburg, 1970). See also I. Barthel, *Über Diätetik und Gesundheitserziehung in den "Medicinischen und Chirurgischen Berlinischen wöchentlichen Nachrichten" von Samuel Schaarschmidt* (med. Diss., Berlin, 1969).

19 Wolfram Kaiser and Arina Völker have surveyed the writings on popular medicine in the *wöchentlichen Hallischen Anzeigen*, published in Halle during most of the century. See Wolfram Kaiser, "Die hallische Universitätszeitung im 18. Jahrhundert," in *Buch und Wissenschaft*, ed. Wolfram Kaiser (Halle, 1982), pp. 3–60; and Arina Völker, "Das populärwissenschaftliche Schrifttum von Johann Juncker," in *Johann Juncker (1679–1759) und seine Zeit (2)*, ed. Wolfram Kaiser and Hans Hübner (Halle, 1979), pp. 41–54.

children, he claimed, depended on not coddling them excessively, and instead on getting them used to a harder, more vigorous life. Hufeland saw three key elements in such an upbringing: daily washing in cold water, weekly bathing, and daily exposure of the children to fresh air.[20] The advantages of giving children this program were twofold. In the first place, the fibers (*Fasern*) of children's bodies, which often are somewhat flaccid, would be strengthened and become less sensitive to external stimuli. Hufeland cautioned that moderation was needed to insure that the fibers do not become too inflexible or totally unresponsive. Secondly, Hufeland played on his favorite theme by intertwining the physical and moral benefits to be expected from his program.

One can be assured that, by means of an upbringing according to these principles, not only the body but also the soul is developed, and that with these methods one can give even to the organs of the soul (*Seelenorganen*) an uncommonly fortuitous orientation, which will make later moral development indescribably easier. Indeed, in my opinion it is an essential part [of moral development].[21]

The immense periodical literature on maintaining health and fostering medical enlightenment was supplemented by a mountain of almanacs, manuals of health, and guides to home medical care. Many of these books were organized around giving readers advice on how to regulate the external influences on health that since antiquity had been known as the "six non-naturals": air, food and drink, motion and rest, excretion and retention, sleep and wakefulness, and emotions. Friedrich Hildebrandt (1764–1816), a professor at Erlangen, published in 1801 a *Taschenbuch für die Gesundheit* (Pocketbook for health) that patterned its treatment of topics on the non-naturals, containing chapters on the air, on dampness and dryness, on warmth and coldness, on food and drink, on excretions, on clothing, on positioning the body (for example in sitting and sleeping), on sleep, on movement and rest, and on the effects of the passions. The advice comprised the predictable amalgam of cultural prejudices and beliefs about nature to be found in all such literature, past or present. In his discussion of the air, for example, Hildebrandt reiterated the standard bias against the corrupting influence of urban life, pointing out that human and animal products make the air in cities much more unhealthy than in the countryside. This makes it mandatory, he continued, that anyone who resides in a city devote "several" hours or at least one hour each day to spending time in fresh air, away from the city's center.[22] Elsewhere, in a

---

20 Christoph Wilhelm Hufeland, "Erinnerung an einige sehr wesentliche, und dennoch sehr vernach-läßigte, Punkte der physischen Erziehung, in der ersten Periode der Kindheit," *Journal des Luxus und der Moden* 7 (1792): 274. In the matter of the proper upbringing of children, Hufeland once again was anticipated by Johann Peter Frank, who laid down practically the same precepts in his *System einer vollständigen medizinischen Polizey*. See Johann Peter Frank, *A Complete System of Medical Police*, ed. and trans. Erna Lesky (Baltimore, 1976), p. xvii. As Lesky points out, undoubtedly Frank was influenced by Rousseau's well-known pedagogical program.

21 Hufeland, "Erinnerung," p. 227.

22 Friedrich Hildebrandt, *Taschenbuch für die Gesundheit auf das Jahr 1801*, 2nd ed. (Erlangen, 1801) p. 29–31. Needless to say, only members of the upper social strata enjoyed the leisure for such prescriptions.

discussion of the effects of heat and cold on the body, Hildebrandt unfurled another favorite European prejudice, arguing that because temperate climates are the most favorable for human life, in such places "mankind achieves its greatest perfection."[23]

Not surprisingly, these books of dietetic advice also featured large portions of middle-class moralizing, because this is probably what made them so successful with readers. Hildebrandt urged his readers to keep to the "golden mean" in living their lives, conducting themselves neither too rigidly nor with excessive self-indulgence.[24] Such moralizing played an even more prominent role in Hufeland's treatise on the prolongation of human life, *Die Kunst das menschliche Leben zu verlängern* (The art of prolonging human life, 1797). The *Makrobiotik*, as the work came to be known in its many subsequent editions, argued that all life, including human life, is the product of a life force (*Lebenskraft*) that modifies and restricts the forces of non-living nature and gives organic beings their unique properties. The aim of prolonging life, consequently, involves maintaining the appropriate level of *Lebenskraft* in the body and preventing the inorganic, non-vital forces present in nature from gaining a dominant influence.

Although Hufeland paid considerable attention to the causes of long life and the means of promoting it, lengthening life was only the ostensible purpose for the *Makrobiotik*. Hufeland's aim was not merely to lengthen his readers' lives, but to enrich them as well. If mere prolongation of our existence was all that mattered in life, he reasoned, we could live longest by simply reducing our expenditure of *Lebenskraft* to the lowest possible level by doing practically nothing apart from minimal physical exercise. Hufeland passionately attacked schemes that were based on this attitude, urging his readers to remember that humanity is called to live an active life. A person "should not merely fill a gap in creation, he should be the lord and sovereign of creation."[25] At the other extreme, Hufeland also disapproved of the argument that a shorter life lived at twice the intensity was worth the same or more as a longer, normal life. He compared such approaches to attempts to ripen fruits in half the time with twice the normal supply of heat and nutrients. Fruit matured in such a manner may achieve an apparent ripeness, Hufeland claimed, but never attain the perfection and finishing they ought to have. Even if a man of thirty could accomplish twice what someone sixty has done, he nonetheless could not have acquired the maturity of the older man. Moreover, Hufeland added, that younger man may have been destined to continue doing useful things for much longer. But his excessive expenditure of *Lebenskraft* would shorten his life and frustrate that destiny.[26]

The notion of accepting mortal destiny lay heavily upon the *Makrobiotik*, as

---

23 Ibid., p. 54.
24 Ibid., p. 10–12.
25 Christoph Wilhelm Hufeland, *Die Kunst das menschliche Leben zu verlängern*, Teil 1, 2nd ed. (Jena, 1798), p. 167. Hereafter referred to in notes as *Makrobiotik*.
26 Ibid., p. 171.

Hufeland repeatedly stressed that in prolonging life attention had to be paid to the purposes and ends that constitute humanity's place in the world. Life could be extended only to its natural and divinely ordained limit, and attempts to lengthen it that opposed our natural destiny were bound to fail. In consonance with his orthodox view of sin as a willful falling away from the ideal of human life, the major emphasis of Hufeland's program was preventive. This was no trivial matter, for he saw a host of evils that could sap people of their moral and physical vigor. Especially dangerous in this regard was love, for excessive occupation with love and lovemaking has several deleterious effects on the body, the principal one being decrease in the supply of *Lebenskraft* itself. "What can decrease the sum of *Lebenskraft* in us more," he argued, "than the waste of that juice which contains [it] in the most concentrated form. . . ?"[27] Hildebrandt also dwelled on this topic in his *Taschenbuch,* pointing out that occasional enjoyment of lovemaking by a mature man would probably do little harm. But because the result of such activities is always a temporary decrease in energy and strength, too frequent an indulgence in it would be harmful. The most desirable form of love, he concluded, is that in which the moral is combined with the physical in the form of a loving, married couple.[28]

Giving people practical advice for living proper physical and moral lives meant guiding them to their rightful place in society as well. To this end, writers commonly added some social perspectives to their valuation of the standard moral and physical virtues. Hildebrandt, sounding a popular theme, held that the occupations of scholars and others who sat for long periods of time were unhealthy. This situation could be remedied if they could take time daily to engage in an activity requiring movement. It would help, he wrote, "if every scholar were at the same time a laborer or farmer," which would permit "the affairs of the scholar" to alternate with "manual labor." Hildebrandt also spoke admiringly of how thick and strong the muscles of a blacksmith were compared to those of a "charming gentleman" (*süssen Herrn*) at court.[29] Hufeland, meanwhile, complained repeatedly that the luxury and immoderateness of the better-off ranks of society removed them ever further from a life of harmony with nature, and would hurt them in the long run. Likewise Hufeland found exemplary the simple, hard working lives of laborers and peasants.[30]

Of course, we should not conclude from such statements that Hildebrandt was urging that scholars be compelled to work the fields or that Hufeland yearned to join the common folk at their labors. The tone of these and other such utterances was elegiac, sighing after a life of natural simplicity that was long (and probably thankfully) gone. Yet Hufeland's and Hildebrandt's readers shared the same sensi-

27 Ibid., Teil 2, p. 11. It should be noted in passing that advice in this section was obviously oriented exclusively toward men, although elsewhere in the medical advice literature (and in Hufeland's own writings) there was plenty of attention paid to women as well.
28 Hildebrandt, *Taschenbuch,* pp. 179–81.
29 Ibid., pp. 205–6.
30 Hufeland, *Makrobiotik,* Teil 2, p. 115.

bility, and could identify with pronouncements that would strike a modern reader as disingenuous, at the very least. Indeed these writings touched quite directly on readers' experiences and beliefs, and reflected that world back to them on every page. Their ability to do so was a measure of their success. Hufeland was a master at this, which is what made the *Makrobiotik* an enormously popular work, one reprinted throughout the nineteenth century and even into the twentieth.

The unmistakable message in such handbooks was of the simple *bürgerliche* virtues of reverence, discipline, simplicity, and avoidance of excesses. The lives that physicians advised their readers to lead were ones of humble acceptance of God's design for human beings in the world. Nature was not to be mastered, it was to be understood and obeyed. Just as important as anything the *Makrobiotik* and other works said about ideal human life, however, was what they said about the physician's role in society. In leading mankind to enlightenment and toward its perfection, the doctor must understand and become involved in the lives of his patients, a situation in which he is simultaneously observer, actor, and judge of a multitude of social relations.

THE ART OF HEALING

In the view of medicine described above, the patient occupied the center of the doctor's attentions. To a large measure this focus reflected the physician's social situation, in which the favor and patronage of influential patients were vital for a successful career.[31] It also reflected the image that physicians attempted to present to the public of themselves as advisors on all aspects of life, not mere healers of sickness. Accordingly, the patient appeared in their writings as an active agent, whose constitution and choices figured essentially in the elaborate rituals that constitute medical practice. Moreover, writers on medical practice did not envision doctors performing their roles along with some generalized and faceless "patient," who acted as an interchangeable foil for the physician's actions. Rather, they treated the patient as a concrete individual, molded by diverse social and general environmental influences, but also possessing something that makes his or her experience of those influences unique. In this situation, they believed the physician must understand and respect the individual as well as that person's position in the surrounding world. This consideration made a significant contribution to how they understood the causes, diagnosis and treatment of disease.

If there was one thing that united writers who upheld the dignity of medical practice, it was their opposition to systems. We need only recall August Friedrich Hecker's denunciation of the "mania for system" (*Systemsucht*) alluded to in the

---

31 For discussions of the role of patronage in medicine, see N. D. Jewson, "Medical Knowledge and the Patronage System in Eighteenth Century England," *Sociology* 8 (1974): 369–85; Ivan Waddington, "The Role of the Hospital in the Development of Modern Medicine: A Sociological Analysis," *Sociology* 7 (1973): 211–24; and Harold J. Cook, "Living in Revolutionary Times: Medical Change under William and Mary," in *Patronage and Institutions: Science, Technology, and Medicine at the European Court 1500-1750*, ed. Bruce T. Moran (Rochester, N.Y., 1991), pp. 111–35.

previous chapter.[32] And knowing as we do their attitude toward the doctor-patient relationship, the reason for this is not hard to discover. By their very nature, systems attempted to base the occurrence of health and disease on the most general physical or chemical principles as, for example, in one late eighteenth-century system that argued that fevers resulted from a lack of oxygen. Such approaches necessarily eliminated the individual patient as an essential factor in order to claim generality for their pathological principles. But it was precisely in the doctor's intimate familiarity with the individual and his or her diverse interactions with the world that writers such as Hufeland and Hecker placed the core of medicine, both in their vision of the medical vocation and in their understanding of disease. The doctor's mission was to heal his fellow men and women, and contribute to their spiritual and physical perfection. This could only be accomplished if the doctor knew the lives, afflictions, sorrows and joys of his patients. Treating people as more or less neutral substrates for detection and manipulation of disease would leave the physician bereft of many of the tasks that comprised the substance of medical practice.

The most basic such task was curing disease. Here too, the tools used by the practitioner in the diagnosis and treatment of diseases reinforced the patient's centrality and individuality.[33] When he is summoned to the patient, the doctor's first task is of course to diagnose the illness. Hufeland's account of this process, a standard one for his day, consisted of two parts: naming the disease and specifying its etiology. The first of these tasks was based upon the symptoms presented for observation. The knowledge obtained in putting a name to the illness is only "historical and empirical," Hufeland wrote, "but it puts us in a position to make ourselves understandable to others, and to consult with other [physicians] about the disease, or to look it up in their writings. . . ."[34] The phenomena of the disease, however, are not the disease itself, only its products. The actual disease is "that definite condition of the forces and matter of the body . . . that so essentially lies at the basis of the phenomena" and is their cause.[35] For example, Hufeland explained, we call an illness dropsy based on its symptoms, but we do not have the true disease until we know that it is a dropsy caused by bodily weakness.

Naming the disease was a complicated and contentious matter. As Johann Peter Frank pointed out in his textbook of medical practice, there were no less than seven different ways of classifying fevers, which yielded largely incompatible schemata of greater or lesser utility for the physician. Indeed the term "fever" itself was somewhat imprecise, Frank observed, because in some cases it referred only to a group of symptoms, and in others it designated a distinctive disease. Yet Frank conceded that such classifications cannot be dispensed with entirely, because

---

32 See Chapter 3, "Criticism and the reform of medical science in the 1790s."
33 On the general method of medical practice in the eighteenth century, see Christian Probst, *Der Weg des ärztlichen Erkennens am Krankenbett*, Sudhoffs Archiv Beiheft 15 (Wiesbaden, 1972).
34 Christoph Wilhelm Hufeland, *System der praktischen Heilkunde*, Bd. 1, "Allgemeine Therapeutik," 2nd ed. (Jena, 1818), p. 177.
35 Ibid., p. 92.

the weight of experience teaches that fevers do display analogous relationships. With good reason, then, one could suppose that an illness that has been identified with a particular kind of fever could be treated according to the same plan.[36]

The second task when confronted with an illness was to formulate an account of its etiology. Often the disease could be identified by bringing into consideration the external causes of the ailment. The investigation of these "remote causes" (*entfernte Ursache*) of disease was a medical tradition reaching back two millennia, and German writers in the early nineteenth century included many of the same causes described in Hippocratic treatises such as *Airs, Waters, Places*. The first, and in many ways the most important, such influence was the air. In his *Handbuch der Pathologie*, the Halle professor, Kurt Polycarp Sprengel (1766–1833), described the morbific influences of the air's warmth, humidity, heaviness and elasticity. High humidity, for example, makes the body's solid parts less sensitive to stimuli, and causes bodily fluids to become more viscous and move slowly. Sprengel also noted that the release of matter into the air from plants, animals and metals could affect health. Echoing an ancient belief, he wrote how dangerous is the air "that is evolved from rotting plant matter in standing waters."[37] Another ancient belief, in the influence of wind direction on health, was also invoked by Sprengel and others. Hufeland, for example, wrote that "higher barometer readings, [and] easterly and northeasterly winds always produce straining of fibers and a tendency towards inflammation."[38]

A second set of standard factors consisted of the characteristics of the local environment. Many of these circumstances were physical, such as the conditions of the air; whether the local water flowed freely or was stagnant in swamps; the condition of the soil; and whether the geography was mountainous or flat, forested or open. But social factors also entered into the balance: the occupations of the people, their dwellings, diet, and lifestyle, and whether they were crammed into cities or spread out over the countryside.

36 Johann Peter Frank, *Behandlung der Krankheiten des Menschen*, Bd. 1 (Berlin, 1835), pp. 23–4. On classifying fevers, see also August Friedrich Hecker, *Kunst die Krankheiten des Menschen zu heilen*, Teil 1, "Allgemeine Grundsätze der Kunst Krankheiten zu heilen," 2nd ed. (Erfurt, 1805), pp. 60–9. Much has been written, principally by Foucault and those influenced by him, about the essentialism of eighteenth-century nosologies and of medical thinking in general. See Michel Foucault, *The Birth of the Clinic*, trans. A. M. Sheridan Smith (New York, 1975), pp. 3–16. But virtually every contemporary handbook of medical practice attested to the insecure and provisional bases of classificatory schemes. With respect to the relationship between nosology and other portions of medical theory, Roger French has pointed out how the nosologies of François Boissier de Sauvages effectively disintegrated pathology into two parts: etiology (the doctrine of disease causation), and nosology (the classification of disease entities). Yet one should not necessarily conclude from this that the majority of writers followed Sauvages's practice. Most German writers, at any rate, underscored the centrality of etiological considerations. Roger French, "Sickness and the Soul: Stahl, Hoffmann and Sauvages on Pathology," in *The Medical Enlightenment of the Eighteenth Century*, ed. Andrew Cunningham and Roger French (Cambridge, 1990), pp. 88–110.
37 Kurt Polycarp Sprengel, *Handbuch der Pathologie*, 3rd ed. (Leipzig, 1802), p. 529.
38 Hufeland, *Enchiridion medicum*, p. 14. Sprengel, however, cautioned doctors against drawing conclusions about the influence of wind from observations made by doctors in other geographical regions. *Handbuch der Pathologie*, pp. 537–8.

In conjunction with these more general points, the physician had to evaluate the peculiarities of the individual that might incline him or her to certain illnesses. These were traditionally known as dispositions (*disposirende Ursache*), and they included a fantastically wide range of considerations. Samuel Gottlieb Vogel (1750–1837), a professor at Rostock and a noted writer on medical practice, claimed that the physician must seek to understand an illness in view of

[the patient's] age, sex, profession, or his other habitual occupations, his entire physical constitution, his entire life and health history from childhood onward, along with the doctors he has seen and medications he has taken, the health of his parents and grandparents, his temperament (*Gemüthsbeschaffenheit*) and style of thought (*Denkungsart*), his relationships and connections, household situation, habits, his lifestyle and diet, the internal and external condition of his home, along with his favorite tastes, his usual companionship, idiosyncrasies, mental powers, properties of the air, clothing, bedding, etc.[39]

In principle, the list of contributing factors was inexhaustible, a point made by that little "etc." at the end. But it is important to note that this epistemology demanded that the physician know his patients as intimately as possible. This was not an account of etiology applicable to someone working in a hospital, faced by rows of patients in a ward. Rather, it reflects the situation of a neighborhood practitioner, whose performance typically takes place in a patient's home.

Although a particular combination of remote causes and dispositions is necessary for the onset of an illness, it is not in itself sufficient. The final ingredient is provided by a group of causes typically referred to as the occasions (*Gelegenheitsursache*), which are specific bodily affects that call forth the disease in the presence of other remote causes. Into this group would fall the traditional "non-naturals" of Galenic medicine, along with other factors such as poisons and contagions.

Out of this multitude of causal agents, the physician has the challenging task of putting together an etiology of the disease, thereby identifying its essential nature. This, however, is only the beginning of his assignment, for once the disease has been determined the doctor must then make a prognosis and choose an appropriate therapy. Vogel cautioned that making an accurate prognosis was one of the most complex and deceptive tasks facing the physician, because so much that could change the prognosis lay hidden from the physician's view or could happen without warning. Yet because it displays full knowledge of the illness and the patient, a correct prognosis is "a doctor's true masterpiece" (*Meisterstück*).[40]

With respect to therapy, the doctor's first efforts should be aimed at producing a causal cure that removes the remote causes of the illness, rather than making a merely palliative cure that treats the symptoms and leaves the underlying causes in

39 Samuel Gottlieb Vogel, *Kurze Anleitung zum gründlichen Studium der Arzneywissenschaft* (Stendal, 1791), p. 109. Elsewhere Vogel presented an exceptionally lengthy set of questions to be asked during the examination of a patient, a list that would surely try the patience of healer and patient alike. See his *Handbuch der practischen Arzneywissenschaft*, 3rd ed. (Vienna, 1801), preface.
40 Vogel, *Kurze Anleitung*, p. 118.

place.[41] Just as in the diagnosis, Hufeland argued, in the actual treatment of the illness the doctor must pay special attention to the patient's unique situation:

> For there is a great difference whether the same disease exists in this or that subject, and this has the most fundamental influence on the form, modifications, and treatment of the disease. Indeed, the fine shadings [of the disease] are determined solely through knowledge and observation of these particularities, and experience teaches us that exactly in this lies the distinguishing mark of the most talented and successful practitioner.[42]

Most of the factors to be considered here also figured in as causal agents: age, sex, individual constitution and temperament, living environment, occupation, the patient's emotional state, and so on. An additional factor, mentioned by August Friedrich Hecker, was the patient's social rank. A healing method must maintain a propriety and decorum appropriate for the patient's place in society.[43]

From the above, it is clear that many writers on medical practice rejected theoretical systems because they failed to account sufficiently for the individuality of patients. Moreover, systems also distorted the way that medical knowledge ought to be constructed and used. Their approach to pathology and diagnosis demanded that the practitioner be above all a careful observer, for only by assembling a natural history of the various causes and symptoms of a patient's illness could he form a proper picture of the situation. The great weakness of systems was their inversion of the proper methods that ought to be applied in medical practice. In contrast to the deductive *Wissenschaften*, medicine could only proceed cautiously along the path of observation, induction, and experience. This point was made in an article on the relationship of medicine to philosophy published in Hufeland's *Journal der practischen Heilkunde*. The author defined two basic types of concepts, "those which arise from the form of thought itself, and are grounded in the faculty of knowledge; and those which are created from our experience."[44] If we examine these two sorts of concepts, he continued, we find that with a priori concepts all of their attributes lie implicit within the concepts themselves: "However, it is entirely different with concepts of experience. In these one finds only what one has previously placed in them. The completeness of such a concept can never be maintained with certainty, since I can never be entirely certain that I have recognized and comprehended every determining condition (*alles Bestimmbares*)."[45] Because medicine, the science of life, qualifies as an empirical science, he concluded, its propositions can never be derived rigorously from first principles.

---

41 Hufeland, *System der praktischen Heilkunde* Bd. 1, pp. 92–3.
42 Hufeland, *Enchiridion Medicum*, p. 7. See also August Friedrich Hecker, *Therapia generalis oder Handbuch der allgemeinen Heilkunde*, 2nd rev. ed. (Erfurt, 1805), pp. 153–62.
43 Hecker, *Therapia generalis*, p. 201.
44 J. M., "Ueber das Verhältniß der Philosophie zur Erfahrung überhaupt, und zur Medicin insbesondere," *Journal der practischen Heilkunde* 17, no. 4 (1803): 31.
45 Ibid., p. 32.

Hufeland joined a host of writers who complained about the tendency to fabricate medical systems. It must be admitted, he wrote on one occasion, that the application of philosophy has been fruitful for medical knowledge in ordering and testing its propositions. But things have gone too far, resulting in what he believed was "an unmistakable partiality for the Speculative, with contempt for the Empirical and Practical."[46] The consequences of this sadly wrongheaded state of affairs arise exactly where it harms medicine the most: in the doctor's ability to observe Nature at the bedside.

Most newer observations are made with preconceived opinions, through the spectacles of a system and without appropriate attention to the manifold phenomena . . . of disease. One sees not what is there but what one wants to see, and one renders, instead of a purely described fact, a commentary on the system with insertion of suitable fragments from the case history and omission of those that are not convenient.[47]

The emphasis placed by Hufeland and others on observation and the cautious collection and digestion of experience left little scope for the deductive theories of medical systems, either in terms of the epistemological value of those systems or in terms of their therapeutic utility. Theory, of course, was indispensable as a foundation; it distinguished the educated physician from the mere empiric. But theory as the foundation for practice had to be distinguished from what is involved in the actual treatment of illness. Hufeland contended that systems are applied to bedside practice in the erroneous belief that practice is a *Wissenschaft* of the sort that natural philosophy is. This he denied strenuously, claiming that whereas medical knowledge was *Wissenschaft,* medical practice was an art (*Kunst*). A similar point about the creative talents of the medical practitioner was made by Johann Georg Zimmermann, whose treatise on medical practice, *Von der Erfahrung in der Arzneykunst* (On experience in medicine, 1763–4), described the importance of genius (*Genie*) to medical practice, a talent that Zimmermann described as the ability to draw correct conclusions about diagnosis and etiology from the myriad circumstances that a physician encounters when first presented with a patient.[48] Other writers took a similar line. Marcus Herz (1747–1803), a prominent Kantian and one of Berlin's leading physicians, also described medicine as a *Kunst.* And just as with any other *Kunst,* only the general rules of medical practice can be learned. The ability to apply those rules to practice requires *Genie.*[49] Samuel Gottlieb Vogel wrote an article for Hufeland's *Journal* in 1795 in which he appropriately referred to this ability as *savoir faire* and assessed its importance to medicine. Vogel stressed at the outset that *savoir faire* could not be equated with knowledge. He noted that there are physicians who incontestably possess the widest theoretical grasp of their discipline who nonetheless are unable to bring

46 *Journal der practischen Heilkunde* 13, no. 1 (1801): 75–6.
47 Ibid., p. 78.
48 Johann Georg Zimmermann, *Von der Erfahrung in der Arzneykunst,* Teil 1 (Zurich, 1763), p. 63.
49 Marcus Herz, *Grundriß aller medicinischen Wissenschaften* (Berlin, 1782), 3–4.

that knowledge to bear when called upon to apply it to healing. Meanwhile, there
are others "who certainly are inferior to them in the requisite knowledge," but
who "exercise their art with more auspicious success and with greater and more
general approval."[50] Nor, Vogel continued, could *savoir faire* be solely the product
of accumulated experience.

Certainly frequent practice and experience teaches much of what belongs to *savoir faire*,
when it is well used; but not all otherwise capable doctors have real experience (*wahre
Erfahrung*) just because they have seen and handled many patients, and even then experience
is not capable of giving all those properties to the doctor that bring good fortune and
prosperity in medical practice.[51]

This repeated emphasis on the art of medical practice and the special talent
required for it reinforced medicine's image as a profession for which one needed a
special calling. But in this case the calling came not from God, but from the
development of innate talent. Through education, those talents would be discovered and allowed to develop, and a properly enlightened system of education
would help each student find his most natural place in the social order. Education
could only do so much, as Marcus Herz noted above. It could not create a talent
for which the potential does not exist.[52] But only through education could the
student's raw talents be shaped into useful skills. This idea extends the ideology of
education that we encountered previously in the discussion of *Bildung*.[53] The idea
that education acts to develop talent is not contrary to education for *Bildung*; it
flows together with it, because acquisition of *Bildung* through education consists –
at least in part – of the maturation of a student's natural talents.

But if education was to perform this function, it had to be the right kind of
education. To arrive at the proper understanding of bedside practice and learn to
perceive his calling as the humble servant of Nature, the student had to be exposed
to the right ideas while still young and impressionable. It would not do for him to
fall prey to the allures of *Naturphilosophie* and other fashionable theoretical systems,
and come to believe that medicine consisted of nothing other than creating
elaborate explanations for life and disease. Rather the student needed to be led to
the bedside in a manner most appropriate for developing his practical talents and
for acquainting him with his future life as a medical practitioner.

THE EDUCATION OF THE PRACTITIONER

Given the role of education in shaping professional identity, it should come as no
surprise that disagreements between physicians concerning the nature of the
medical profession often became debates over the content of medical education.

50 Samuel Gottlieb Vogel, "Einige Bemerkungen über das Sçavoir [sic] faire in der medicinischen
  Praxis," *Journal der practischen Heilkunde* 1, no. 3 (1795): 296–7.
51 Ibid., p. 297.
52 See Zimmermann's comment on this point in *Von der Erfahrung*, Teil 1, p. 23.
53 See chapter 2, "Responses to utilitarian reform."

This is what took place in the wake of the 1804 publication of Johann Christian Reil's *Pepinieren zum Unterricht ärztlicher Routiniers als Bedürfnisse des Staats nach seiner Lage wie sie ist* (Pepineries for the instruction of medical routiniers according to the needs of the state in its current situation). Reil advocated the creation of a group of medical auxiliaries or "Routiniers" as the backbone of a rural health care system. But alongside his delineation of this class of healers, he took the opportunity to describe how physicians differed from Routiniers and how their education should be designed accordingly. Reil's view of physicians centered on their free possession of *Wissenschaft,* the cultivation of which must be unencumbered by any reference to its potential application. "To the student," Reil wrote:

> *Wissenschaft* itself is the goal of its attainment, which he may not sully with any sidelong glance toward its external use. He seeks to develop it in himself, to identify his spirit with it, and to cultivate [his spirit] to become the living and indivisible organ [of *Wissenschaft*]. Therefore is his teacher not so much an instrument of training as he is an example of how the spirit must develop *Wissenschaft* in itself.[54]

In contrast to physicians, whose task was to uncover nature's most profound truths, Reil characterized Routiniers as mere "psychological automatons," who are aware of the rules according to which they function, but who do not understand the principles on which those rules are grounded.[55]

By identifying physicians with the pursuit of *Wissenschaft* and specifying how their education should be structured, Reil gave his numerous opponents an opportunity to articulate their own views of the profession and medical education. A number of commentators took issue with Reil's claim that a "natural attraction" existed between the university-educated physician and the wealthier classes. Any care that the physician might give *gratis* to the poorer members of society, he had maintained, could only be freely chosen and must not be coerced by the state.[56] Reil's intention had been to emphasize the essential freedom that must inhere in the physician, but some of his readers interpreted this as a renunciation of professional vocation. One critic wondered whether Reil was joking, while another, who took him seriously, angrily denounced his apparent callousness:

> These so-called *wissenschaftliche* doctors [of whom Reil speaks] are in reality the elegant doctors, who repair from their studies only to the perfumed chambers of the rich and powerful. Perhaps now and again they drive in their carriages to an estate in the country, and at best [they go] to the less powerful when it is not going well with the routinier's treatment, or they are called in to prescribe the final stimulant when Death has drawn back to butcher its victim.[57]

54 Johann Christian Reil, *Pepinieren zum Unterricht ärztlicher Routiniers als Bedürfnisse des Staats nach seiner Lage wie sie ist* (Halle, 1804), p. 30.
55 Ibid., pp. 63–4.
56 Ibid., pp. 9–10.
57 See the review in the *Medicinisch-chirurgische Zeitung,* 3 January 1805, p. 5; and "Auch ein Vorschlag ärztliche Routiniers zu bilden," *Allgemeine medicinische Annalen* (1807), cols. 936–7.

Significantly, many critics saw the problem as a question of education, and transformed Reil's proposal into a debate over the quality of that education. In doing so, some simply ignored the details of Reil's plan for training routiniers and attacked the current medical curriculum, saying that it was failing to train adequately prepared practitioners, and instead was filling students' heads with a lot of speculative nonsense.[58] Even those critics who spoke directly to Reil's proposal based their arguments on educational matters. They raised questions about whether the routinier's training would allow him to substitute adequately for the fully educated physician. Hufeland in particular took this line after Reil, in dedicating his book to him, had urged Hufeland to make a public response to his ideas. The difference between real doctors and routiniers, Hufeland claimed, is that the former combine scientific knowledge with practical experience, whereas the latter have only their craft skills and experience. This being a much less solid basis than that possessed by the doctors, routiniers are more likely to fall into errors of judgment and give unsatisfactory treatment.[59] Rather than create an officially sanctioned class of inept practitioners by training routiniers in Pepineries, Hufeland argued, the state's task was to improve the currently available medical education and practice. To this end, he envisioned two general approaches.

First, since according to Hufeland there would always be routiniers – by which he meant less talented medical students and others lacking the proper education – the problem became one of channeling their activities and limiting the damage they could do. He distinguished two types of routiniers, the first of which consisted of routiniers who substituted high levels of talent and experience for the scientific knowledge of physicians. Individuals in this group who demonstrated great promise could be allowed to take the state examinations and be installed alongside the doctors with full right to practice medicine. The second group, comprised of practitioners lacking in both knowledge and ability, could still be valuable in extending the physician's reach out among the peasantry and urban poor. These routiniers could be assigned as assistants to physicians, providing them with additional eyes and ears and performing the simplest treatments, such as bloodletting, bathing, and bandaging.[60]

But the problem of routiniers was not merely one of increasing the number of medical personnel in Prussia. If it was true that physicians' education gave them a practical advantage over routiniers, then obviously that education had to be of the right sort. Consequently, as a second solution to the problem of adequate health care, Hufeland also wanted medical curricula structured to prevent the graduation of virtual routiniers by the universities. From Hufeland's standpoint, one of the universities' chief flaws was their combination of teaching and research. Hufeland

58 See, for example, the *Allgemeine Literatur-Zeitung*, 10 November 1804.
59 Christoph Wilhelm Hufeland, "Ueber Aerzte und Routiniers," *Journal der practischen Heilkunde* 21 (1805): 10–12.
60 Ibid., pp. 17–20.

echoed criticisms published in other reviews of Reil's book, lamenting the current arrangement that permitted university professors to ignore the division between teaching and research, so that impressionable young men are all too easily led astray by their professors' theories and hypotheses. It was absolutely essential that universities prevent such things from happening by keeping students away from all "speculative and transcendental instruction." "This is all the more important," Hufeland continued,

since the youthful temperament and its vivid fantasies find it much more comfortable and pleasant to speculate than to learn diligently and mechanically. . . . So very much depends on the first orientation that the intellect receives, and it is extremely difficult, as I know from frequent experience, that a young man, who at first is used to transcendental reasonings and contempt for experience, should afterwards receive that pure sense for observation of Nature, practical talent, and taste for empirical knowledge which alone . . . constitute the doctor.[61]

All this is perpetuated by the combination of teaching and research in universities. To prevent it, Hufeland urged that academies of science assume sole responsibility for research and leave teaching to the universities.

Where Reil emphasized the cultivation of *Wissenschaft* in students, Hufeland underscored those elements of the curriculum that could best prepare students for their vocation as healers. In light of the overwhelming importance he attached to careful observation of patients, appreciation of their situations and histories, and *savoir faire* in dealing with them, Hufeland saw clinical training as the essential portion of medical education. As fundamental as clinical training was, however, it had to be carried out carefully to succeed. It was not sufficient to run students through a hospital, lecture them on a few noteworthy cases, and release them on the public. The clinic had to be fashioned so as to teach students the proper way to think and act; it had to reflect the right ideas about medicine. This meant that students should work in a dispensary or polyclinic, in which patients were cared for in their homes, and the students would learn how to become the careful observers they were supposed to be. Shortly after his arrival at Jena, Hufeland had set up such a clinical course, and he duplicated it when he moved to Berlin. On both occasions, he published programmatic essays in the *Journal der practischen Heilkunde,* describing the structure and especially the advantages of polyclinical training.

Hufeland began by setting out the advantages of polyclinics over hospital clinics. The biggest drawback of hospitals is the welter of facts and images they present to students. Given that the student's most important task as a future physician is learning how to make exact and careful observation of nature, "the natural result must be that his head is filled with a chaos of sensory impressions and recipes; but

61 Ibid., p. 16.

without order, without purposeful connections."[62] Furthermore, polyclinics offer students the opportunity to treat patients directly, whereas in hospitals they are only passive onlookers to the work of the staff doctors.

But far and away the decisive advantage of polyclinics over hospital clinics in Hufeland's eyes was the fact that they would expose students to "real" medicine. In hospitals, he claimed, everything – diet, exercise, light, temperature, medication – stands under the complete control of the physician. However that is certainly not what the young physician will face when he enters practice.

> In the hospital, the young doctor becomes acquainted with things as they should be. In the clinical institute, [he learns] them as they really are in the world, and as he will find them in the future. Instead of everything being carried out at the physician's nod with the greatest punctuality, the self-interest and prejudice of the patient and his relatives, the want and misery, and countless other circumstances put a multitude of hindrances in his way.[63]

The student's success as a future practitioner depended crucially on learning to cope with these situations, and the sooner he became acquainted with them, the better off he would be. But it was not only for reasons of becoming familiar with the daily exigencies of medical practice that Hufeland favored polyclinics so decisively; they also conformed more closely to the contours of medical knowledge. Polyclinics allow illness to be studied in the circumstances in which it arose, whereas by institutionalizing patients, hospitals tear apart the complex fabric by which a patient and his or her sufferings are understood. Hufeland believed that the diagnosis and treatment of disease could only occur in a situation where the physician can comprehend the patient in his or her entire environment: social, moral, and physical. As useful as they may be for caring for the poor and for research – benefits that Hufeland readily granted them – hospitals remove the patient from the setting that caused the illness and alter the face of the disease, thereby preventing the physician from studying it properly. Not without reason, therefore, did Hufeland declare himself to be "a little mistrustful" of results reported from hospitals.[64]

Hufeland's program for clinical education found much favorable response among his colleagues. One writer in the *Allgemeine medizinische Annalen* noted that Hufeland's arguments had settled the question of whether hospital clinics or polyclinics were better for students decisively in favor of the latter. The writer's

---

62 Christoph Wilhelm Hufeland, "Nachrichten von der medizinisch-chirurgischen Krankenanstalt zu Jena, nebst einer Vergleichung der klinischen und Hospitalanstalten überhaupt," *Journal der practischen Heilkunde* 3 (1797): 533. If anything, Hufeland's insistence on the advantages of polyclinics actually increased over time, even though he was appointed to the position of director of the Charité hospital after moving to Berlin. After the University of Berlin opened in 1810, Hufeland described the polyclinic he led there in "Ankündigung des königlichen poliklinischen Institut auf der Universität zu Berlin nebst den Gesetze derselben," *Journal der practischen Heilkunde* 31 (1810): 1–56.

63 Hufeland, "Nachrichten von der medizinisch-chirurgischen Krankenanstalt zu Jena," p. 536.

64 Ibid.

only regret was that in polyclinics students work with poor patients, and therefore do not have a chance to learn the ways and faults of the better off patients on whom their future success would depend. He suggested that instead of working in polyclinics students should spend time as assistants to older, established physicians.[65]

The intimate relationship between polyclinics and medical theory that lay behind Hufeland's program was made fully explicit by the Würzburg professor Philipp Joseph Horsch (1772–1820) in 1808. The most important thing that students draw from their experience in the polyclinics, Horsch asserted, is the combined insight of a bedside practitioner and a public health official. On the one hand, the students' involvement in diagnosing individual patients gives them a chance to reflect upon the particularities of illnesses, whereas on the other hand the clinic's cases can be assembled and compared to reveal the "general influences upon the illnesses of the people." This demands that the clinic have an extensive practice based not on a selection of cases according to arbitrary criteria – an indirect slap at hospital clinics – but as they actually present themselves in the community.

The same fruitful combination of individual and general perspectives that polyclinics offer in diagnosis aids the student in prognosis and treatment of illness as well. Horsch laid out the usual assortment of considerations that polyclinical practice brings within the student's purview: distribution of the population by age and sex; social hierarchy and trades of the people (especially the trades, he added, because some are well known to decrease a population's health); "the position of their physical and moral cultivation"; lifestyle and eating habits; physical characteristics of the city; properties of the local soil, agriculture, and climate; and local illnesses and cycles of disease. As Hufeland had done, Horsch stressed that the decided advantage of polyclinics as teaching facilities is that they allow patients to be treated and understood in their real situations, not artificial ones.[66]

Horsch cautioned that students must not be exposed to polyclinical practice too early in their studies. Rather they should complete their course of theoretical subjects and then take a clinical course in a hospital. Echoing a point that had been made previously by the Göttingen professor Karl Gustav Himly (1772–1837), Horsch declared that hospitals offer easier observation of patients under constant circumstances.[67] Therefore the course of the illness is not so easily disturbed, and the student gets a purer view of it. A polyclinic is no less favorable for observation, Horsch admitted, "but with such a comprehensive plan of practice it would lose too much time [giving students] the first introduction to the art of observation,

---

65 *Allgemeine medicinische Annalen* (1810), cols. 1039–44.
66 Philipp Joseph Horsch, *Beobachtungen über die Witterung und die Krankheiten in Würzburg im Jahr 1807. Nebst einer ausführlichen Nachricht von der klinischen-technischen Bildungsanstalt des Arztes als Kliniker und als Staatsdiener* (Würzburg, 1808), pp. 12–13.
67 See Karl Himly, *Verfassung der öffentlichen medizinisch-chirurgischen Klinik zu Göttingen* (Göttingen, 1803), p. 11.

and therefore be hindered in the full realization of its goal. Observation is complicated by numerous external circumstances in the private practice [of the polyclinic], which do not exist at all in the hospital."[68] Thus in Horsch's scheme polyclinics provided the culmination to the student's education, where the medicine he has learned thus far in its formal and idealized aspect is given a concrete shape.[69]

The final advantage that Horsch saw in polyclinical instruction recalled the direct interest of state governments in the establishment of clinical facilities. He pointed out the benefits accruing to the general welfare from polyclinics more explicitly than Hufeland did, claiming that polyclinics not only train healers of individual disease, they also prepare physicians who are attuned to the health problems of the population as a whole. Horsch saw these two sides of medicine as inseparable. With practically the same breath he spoke of how polyclinics demand of their trainees "activity out of love of humanity and sympathy for one's patients," while at the same time training them to be servants of the state.[70] Thus the physician's clinical education would help him to identify his professional role simultaneously with state and society.

CONCLUSION: THE HEALING ART AND PROFESSIONAL IDENTITY

At first glance, the three facets of professional identity examined here – the medical vocation, the epistemology of medical practice, and the organization of clinical education – would appear to be intimately linked and mutually supportive. Each contributed to a sense that the doctor's role was one of service as advisor and comforter to people living in relatively small, stable, and tightly knit communities. The dignity of the medical profession rested on the sense of sacrifice and devotion displayed by its members, virtues cultivated through university study and clinical training. Along with the *Naturphilosophen*, Hufeland and like-minded writers saw university medical education as conferring *Bildung* upon students, but their understanding of it gave far more shading to duty than did physicians who saw themselves as Schelling's compatriots. The cozy sense of community and social hierarchy articulated by Hufeland, Hildebrandt, and Vogel captured the social conservatism of the German middle classes.

Yet there is something quite paradoxical about the situation in which such views were formulated. For if they repeatedly underscored the importance of the patient in all his or her uniqueness as the focal point of medical knowledge and

68 Horsch, *Beobachtungen,* p. 19.
69 Here too, Himly offered a similar perspective. Himly, *Verfassung,* pp. 13–18. It should be added that the advantages Hufeland and Horsch saw for polyclinics did not find universal assent. Among others, the Leipzig professor Ernst Benjamin Hebenstreit wrote in his *Lehrsätze der medicinischen Polizey* (Leipzig, 1791), p. 221, that stationary hospital clinics were much to be preferred over polyclinics for education of students.
70 Horsch, *Beobachtungen,* pp. 13ff.

action, they nonetheless made their arguments and offered their advice in the print media, assuming roles as writers in the public sphere. That is, they displayed their epistemology and gave advice to readers of whom they had no direct personal knowledge. And such writings were not merely forms of advertising, as perhaps could be argued for dietetic writings of earlier times.[71] The public sphere, as it was constituted in the late eighteenth century, had become far too important to remain in such a secondary role. Instead it was, as this and the preceding chapter have shown, the main arena in which questions over the nature of the medical profession were thrashed out. Patronage still counted for a good deal to individual physicians, and success as a writer did not invalidate the need to cultivate influence and sponsorship on a personal level. But the profession as a whole depended on the public to render judgment on its status and worth.

From an entirely different direction, the intrusion of state interests also put physicians in a paradoxical situation. This is seen most clearly in Horsch's description of the Würzburg university clinic, which would train both bedside healers and public health officials. Horsch's efforts to combine these functions remind us of the growing importance of the profession's identification with government and rational administration. Yet although both were vital to the profession, the two roles could not sit together so comfortably. The bedside healer, acting in a concrete social setting with individual patients, would tend to highlight the patient's contribution to the occurrence of illness. The public health official, however, would act as a bureaucrat from exactly the opposite motivation – to strip away the encrustations of individuality to uncover larger patterns extending over society as a whole. Whatever their long-term incompatibility, however, Horsch himself apparently saw no difficulty. He clearly hoped to have it both ways, with physicians retaining their former status, privileges, and mission through their identification with the learned culture of the higher university professions, but also attaching themselves to the new world of enlightened administration and bureaucratic rationalization.

The temptation is strong to see the professional ideology and epistemology portrayed here as basically conservative, resting on an idealized view of a hierarchical society in which there was no public sphere, personal service found its appropriate reward, university-educated physicians were treated as gentlemen, and state bureaucracy was a comfortably insignificant irritant. And indeed it was conservative, paying as it did little regard to the forces that were transforming German society and its culture. Yet although socially and culturally conservative, the ideology articulated by Hufeland and others also manifested an important novelty. In contrast to the image of medicine as a learned estate formulated at mid-century by Friedrich Boerner in his *Nachrichten*, by 1800 writers on the profession had begun to lay considerable weight on its social function. The

---

71 See, for example, the description of medical advertising in seventeenth-century London in Harold J. Cook, *The Decline of the Old Medical Regime in Stuart London* (Ithaca, N.Y., 1986), pp. 35–45.

differences should not be drawn too starkly; functional considerations were by no means absent in 1750, and it was still true that in 1800 the profession could surrender its claims to learnedness (or as it was more commonly called by then, *Wissenschaft*) only at some peril of its status versus other, unlettered healing occupations. Yet the center of gravity had clearly shifted.

In the new and still quirky world of corporate professional privilege and practical utility that university medical education had to satisfy, the polyclinic found its place. It embodied and transmitted an entire cosmology of medicine, both at the level of the physician's own identity and at the level at which he understood disease. It allowed the physician to be educated at the university as a man of *Wissenschaft*. At the same time, as a host of writers repeatedly stressed, *Wissenschaft* could never be permitted to remain the ultimate end of medical education, and the polyclinic performed that crucial symbolic and practical role of moving the student out of the university and into his socially constituted role as healer.

5

Breaking the shackles of history: The Brunonian revolution in Germany

For all the real disagreements – especially regarding medical education – that existed between the *Naturphilosophen* and those who believed medicine to be a vocation to healing, in a curious way the two groups could tolerate each other fairly well. That is because both implicitly accepted a degree of separation between theory and practice. For their part, the *Naturphilosophen* were not especially interested in designing their theories to provide useful guides to practice. Even a theorist who did seek to close such links, such as Johann Christian Reil, contented himself with alluding only in the most general way to the therapeutic implications of the system described in "Von der Lebenskraft," recognizing that a real unification of theory and practice lay somewhere in the future. Until such a time should arrive, Reil readily accepted the "empirical" methods of practice advocated by Hecker and Gruner.[1] On the other side, Christoph Wilhelm Hufeland too claimed on occasion to see a future when medical practice would become an applied science, although he held deep misgivings over its desirability. Hufeland's image of that future therefore tended to be far more remote than Reil's. These doubts about a unified science of medicine did not prevent Hufeland from attributing some value to theory, and he proclaimed medical theories welcome for their service in broadening physicians' perspectives on the phenomena of disease.[2]

Although neither of these groups chose the most radical of the possibilities offered in the 1790s, other physicians did. This chapter will describe how Brunonianism, the single most important medical movement of the 1790s, attempted to bridge the gap between theory and practice by presenting a single unified system of medicine.[3] The movement deserves our close scrutiny, for the commotion it

---

1 See, for example, Johann Christian Reil, *Ueber die Erkenntniß und Cur der Fieber* Bd. 1, 2nd ed. (Vienna, 1800), pp. 17–19.
2 Christoph Wilhelm Hufeland, "Bemerkungen über die Brownischen Praxis," *Journal der practischen Heilkunde* 1797, 4: 118-141, esp. pp. 119-120.
3 The system is variously named "Brunonianism," based on the Latinized version of Brown's name, and "Brownianism." The former is more common in the English historiography, the latter in the German (*Brownianismus*). For a general history of Brunonianism in Britain and Germany, see Guenter B. Risse, *The History of John Brown's Medical System in Germany During the Years 1790–1806* (Ph.D. diss., University of Chicago, 1971). An interesting and provocative discussion of the place of

caused in Germany was enormous. One could scarcely open a general-interest medical periodical in the decade after 1795 without finding a reference to the theoretical system based upon the ideas of the Scottish physician, John Brown (1735?–88). The debate over the merits of the system convulsed the medical community. Moreover, as had been true of *Naturphilosophie*, Brunonianism participated in the cultural trends of the day. It received extensive coverage in the general literary reviews, feeding the interest of the broader educated public and touching even the Olympian heights of Weimar, where Goethe felt himself called to peruse Brown's *Elementa medicinae*.[4]

The timing of the Brunonian movement is crucial for understanding it, because virtually no one in Central Europe paid any attention to Brown's *Elementa* when he first published it in 1780. It was not as though German physicians were unaware of the British medical literature, for several medical reviews provided ample coverage of British works. Besides, Brown's treatise was written in Latin, making it more accessible to German readers. In spite of these advantages, and the brief flurry of interest among British physicians for Brown's ideas, they made no impression at all among the Germans until 1795.

Several factors can be cited to explain this delay. First, there is little question that German receptivity for Brown's ideas was heightened by the interest in *Naturphilosophie* that began to blossom shortly after the first introduction of Brown's theory into German-speaking Europe. Among physicians schooled in Schelling's philosophy, Brown's view of life as a dialectical process appeared to arise from the same insight into Nature as their own.[5] Although the connections between the two movements were significant – both in terms of intellectual fructification and personal contacts – we should guard against seeing German

Brunonianism in the evolution of modern medical theory can be found in Thomas Henkelmann, *Zur Geschichte des pathophysiologischen Denkens: John Brown (1735–1788) und sein System der Medizin* (Berlin, 1981). Nelly Tsouyopoulos, *Andreas Röschlaub und die Romantische Medizin* (Stuttgart, 1982) focuses on the work of the leading German Brunonian and provides a useful exposition of his doctrines. My own interpretation of Röschlaub differs in certain respects from the one offered by Tsouyopoulos. Somewhat less helpful is Hans-Joachim Schwanitz, *Homöopathie und Brownianismus 1795–1844: zwei wissenschaftstheoretische Fallstudien aus der praktischen Medizin* (Stuttgart, 1983). For British and European perspectives on Brunonianism, see *Brunonianism in Britain and Europe*, ed. W. F. Bynum and Roy Porter, *Medical History*, suppl. 8 (London, 1988).

4 Goethe wrote to Schiller that he found the book to be "animated by an exquisite spirit," but also difficult to understand, so he laid it aside for more pressing matters. Letter dated 19 March 1802, published in *Der Briefwechsel zwischen Schiller und Goethe*, letter 852 (Munich, n.d.), pp. 759–60.

5 On the connections between the Romantic movement and Brunonianism, see especially the articles by John Neubauer, "Dr. John Brown (1735–1788) and early German Romanticism," *Journal of the History of Ideas* 28 (1967): 367–82; and idem, "Novalis und die Ursprünge der romantischen Bewegung in der Medizin," *Sudhoffs Archiv* 53 (1969): 160–70. Risse has emphasized the place of Brunonianism as part of the general domination of medicine by philosophy in Guenter B. Risse, "Kant, Schelling, and the Early Search for a Philosophical Science of Medicine in Germany," *Journal of the History of Medicine and Allied Sciences* 27 (1972): 145–58; idem, "Schelling, Naturphilosophie, and John Brown's System of Medicine," *Bulletin of the History of Medicine* 50 (1976): 321–34; and idem, 'Philosophical' Medicine in Nineteenth-Century Germany: An Episode in the Relations Between Philosophy and Medicine," *Journal of Medicine and Philosophy* 1 (1976): 72–92. Tsouyopoulos has an extensive review of the historical literature in *Andreas Röschlaub*, pp. 10–52.

Brunonianism as simply an offshoot of *Naturphilosophie*. In certain crucial respects, the two movements differed greatly. *Naturphilosophie* was no more than what its name implies: a system of natural philosophy. It never attempted to speak seriously to medical practice. Brunonianism, by contrast, addressed clinical medicine, and took the unification of theory and practice as its main objective. Unlike *Naturphilosophie*, then, Brunonianism was a movement for reform of the medical profession. The difference between the groups can also be seen in the reaction they met from opponents. *Naturphilosophie* was criticized for being ridiculous, useless, unintelligible, and damaging to the characters of young men. Brunonianism was condemned as a threat to the medical profession as a whole, a dangerous doctrine that had to be put down at all costs.

The phenomenon of Brunonianism must also be seen as one manifestation of a larger conflict that was developing in the universities over the nature of *Wissenschaft*. The German Brunonians followed Reil in attempting to fashion their system on the principles of Kant's critical philosophy; but where Reil had remained content with the preliminary outline sketched in "Von der Lebenskraft," the Brunonians created a system with direct and obvious implications for medical practice. But the Kantian model of *Wissenschaft* was not the only one available, and opponents of the system also had their learned resources to draw upon. As we shall see, the opponents of Brunonianism held a conception of medical *Wissenschaft* that had more in common with history than with natural sciences such as physics. Thus while one group of physicians attempted to destroy established medicine through philosophical criticism, another group used the historical *Wissenschaften* to reinforce it, thereby laying the foundations for a new medical discipline: the history of medicine.

Finally, the Brunonian movement must also be seen as part of a general revolutionary spirit that infiltrated German society in the 1790s, carried in by the revolution in France and the Jacobin uprisings in western Germany. Like the years 1848 and 1968, the 1790s were a time when political revolution, with all its thrills and terrors, was a palpable presence in everyday life. Brunonian medicine became the banner under which scores of young, disaffected medical students marched, young men who believed their prospects in the established profession and in bourgeois society were unappealing. If we fail to bear this revolutionary mood in mind, even the most thorough discussion of Brunonianism within its professional and university contexts will not suffice to capture fully what the movement represented to its followers and foes in its first few years.

In what follows I want to address two problems. First, how did Brunonianism insert itself into the German medical and university world of the 1790s, and how did it propose to satisfy the different demands of *Wissenschaft* and practical efficacy? Second, and more importantly, why did it engender such ferocious opposition before disappearing as a unified movement between 1805 and 1810? Why, in other words, was Brunonianism perceived to be so dangerous to the German medical establishment? As the following discusion will demonstrate, Brunonianism brought German physicians face to face with the implications of the Enlightenment ideology that many of them had been championing. At issue was the character of medicine as a learned profession.

PRELUDE TO REVOLUTION

The storm that overtook the German medical community in 1795 arose almost from out of nowhere. A reader of the periodical literature in the early 1790s, even one who kept a close eye on developments, would have had not the slightest inkling of the approaching turmoil. To be sure, controversy abounded, as it always did in medicine; nonetheless, this was controversy mostly among physicians themselves, confined to the safe environs of professional periodicals. Rarely did medical disputes reach the pages of the general circulation press, and when they did they seemed to generate little or no interest.

Among the periodicals through which the educated reader could keep abreast of the latest cultural and political goings-on, the *Teutscher Merkur* was one of the more influential and prestigious. Edited by the novelist, poet and critic Christoph Martin Wieland (1733–1813), one of Weimar's resident luminaries, the *Teutscher Merkur* had originally been launched in 1773 as a journal of literature and art criticism. Wieland, a perspicacious journalist who realized that a successful publication could offer more than debates over classical aesthetics, had gradually modified the contents of his magazine over the years. By the 1790s, alongside his traditional offerings Wieland was publishing historical essays and articles of contemporary political interest, including reports from revolutionary Paris.[6] Medicine, however, had seldom found itself among the journal's subjects.

Consequently it must have been all the more shocking to readers when Wieland led off his issue of August 1795 with a devastatingly critical review of the state of medical knowledge titled "Ueber die Medicin. Arkesilas an Ekdemus." This article, which introduced many of the issues that would become so prominent in the coming conflict over Brunonianism, was written pseudonymously by Johann Benjamin Erhard (1766–1827), a physician and Kantian philosopher.[7] At the opening of the dialogue Erhard, taking the voice of Arkesilas, an ancient Skeptic, has just finished demonstrating the shortcomings of philosophy to a young friend, Ekdemus. Ekdemus has proposed the study and practice of medicine as an alternative to philosophy where he may accomplish useful things for humanity, and find

---

6 Victor Lange, *The Classical Age of German Literature 1740–1815* (New York, 1982), pp. 98–100.
7 The article was unsigned, although it was attributed to Erhard in Johann Benjamin Erhard, *Über das Recht des Volks zu einer Revolution und andere Schriften,* ed. Hellmut G. Haasis (Frankfurt, 1970), p. 235. Evidence for the attribution was not given by Haasis, but there is good reason to believe it is correct. The most convincing confirmation comes from an article written by Erhard in 1799 for one of the leading Brunonian medical journals. The style of this article matches quite closely that of the article in the *Teutscher Merkur,* and it repeats many of the same arguments, in places almost word for word. See Johann Benjamin Erhard, "Ueber die Möglichkeit der Heilkunst," *Magazin zur Vervollkommnung der theoretischen und practischen Heilkunde* 1 (1799): 23–83.

honor and reward. Arkesilas, however, will dissuade Ekdemus from these fantasies by proving that medicine accomplishes nothing useful. "And when I have proven this," he added, "I am confident that you will also no longer value the honor of medicine, which is based merely on the ignorance of the masses. Thus there remains to medicine no advantage over philosophy other than it more often makes one wealthy. But this advantage it shares with swindling and usury."[8]

Erhard's attack focused on what he called the "uncertainty" of medical knowledge and its failure to measure up to the criteria of a philosophical *Wissenschaft*. He located the central problem in doctors' lack of a clear idea either of illness in general or of particular diseases. Ask any physician, Erhard urged, to describe the internal condition of the body during an illness: "He will name all the phenomena (*Symptomata*) which the illness presents, and perhaps also claim that the breast or liver is the seat of the illness. But not one word [will he give] over the internal changes that must occur in order for these phenomena to be present."[9]

This lack of any definite connection between symptoms and the disease they represented had serious consequences for medical practice. Many of the physician's bedside activities depended on interpretation of a patient's symptoms, first for identifying the disease, then for determining its probable course, and finally for formulating a prognosis and taking remedial action. Diagnosis rested on the doctrine that symptoms could be used to unearth the causes of illness, whereas prognosis and therapy derived from the belief that each disease followed its own unique course of development in the body, and this development could be traced through a progression of symptoms. For this procedure to be successful it was vital for physicians to distinguish those symptoms that were expressions of the illness itself from symptoms that were merely accidents or the result of the illness's appearance in the body and changes in it. In semiotics the former group of symptoms were commonly called the *Indicans,* and the latter were the *Contraindicans.* Erhard rejected this entire method. Because physicians have no idea of the essence of illness, either in general or in particular, he wrote, the identification of the *Indicans* is completely arbitrary.[10]

Along with semiotics, Erhard denounced another venerable portion of bedside practice, the taking of case histories. Doctors are not satisfied with knowing what is wrong with the patient at the moment, he wrote. They must go further, subjecting patients to an embarrassing inquisition into their past illnesses and their personal lives. The reason for this ritual, he asserted, rested on the fact that neither the patient nor the doctor knows what is really wrong: "For if the patient could describe the condition exactly and the physician recognize it, they would not need the past conditions. If the patient is truly healed from past illnesses, then knowledge of them is mere curiosity; if this is not the case, then the illnesses are part of the present condition."[11]

8 "Ueber die Medicin. Arkesilas an Ekdemus," *Der neue teutsche Merkur,* August 1795, p. 338.
9 Ibid., p. 340.
10 Ibid., pp. 344–6, 352–8.
11 Ibid., p. 346.

Erhard also discounted the allegedly empirical grounds on which physicians believed in the effectiveness of their therapies. He compiled a list showing how various writers had cured a single disease with the most diverse assortment of drugs imaginable, and conversely, how a single drug was credited with therapeutic powers in a staggering array of illnesses. As long as the nature of illness is not better understood, he concluded, "experience fundamentally will teach nothing more than that one can ingest certain substances without dying."[12]

Erhard attacked every area of medical knowledge so vigorously that some rejoinder from the medical community was obviously called for, despite Wieland's declared reluctance to open the doors on a potentially tiresome literary feud. Two months later, the response came from an outraged Hufeland.[13] Hufeland's first objection to the article was also his most significant: the *Teutscher Merkur* was not an appropriate place for such a criticism of medicine to be published.

A complaint must be brought before that forum that has knowledge of the matter. It would have been entirely appropriate in a medical journal. . . . But here, where it is brought before the larger public that can only read it but not judge it, here it can only do damage (through agitation of unresolved doubt and erroneous opinion) but not be useful.[14]

Heaven help the poor doctor, Hufeland sighed, who now had to practice in a town where people read the *Teutscher Merkur.* Alongside his usual struggle against illness, he would now also have to overcome the doubts and objections of his patients.[15] So upset was Hufeland by this point that he returned to it later on, again mentioning the publication of this article in Wieland's journal as evidence of the author's merely mischievous intention.

There was more to Hufeland's carping on this issue than first meets the eye. He was not simply trying to uphold the shattered dignity of his profession before what he believed would now be a thoroughly skeptical public. More significantly, his objection rested upon his view of medical knowledge. For Hufeland, as we saw in the preceding chapter, medical practice must be based on knowledge that does not aim at philosophical comprehensiveness. Medical knowledge instead must attempt to understand the particularities of life.[16] This understanding of everyday experience can develop only through experience itself, and the portion of medicine in which a doctor's experience makes itself felt most crucially is semiotics, the very focus of Arkesilas's criticism. How, Hufeland might have asked, can the public judge a doctrine when the only knowledge of it comes through experience with it? The public's lack of medical experience quite literally made it incompetent to judge the state of medical knowledge.

With the same intention in mind, Hufeland also attempted to demonstrate that his opponent could not have been a physician, by using examples from the article

12 Ibid., pp. 358–9.
13 Christoph Wilhelm Hufeland, "Ein Wort über den Angriff der razionellen Medicin im N.T. Merkur. August 1795," *Der neue teutsche Merkur,* October 1795, pp. 138–53.
14 Ibid., p. 139.
15 Ibid., p. 141.
16 See the section titled "The art of healing" in Chapter 4.

that he thought betrayed Arkesilas's ignorance of medicine. One such example is particularly striking and testifies to how remarkably far apart Hufeland and Erhard were over the nature of medical knowledge. Hufeland returned to the list presented by Arkesilas of the numerous drugs that were said to cure a single disease. Arkesilas had argued that such a variety of medicaments proves the ignorance of physicians. Hufeland, by contrast, saw no problem whatsoever, and turned the point against Arkesilas, saying it only proved *his* ignorance.

It is truly sad to see someone take it upon himself to judge medicine who does not even know that entirely opposite causes often bring forth the same effects, hence illnesses, and therefore the same illness can be cured with opposite treatments, while illnesses that appear to be entirely different can be treated with identical methods.

"Admittedly," Hufeland concluded, "an empiric would judge things in this manner, but therein lies the difference and advantage of rational medicine over empiricism."[17]

"Rational" medicine meant two things for Hufeland. First, it denoted that medicine was not some handicraft like surgery, but instead a learned discipline. A physician read and studied widely in order to train his mind and to attain the broadest possible perspectives on natural phenomena. Second, rational medicine stipulated that a physician consider disease and patient in all their complex concreteness. Opposite causes could well produce the same effect because they acted on a patient who reacted to those external causes in accord with his or her unique constitution, temperament, and situation. Any attempt to isolate a single, predominating cause or to treat the processes of life mechanistically could only lead to a debased sort of medical practice. Hufeland believed the only alternative to his conception of medical knowledge was the rawest form of medical empiricism, in which one treats illness without any theoretical guidance whatsoever. And he clearly believed Arkesilas was advocating such empiricism against what Hufeland called "razionellen Medicin."[18]

Erhard, for his part, might well have thrown up his hands in frustration, for Hufeland's reply described a variety of causation that Erhard had specifically claimed was no clear notion of causation at all. In his reply to Hufeland, which Wieland published several months later, Erhard could only protest that Hufeland had completely misunderstood him – which appeared true enough – and that he was advocating anything but empiricism. Quite to the contrary, Erhard called for medicine to develop the same "laws derived from experience" that physics had.[19]

Hufeland's standard of medical knowledge placed the public outside the circle of competence for judging or criticizing medicine, in essence defining a kind of

17 Hufeland, "Ein Wort über den Angriff," pp. 144–5.
18 If nowhere else, this point was clearly implied by the title of Hufeland's article: "Ein Wort über den Angriff der razionellen Medicin" ("A word on the attack against rational medicine").
19 "An Hrn. Rath D. Hufeland in Jena, über dessen Wort im N.T. Merkur 1795. 10. St. S. 168. Vom Verf. des Arkesilas," *Der neue teutsche Merkur,* January 1796, pp 76–92, quoted on p. 89.

expertise that belonged solely to medical professionals. Erhard's standards, on the other hand, appealed to reason rather than an expert's experience, and thus were grounded on the very ideological foundations of the public sphere. This gave him, as he told Hufeland in his reply, every right to publish his criticisms in the *Teutscher Merkur*. "Since I consider medicine as a matter belonging to mankind in general and not to a particular guild, I did not need to choose any other journal than one ... that has a thinking public."[20] Erhard further challenged Hufeland to explain what he intended by arguing that Arkesilas was not a doctor. Characteristically, he did not parry Hufeland by claiming he too was a physician, but by contending only that Hufeland's attack on his credentials did not pertain to the criticisms he had advanced. Erhard also turned Hufeland's weapon of professional credentials against him. He chided his opponent for signing his own name to his reply, when urbanity demanded that Hufeland choose a classical pseudonym like his own. Such a choice would have permitted Hufeland to defend medicine on no other basis than the merits of the arguments presented. Instead, Hufeland had seemingly attempted to let his authority carry the day for him. "To squash a young man with the weight of your name, as you would smash a fly," Erhard wrote sweetly, "certainly could not have been your intention."[21]

Behind this whole exchange over credentials and professional authority lay an important point. Hufeland's standard of medical knowledge excluded more than just the public from competence in medical affairs; it also excluded a "young man" such as Erhard. Of course it was necessary for an aspiring physician to study medicine systematically to acquire an idea of its guiding principles, but having completed a course of studies did not qualify a graduate as an accomplished medical practitioner. Only after spending years accumulating experience at the bedside would the now mature doctor have acquired sufficient knowledge of medicine to become a true physician and healer. In effect, Hufeland's conception of medical knowledge legitimated a hierarchy within the profession that placed younger physicians in a disadvantageous position, to say the least.

Erhard's attack on the accepted foundations of medical knowledge consequently presented far-reaching implications for the structure of the profession as well. He recognized this quite clearly, and in his first article Arkesilas took several opportunities to deride the institutions through which the medical powers exercise their control. For instance, many people are attracted by the alleged freedom of thought that physicians have, but Arkesilas, speaking to Ekdemus, ridiculed this notion by pointing to the kinds of examinations he would have to undergo at the hands of the medical establishment.

Can you really suppose that freedom of thought could be tolerated in a *Wissenschaft* which cannot maintain its rights on the basis of either reason or experience, and which nonetheless presumes to recognize masters and journeymen? After what has been said, how could

20 Ibid., p. 76.
21 Ibid., pp. 78–9.

the examinations conducted by doctors be anything other than inquiries into whether [the candidate] knows by heart their errors, opinions, and things that do not belong to medicine at all?[22]

Probably most outrageous of all to established physicians was Erhard's critique of the subjects that medical students were required to take, among which he chose anatomy for special emphasis. In selecting the one subject usually considered most central to medicine, Erhard was attacking by implication the entire medical curriculum. He willingly conceded to anatomy an important place in the study of natural history and physiology. Its supposed value for medical practice, on the other hand, he branded a "baseless deception." Erhard pointed out that many writers compare medical practitioners to watchmakers when defending the utility of anatomy for practice, a comparison that simply does not work. Watchmakers open up watches and remove individual parts for repair or replacement, something that physicians are unable to do. Although anatomy may yield knowledge of the seat of illness in some cases, Erhard concluded, it never can tell physicians what the cause of illness is.[23]

If professional ideology, clinical epistemology, and medical education formed a tightly knit triad in Hufeland's conception of medicine, so too did they for Erhard. For him, the public use of reason took on its most radical coloration, thereby highlighting for all to see the democratizing implications of Enlightenment ideology. Such implications had been there all along, but perhaps it took the environment of the 1790s to bring them to the surface against the resistance of more didactic and authoritarian strains of Enlightenment thought. In Erhard's view, there was no professional mystery, no art to medical practice requiring special talent and years of experience at the bedside. Before a tribunal composed of the "public" itself, Erhard in essence ceded to that public the right to judge medicine and medical practitioners, an action likely to find a sympathetic reception in such a forum. That of course is what made this remarkable essay so dangerous, raising a threat to the profession that Hufeland for one did not fail to apprehend.

HISTORICAL EPISTEMOLOGY AND PROFESSIONAL AUTHORITY

One of the most damaging strategies in Erhard's article in the *Teutscher Merkur* was his appropriation of Kantian philosophy as the standard for measuring the claims of medical knowledge and finding them inadequate. As we have already seen in the writings of Reil and Carl Christian Erhard Schmid, Kant's critical philosophy had by the 1790s come to define the epistemological conditions of academic *Wissenschaft* in Germany. Erhard's use of such epistemological criteria, therefore, could well be taken – as surely he intended it to be taken – as denying to medicine the status of *Wissenschaft*.

22 "Ueber die Medicin," p. 370.
23 Ibid., pp. 371–2.

Yet Kantian critical philosophy and its elaborations by Fichte and Schelling were not the only accepted forms of university *Wissenschaft* in the 1790s. Although one might easily receive that impression, judging from Kant's own influence and the tremendous appeal of movements such as *Naturphilosophie,* it was in fact countered by another type of scholarly pursuit based on epistemological premises that diverged sharply from Kant's: history. Over the course of the eighteenth century, philologists and historians had developed a method and epistemology for their disciplines that gave them a theoretical foundation quite different from the type of demonstrative construction from first principles that marked philosophy. For our purposes, what is significant about this historical epistemology is its resemblance to the method of medical practice advocated by Hufeland, Gruner, and Hecker. Moreover, beyond simple resemblance, the historical record itself was appropriated to provide a measure of justification for that method. As one final element for understanding the impact of the Brunonian revolution, therefore, let us examine this alternative conception of *Wissenschaft.*

Up until the eighteenth century, history had for the most part served as an exemplary or didactic tool for other disciplines. The historical record provided a reservoir to be drawn upon for illustrating or demonstrating the truth of a principle in theology, law, or political theory. For this reason, histories were "ahistorical"; that is, they did not attempt to explain historical events in any particular temporal framework or account for change over time. What counted were the principles being advocated, and their truth did not depend on their history. During the Enlightenment, this attitude gave way to a belief that history ought to unearth the patterns of past phenomena and the reasons for change over time. Instead of using history to supply illustrations for arguments that were not themselves historical, scholars began to argue that it should seek to develop an understanding of the causes and effects of past events. To separate their endeavors from previous historical scholarship, they gave it a distinctive name: pragmatic history.[24]

There remained the question of what sort of understanding pragmatic history could present. Seventeenth-century rationalists had criticized historical scholarship as a source of hazy heuristic aids for discovering truths that philosophical methods provided in a more satisfactory manner. History was at best a second-rate form of knowledge that was not capable of revealing the objective truths of the world. For their part, Enlightenment historians accepted the thrust of this argument. Historical knowledge, they agreed, could not arrive at universal truths because all history was written from a particular standpoint. However, to historians the inability to find objective purchase from which to survey the past was not their weakness, as it was to philosophers, but their strength. For historical knowledge constituted knowledge of particulars, of life as experienced. More than that, however, the

---

24 Peter Hanns Reill, *The German Enlightenment and the Rise of Historicism* (Berkeley and Los Angeles, 1975), pp. 45–9.

contact that comprises historical knowledge is not passive reception of an object through the senses. It is an active intuition of the object, a process requiring reason and the imagination in addition to the senses. To Enlightenment historians, according to Peter Hans Reill, "historical understanding is an understanding of the spirit, or *Gemüthe,* an act of reexperiencing or seeing again, though from a different vantage point. It is not the apprehension of a mechanical cause-and-effect relation."[25] Most importantly, historical writing attempts to recreate the conditions of an event. It does not deny the notion of causation; instead it attempts to examine and account for causation within specified historical contexts.

This conception of historical methodology shared two essential points of identity with the medical practice of Hufeland and other eighteenth-century physicians. First, both groups regarded theirs as a necessarily subjective activity, but one guided by theory. Practitioners of both groups attempted to tread a narrow path between practice as mere application of theoretical principles on the one side and total renunciation of theory on the other. To fall into believing that historical or medical practice was no more than applied theory would be untrue to what they believed distinguished them from the philosophers, whereas a misstep in the other direction would reduce medical and historical knowledge to a completely subjective condition in which a historian or a physician knows only what he has experienced himself. As university scholars and men of *Wissenschaft,* neither physicians nor historians could allow themselves to admit that possibility.

The second point of contact between history and medicine was the contention that the understanding of the particular was an intuitive, commonsensical apprehension of an object in all its complex relationships with its surroundings.[26] Such an understanding demanded above all experience with it. The historian immersed himself in the past via his thorough study of it and via his imagination. The physician immersed himself in his object, illness, through repeated contact with it at the bedside, and by study of other physicians' reports of their experiences.

Case histories, the medium used by physicians to communicate their practical experience with illness, provided a striking embodiment of physicians' historical methodology. Their basic form, a chronicle of symptomatic developments, was designed to allow the reader to join the writer at the bedside and recreate the experience of watching the disease unfold and change. Case histories also put the events in a proper network of relations by recounting the natural historical details of a case: descriptions of the patient, the patient's surroundings and occupation, weather conditions, past illnesses, etiology, and so forth. The wealth of information collected in published case histories brought a far greater world of experience to a physician than he could ever hope to gather in the course of his own practice. The overwhelming importance of case histories to medical practice is indicated

---

25 Ibid., p. 110.
26 The points of epistemological contact between history and medicine have also been described by Carlo Ginzburg in "Morelli, Freud, and Sherlock Holmes: Clues and Scientific Method," *History Workshop* 9 (1980): 5–34.

by the use made of them by late eighteenth-century medical journalists. When Hufeland began publishing his *Journal der practischen Heilkunde,* he could think of no better way to advance medical practice than to devote the bulk of each issue to illustrative or unusual case histories sent in by contributors.

Despite the pronounced similarities between the practices of history and medicine, physicians seem to have taken little notice of them before the 1790s. History was used for exemplary purposes to lionize a writer's heroes and attack his enemies. By the early years of that decade, however, physicians had begun using history in a new way, as a source of authority to justify what they took to be proper medical practice. These writers used the historical record to demonstrate that progress in medical knowledge through the ages had always occurred at those times when physicians remained most true to the spirit of careful bedside observation and gradual accumulation of experience. In effect, they appropriated the methods of the historians to write histories demonstrating the triumph of historical method, as applied to medical practice.

What is more, they did it quite deliberately. The most important of the new historians of medicine was Kurt Polykarp Sprengel (1766–1833), a professor at the University of Halle. Sprengel's major historical treatise, the *Versuch einer pragmatischen Geschichte der Arzneikunde* (Essay at a pragmatic history of medicine, 1792–9), was a mammoth, five-volume narrative of the history of medicine from earliest recorded history through the most recent times. Sprengel's work was no mere chronological collection of medical anecdotes. He understood perfectly well what the latest developments in history were about, and he applied the program of the pragmatic historians to his own work. History of medicine, he wrote, can only be understood as a part of the history of culture. His task as a historian was therefore to describe not only the medical doctrines of the past, but also the cultural conditions that gave rise to them. Sprengel expected the same benefits from his endeavor as other historians claimed for pragmatic history:

Modern historians name a history pragmatic when it makes us wise (*klug*). And it makes us wise when it gives us an occasion for considering the stepwise development of human understanding, for better comprehension of medical doctrine, for using even the fruitless efforts of the past to uncover truth, and for correcting our own systems.[27]

Concomitant with what he believed to be history's pragmatic function, Sprengel argued that the history of medicine taught a clear lesson to physicians, a lesson that tied the medical practice of his time to all previous ages. As Sprengel put it in the introduction to the second edition of the *Versuch,* the lesson is that "medicine loses by connecting itself to any school-philosophy, and it gains only through cultivation of the study of experience."[28] Another medical historian, August Friedrich Hecker, expressed the same attitude in his short history of

27 Kurt Polykarp Sprengel, *Versuch einer pragmatischen Geschichte der Arzneikunde,* Bd. 1, 2nd ed. (Halle, 1800), pp. 6–7.
28 Ibid., p. iv.

medicine, *Die Heilkunst auf ihrem Weg zur Gewißheit* (Healing on the path to certainty, 1802), declaring proudly that medical practice has steadily approached the highest degree of perfection to which it can aspire through its ever-widening collection of experience.[29]

Sprengel and Hecker's use of pragmatic history seems almost retrograde, a return to the time when history was simply a tool for arguing ahistorical dogmas. In part this contention is justified by the fact that Sprengel and Hecker were physicians, not historians, and they used history to make certain points about medicine. At the same time, however, Sprengel and Hecker did manifest the new methods and aims of historical scholarship. They used history not merely to illustrate their points about medical practice and theory, but instead as a running argument for them. History itself became the basis for contending that medicine had progressed when it adhered to certain doctrines.

Clearly, one important impulse toward the writing of history of medicine came from the transformations undergone by the profession during the final decades of the eighteenth century. History legitimized a certain view of the profession, and it helped physicians fend off the criticisms of Kantians such as Erhard. Just as important as this function, moreover, was the fact that history gave medicine its anchor in the glorious legacy of classical Greece. The second half of the eighteenth century witnessed a growing fascination – and indeed, obsession – with ancient Greek literature and art on the part of educated German elites.[30] Such preoccupations became the centerpiece of an educational reform preached by a group of pedagogues who argued that contact with the Good, the True, and the Beautiful through mastery of the Greek language and literature was the surest route to acquisition of *Bildung*. That was no trifling benefit, because *Bildung,* as we have seen time and again, functioned as an indispensable marker of social status. The neoclassical revival thus contributed to the reinforcement of social elites at a time of a radical democratic challenge.

For medicine, the neoclassicist movement could mean only one thing: the triumph of Hippocratic medicine. Hippocrates became the symbol of all that physicians saw as good and true in medicine. He was hailed as the patron of the divine arts of bedside practice, of observing illnesses carefully with an unprejudiced eye and letting Nature speak for herself; of the understanding of semiotics, by which Nature's language is translated; of trusting in Nature's own healing powers instead of the futile machinations of witless physicians; and of comprehending the world in such a way that the individual is seen in the totality of his or her relationships.[31] So powerful an icon was Hippocrates to medical historians that

29 August Friedrich Hecker, *Die Heilkunst auf ihrem Weg zur Gewißheit,* 2nd ed. (Erfurt, 1805), p. 3.
30 For nice review of the neo-classical revival in Germany after 1750, see Suzanne L. Marchand, *Archaeology and Cultural Politics in Germany, 1800–1965: The Decline of Philhellenism* (Ph.D. diss., University of Chicago, 1992), chapter 1. Also helpful are Friedrich Paulsen, *Geschichte des gelehrten Unterrichts,* Bd. 2, repr. of 3rd ed. (Berlin, 1921), pp. 9–47, 191–247; and Eliza M. Butler's brilliant and idiosyncratic *The Tyranny of Greece over Germany* (New York, 1935).
31 Sprengel, *Versuch einer pragmatischen Geschichte,* Bd. 1, pp. 383–427.

Sprengel and Ernst Gottfried Baldinger published a "profession of faith" to Hippocrates, a sort of Hippocratic Oath for physicians of the neoclassicist religion:

I believe Hippocrates [was] a man of extraordinary talents, [and] can be called the creator of rational medicine. . . . [H]e separated medicine from speculative philosophy, and was the first to make it a concern of healthy human understanding. Therein the best physicians of all times and peoples have followed him, and we too must follow him, if we strive for the glory of being true physicians.[32]

Sprengel and the other medical historians took care not to exalt Hippocratic teachings to the status of an inviolable canon of sacred writings; quite the opposite. They acknowledged that the Hippocratic writers had made mistakes and had held false beliefs. Indeed, their histories treated quite harshly those physicians who attempted to transform Hippocratic doctrines into a dogmatic system, as Hippocrates' immediate followers had done, along with what they called the dogmatism displayed by Galen and, more recently, Thomas Sydenham (1624–89). What interested them rather was the *method* of medical practice taught by the Hippocratics. For them it was the enunciation in medicine of the same spirit by which a past culture had for one brief, glorious moment seized upon Truth. By showing medicine's roots in classical antiquity, history at the same time displayed the profession's divine inspiration.

This was the theme articulated in 1801 by Karl Joseph Hieronymus Windischmann (1775–1839), a young physician who would later become professor at the University of Bonn. In an article published in Hufeland's *Journal*, Windischmann bemoaned what he regarded as the disintegration of a truly unified view of the world. Corresponding to the analytical spirit of the modern age, he declared, each individual science has proclaimed its independence and has begun touting itself as the basis for the ultimate system of medicine. The result could only be a sadly one-sided view of Nature that contrasts wretchedly with the ancient Greeks' sympathy for the sublime unity of life. Windischmann argued that the analysis of knowledge into tiny, meaningless specialties was not their way; the Greeks strove rather to come to a synthetic understanding of Nature. They saw it as the product of one primitive force, and consequently were able to understand the essential workings of Nature as no others have.[33] He concluded in another of his writings

32 "Des Herrn Kurt Sprengel zu Halle, und E. G. Baldingers Hippokratisches Glaubensbekenntniß," *Neues Magazin für Aerzte* 16 (1794): 468.
33 Karl Joseph Hieronymus Windischmann, "Ueber die gegenwärtige Lage der Heilkunde und den Weg zu ihrer festen Begründung," *Journal der practischen Heilkunde* 13 (1801): 9–72. The themes of the synthetic quality of ancient culture versus the analytic tendencies of the contemporary age were common ones at this time. They were prominent in Friedrich Schiller's famous essay, "Ueber naive und sentimentalische Dichtung" ("On Naive and Sentimental Poetry," 1795–96), which contrasts the ancients' spontaneous, naive apprehension of nature with the reflective mode of the moderns, which treats nature as a mere object. Although not employing the terms "synthetic" and "analytic," Schiller plainly was referring to the same characteristics that Windischmann pointed to. See Friedrich Schiller, "On Naive and Sentimental Poetry," in *German Aesthetic and Literary Criticism*, ed. H. B. Nisbet (Cambridge, 1985), pp. 185–232, esp. pp. 188–91. Schiller placed the same issues at the center of his "Ueber die ästhetische Erziehung des Menschen" ("On the Aesthetic Education

that "a sharp boundary is to be drawn between those base and common abilities of which our age is full, and the true and divine art, in which the ancient world and above all the Hellenes partook."[34]

Although Sprengel, Hecker, and other writers of medical history disclaimed any intention of establishing an orthodoxy of Hippocratic teachings, their trumpeting of his methodology necessarily carried with it a stubborn insistence on certain concepts. First, in their view all true medical theories accepted semiotics as a diagnostic and therapeutic guide. A still more essential pillar of the method was belief in a healing power of Nature. The Hippocratics had taught that in many cases the patient's own restorative powers could heal sickness, whereas the physician's job was to support Nature's work through his own ministrations. This doctrine was substantiated by observation of the progression often displayed by diseases through a stage called "crisis," in which the body visibly expels a disease-causing agent through sweating, vomiting, or some other release of material.[35]

The eighteenth-century apologists for Hippocratic medicine did not believe that every disease resolved itself during a crisis produced by Nature's healing power, and Hecker ridiculed doctors who sit passively at the bedside, waiting for the onset of a crisis while their patients expire.[36] Nonetheless, any acceptable medical theory had to ascribe some restorative action to Nature, along with upholding the rest of the Hippocratic method. Every new theory consequently was subjected to a test of conformity with Hippocratic teachings, and the judgment rendered on these theories was often reduced to variations on a favorite aphoristic saying: "What is good in the theory is not new, and what is new in it is not good."

At the same time that history reinforced the methodological claims of medical practitioners, it also supported the profession's hierarchy of experience. Experience taught the same lesson, whether it was in medicine or history. One could understand the course of medical history or the course of a disease only through direct and repeated contact with the object of interest. Sprengel, for one, denounced as hopeless any attempt to deduce a unified history of medicine from "pure reason," before the sources had been thoroughly researched.[37] Needless to say, the same held true for bedside practice as well.

But although history may have provided physicians with an epistemology

of Man," 1794–5), where he made the following comment: "Why was the individual Greek qualified to be the representative of his time, and why may the individual Modern not dare to be so? Because it was all-uniting Nature that bestowed upon the former, and all-dividing Intellect that bestowed upon the latter, their respective forms." Friedrich Schiller, *On the Aesthetic Education of Man, in a Series of Letters,* trans. with an introduction by Reginald Snell, "Sixth Letter" (New York, 1965), p. 39.
34 Karl Joseph Hieronymous Windischmann, *Versuch über den Gang der Bildung in der heilenden Kunst* (Frankfurt, 1809), p. 3.
35 On the history of the healing power of Nature, see Max Neuburger, *Die Lehre von der Heilkraft der Natur im Wandel der Zeiten* (Stuttgart, 1926).
36 Hecker, *Die Heilkunst auf ihrem Weg,* p. 110.
37 Sprengel, *Versuch einer pragmatischen Geschichte,* Bd. 1, p. 14.

appropriate to medical practice, it contributed nothing to the reintegration of physiology and pathology with the rest of medical teaching. Sprengel would certainly not have wanted to deny that physiology and pathology properly belong in medicine; in fact, he wrote a major textbook of pathology. Morevoer, those disciplines constituted the link between medicine as a *Wissenschaft* and natural philosophy, thus distinguishing physicians from healers of lower social rank. Even Hufeland repeatedly underscored the importance of the theoretical subjects for medical education, though merely as propaedeutic for bedside practice.[38] However, for those physicians who felt that a true *Wissenschaft* of medicine ought to link theory and practice, this probably did not suffice. As we have seen, it certainly did not satisfy Erhard. And it also did not suffice for a group of dissident physicians who began preaching the medical theory of an outcast Scottish physician by the name of John Brown.

THE COMING OF THE BRUNONIAN REVOLUTION

The heart of the medical system described by John Brown in his *Elementa medicinae* (1780) lay in his view of life as an enforced rather than a spontaneous condition. Brown rejected the common eighteenth-century viewpoint – held by his teacher, William Cullen (1710–90), among many others – of life as the product of some fundamental force. He claimed instead that life only occurred as a result of stimuli impinging on matter possessing a quality Brown called "irritability." The activity resulting from the interaction of the two factors constituted life, and in the absence of either factor – the stimulus or the irritable material – life could not be present. Brown further proposed that organic bodies have only a finite amount of irritability, and external stimuli can cause it to be used up. In cases of extreme amounts of stimulation, he believed, irritability can actually sink to zero, resulting in death. On the other hand, when the quantity of external stimuli diminishes, total stimulation also declines, which allows irritability to be replenished. At all times, irritability reacts gradually to the quantity of external stimuli so as to restore a constant level of stimulation.[39]

This conception of physiology had direct relevance for pathology and therapy. Because life consisted of the stimulation produced by an external stimulus acting on excitable matter, Brown regarded the condition of health as a balanced relationship between the two. Should there be a marked change in the level of external stimuli, the balance would be upset, and the individual would suffer from either over- or understimulation. Brown appeared to assume that irritability could not immediately adjust to large changes in external stimuli, and it was during those

38 See Christoph Wilhelm Hufeland "Ueber Aerzte und Routiniers," in *Journal der practischen Heil-kunde* 21 (1805):10–12; and idem, *Eine Wort an meine künftigen Zuhörer als Ankündigung meiner auf Ostern anzufangenden Vorlesungen* (Jena, 1793).
39 Summary descriptions of Brown's theory are presented in Karl Rothschuh, *Konzepte der Medizin in Vergangenheit und Gegenwart* (Stuttgart, 1978), pp. 345–50, and more extensively in Risse, *History of John Brown's Medical System*, pp. 101–34.

periods of disequilibrium that illness occurred. Brown called the condition of overstimulation "sthenia," and the opposite condition "asthenia." Because external stimuli varied only in quantity and never in quality, Brown argued, all diseases could be classed as either sthenic or asthenic. These comprised the two basic types of illness in Brown's scheme.[40] Treatment was correspondingly simple. One had only to diagnose the disease to determine the proper treatment, which consisted either of increasing or decreasing the total quantity of stimuli supplied to the patient, by means of diet, exercise, or medicaments. Brown especially favored the use of brandy and opium, which he saw as strengthening agents for asthenic diseases.

The distinctiveness of Brown's theory is that it drew clear diagnostic and therapeutic consequences from a simple, unified pathological principle. Furthermore, Brown's pathology did not posit illness as a specific entity or distorted function inherent in some portion of the body, but as a general relationship between the organism and the environment. Brunonian doctrine therefore fulfilled Erhard's call for a medical practice based on the "real" causes of disease rather than on divination of the meaning of symptoms. Along with Erhard, the Brunonians could tear down the entire edifice of accepted medical practice – nosology, prognosis, the doctrines of crisis and critical days, therapeutic indications and counter-indications. However, where Erhard had offered only criticism, Brunonianism offered an alternative. Brunonianism now stood ready to complete what Erhard had begun, and to inaugurate a revolution in German medicine.

Therein, of course, lay its appeal, and in Germany Brunonianism became a symbol for overthrow of the medical establishment. The first writer to introduce Brown's doctrine in the 1790s, Melchior Adam Weikard (1742–1803), used his outline of the system, published in 1795, as a platform from which to hurl bombs at the university medical faculties.[41] Invoking the primitivism that had proved so potent in Rousseau's social commentary, Weikard likened contemporary university medicine to a young child of nature (*Naturmädchen*) who has been removed from the purity and innocence of the countryside and who, once in the city, enters into elegant society. Predictably, in such surroundings she becomes accustomed to "luxury" and "coquetry," and surrenders her former virtue(s) to the corrupting influence of admirers. Only by means of the Brunonian system, Weikard proclaimed, could the maiden be purified of such decadence and corruption, and

40 Brown also defined a third condition, called "indirect asthenia," which would occur when the level of overstimulation became so extreme that it threatened to exhaust the body's supply of irritability. This would lead to a kind of prostration and weakness that resembles direct asthenia in its symptomatic manifestation, but in fact would require entirely different treatment.
41 Weikard in fact was not the first person to introduce Brown's ideas into Germany, and the occasion of their introduction is a story in itself. In 1790, a plagiarized version of Brown's theory was published in the French *Journal de physique* by the Göttingen physician, Christoph Girtanner. Girtanner, who had learned of Brown's system while traveling in Edinburgh, was even cheeky enough to declare that "his" ideas had found a favorable reception in Edinburgh when he had presented them there. The story is recounted by Risse in *History of John Brown's Medical System*, pp. 137–56.

restored to her original simplicity. "Admittedly the majority of elegant men from the city will forsake the unadorned maiden," he added "but in her simple, natural state she will also find sincere suitors who will prevail by far over the gallant dandies (*Fats*)."[42]

If it accomplished nothing else, Weikard's inflammatory denunciation of the university medical faculties ensured that the German debut of Brunonianism would be accompanied by raucous controversy. The response from the other side was swift and it matched Weikard's polemics thunderbolt for thunderbolt. In fact, the first review of the new Brunonian literature, published in the *Allgemeine Literatur-Zeitung* late in 1795, considerably surpassed Weikard's rhetoric, establishing its own standard of excess. The reviewer claimed that Brown had developed his system based on the effects of wine on his own person, which admittedly were sometimes extremely invigorating, but on other occasions so depressing that Brown could be found lying drunken in the streets. This in itself was reason enough not to take Brown's ideas seriously. "Of such a system," the reviewer scoffed, "which from the beginning was the object of derision, not much could be expected."[43] Nor was Weikard, Brown's evangelist to the German people, spared the reviewer's abuse. He pointed out that it was only to be expected that the universities would be a mote in Weikard's eye, since in his autobiography Weikard had admitted to never having enjoyed a rational academic education or having studied his profession systematically:

All such men rail at university education because they do not know it, and hold it for mere scholastic nonsense and useless formalisms because they have learned something without it. But they prove through their own example that they lack what only a university education can give: orderly thinking, a systematic connection of materials, and thorough knowledge.[44]

Such language warmed the debate over Brunonianism by several degrees, but in truth the Brunonians needed little prompting from the other side to present their mission not just as a reform of medicine, but as a complete revolution and the inauguration of a new era. Just as the Jacobins had leveled the ramshackle institutions of the ancien régime in pursuit of a purer society, so too would Brown's partisans overturn the German medical profession. One reviewer of a Brunonian treatise caught the contemporary mood quite vividly: "While the political systems of our age have been shaken by powerful revolutions, no less significant changes have threatened the scientific [systems]. . . . Everywhere, one sees contemporaries striving, only too often with youthful impetuosity, not so much to repair the aging structure [of science] as to erect a new one on the ruins of the old." This spirit of revolution, the reviewer went on, has freed science and medicine from their servitude to the past. The former bonds of authority have

42 Melchior Adam Weikard, *Entwurf einer einfachen Arzneykunst, oder Erläuterung und Bestätigung der Brownischen Arzneylehre* (Frankfurt, 1795), pp. vii–viii.
43 *Allgemeine Literatur-Zeitung*, 12 October 1795, col. 73.
44 Ibid., 13 October 1795, cols. 86–7.

dissolved, and a new freedom of inquiry has taken their place: "The time is past when one can stamp out the sprouting of new ideas with political or scientific dogmas, or cripple the spirit of investigation with fiats such as 'the True is old, and the New is untrue.'" As far-reaching as these revolutionary changes have been in themselves, the reviewer explained, even more significantly they have cleared the way for the dramatic and epochal introduction of Brunonianism into Germany.

Finally there was brought to the site of battle a system which first had to wander through southern Europe before exerting an influence on Germany, an influence that perhaps it will never enjoy in its northern fatherland. Never was there contrived a system that shook the existing medical theories so deeply to their foundations, started out from so few ideas, and in its simple progress was so similar to the course of Nature (which it describes) as Brown's system.[45]

Such language, although uncommon in supposedly impartial reviews, filled the pages of many a preface to works on Brunonian medicine. Brunonianism found its most enthusiastic following among the alienated generation of young people born in the 1770s, the same generation from which the early Romantics and *Naturphilosophen* came, who experienced the French Revolution as adolescents or young men. In this regard it was hardly accidental that Brunonianism appeared at just the time when medical enrollments at German universities were at the highest levels they had ever reached, and this after more than a decade of sharp increases.[46] In 1795, there were, comparatively speaking, a lot of young physicians or medical students in Germany. Weikard, although himself anything but a young man, nonetheless appreciated the attractiveness of Brown's ideas for younger physicians. Anyone knowing the German medical profession, he declared, could have predicted the defenders of Brunonianism would be those who practiced not merely out of published compendia, but with a "penetrating spirit," as well as "younger, unbiased doctors whose earnest intention it is to distinguish themselves in their medical practices."[47]

The revolutionary appeal of Brunonianism was not lost on its numerous detractors either, which they unhesitatingly blamed on the contemporary mood. Hecker, indulging in his customary hyperbole, called Weikard's writings "literary sansculottism." Hufeland, for his part, maintained a more dignified reserve, reacting to the Brunonians' revolutionary rhetoric less stridently, but no less pointedly. "We assure these gentlemen," he declared on one occasion, "that we detect not the slightest need for a revolution."[48]

45 *Medicinisch-chirurgische Zeitung*, 4 January 1798, pp. 9–11.
46 On the increasing population of medical students toward the end of the eighteenth century, see Chapter 2.
47 Quoted in *Journal der Erfindungen, Theorien, und Widersprüche in der Natur- und Arzneywissenschaften* 3 (1795): 115–6.
48 August Friedrich Hecker, "Auch eine Geschichte des Brownischen Systems," *Journal der Erfindungen, Theorien, und Widersprüche in der Natur- und Arzneywissenschaft* 4 (1796): 92; and Hufeland, "Bemerkungen über die Brownische Praxis," p. 129.

Other older physicians berated their younger colleagues for being so vulnerable to the allures of deceptively simple systems and for their unwillingness to learn medicine the hard way, through experience at the bedside. Noteworthy in this regard was the claim made by the reviewer in the *Allgemeine Literatur-Zeitung* that Brown had had "little experience" when he developed his theories.[49] Hufeland's reply to Erhard in the *Teutscher Merkur* implied the same thing, and he also used it against Andreas Röschlaub (1768–1835), a leader of the German Brunonians, stating that Röschlaub had had little practical experience when he took up Brunonian ideas, whereas his own approach to medicine grew out of years of practice.[50] Another writer blamed the friction between older and younger physicians on both sides, with older doctors not taking their young colleagues seriously and being too content to remain in the ruts of their established methods, and young doctors being unwilling to pay experience its proper due. Although the writer urged compromise on both sides, he added "but in particular the young doctors should be more deferential."[51] Compromise, apparently, was desirable, but submission to authority was even better.

The same dismissive attitude toward young medical practitioners carried over into guides for medical practice. The Heidelberg professor Franz Anton Mai (1742–1814) wrote one of the most popular of these manuals, a five part work entitled *Stolpertus, ein junger Arzt am Krankenbett* (1777–1807). In each installment of his book, Mai took a fictitious young colleague by the name of Stolpertus (*stolpern* means "to stumble") through some of the more perplexing difficulties facing the practitioner, advising beginners on how to interview patients so as to get the most information possible; how to treat women; how to select medicaments carefully, not putting too much reliance in their own powers as physicians; and much more. Although Mai wrote his book with considerable good humor and self-deprecating concessions to the mistakes of his own past, his tone expressed the conviction that he was now in a position to pass judgment on those mistakes and those of younger physicians in general.

Among the more serious mistakes that Mai saw younger doctors making was giving themselves over entirely to Brunonianism and rejecting the medical practice of their elders. He characterized the typical young Brunonian zealot as consumed with self-love, and described the consequences of his narcissism:

All of his actions carry the stamp of this most beloved temptress; at the bedside, in his study, in consultations, everywhere she peeks out, like the ass under the lion's skin. The young doctor never wants to learn of his mistakes, and should another, more experienced doctor take it into his head not to underscore the young doctor's opinions at the bedside, then does his breast swell and his head burn. . . .

49 *Allgemeine Literatur-Zeitung* 12 October 1795, col. 73.
50 Christoph Wilhelm Hufeland, "Des Herausgebers Erklärung an das Publikum über sein System der practischen Heilkunde und einige von ihm herauszugebende Schriften," *Journal der practischen Heilkunde* 7 (1799): 185.
51 "Über Collegialität der Ärzte," *Allgemeine medicinische Annalen* (1806), col. 1,140.

I had the pleasure [Mai continued] of knowing such a medical Don Quixote, who still had university lather behind his ears, and who nonetheless, at least with his mouth, cut down all illnesses like marionettes. Armed with the fool's cap of his self-love, ... he rode unashamedly over all his honorable, meritorious colleagues, and through this raving display he robbed himself of an indispensable aid, of which every reasonable young doctor should make use, if ... he truly wants to be useful to his fellow citizens.[52]

As the rhetorical denunciations from both sides makes clear, the conflict over Brunonianism was deeply embedded in a wider generational conflict. Much of the language accompanying Brunonianism repeated the clamor that resounded elsewhere through German public life in response to the French Revolution. Young people marched in the streets, exuberantly singing the *Marseillaise;* their parents covered their ears and scurried for safety. It was an opportunity for new beginnings. But within the medical profession, the generational conflict acquired still more significant meanings. There, breaking the shackles of history meant much more than clearing the ground of past ruins and starting afresh. Brunonianism meant eliminating history itself as a methodology and as a justification of medical practice. It also meant toppling the hierarchical structure of medicine that treated young physicians as second-class doctors.

THE FRUITION OF THE BRUNONIAN SYSTEM

Melchior Adam Weikard, having inaugurated the Brunonian movement in Germany, tirelessly continued to proselytize for it. For the next few years after 1795, he spread the gospel through published guides to Brunonian practice, translations of treatises by major Italian followers of Brown, and a Brunonian medical journal. Despite Weikard's endeavors, however, there was more bluster than substance to the movement. Although the critique offered by Brunonians of contemporary medical theory and practice, especially the latter, was powerful enough, it had not yet become clear that Brunonianism presented a satisfactory alternative. The problem was that young physicians who rejected the medical *Wissenschaft* of established physicians had not rejected the notion of a unified system of medicine. Like Erhard, they looked to philosophy to supply the operative rules of a medical *Wissenschaft* that would replace the current doctrines.

Brunonianism was not yet such a system, for it lacked an adequate grounding in philosophical analysis. Brown himself had been mainly interested in reforming medical practice, and he developed his pathological theory only far enough to suggest a justification for his methods. Nor was Weikard interested in developing it systematically as a university *Wissenschaft.* From his viewpoint, the last thing he would have wanted was a theoretical system resembling the refuse churned out by the medical faculties. Weikard fully appreciated the challenge posed by Brunonian

52 Franz Anton Mai, *Stolpertus ein junger Arzt am Krankenbette,* Bd. 3, "Stolpertus ein junger Browni-aner am Krankenbette von einem patriotischen Pfälzer" (Mannheim, 1798), pp. 162–3.

medicine to existing doctrines, but he would not be the one to press that challenge home in medical theory.

In addition to the lack of a sufficient theoretical grounding, Brunonianism also lacked an adequate practical basis. If Brunonian medicine was to be a true union of theory and practice, then experiences with it had to be collected and explained in terms of theory. It would not be enough for Weikard to publish articles from contributors saying they had tried it and found their patients recovered. This piling up of individual examples would merely reproduce the type of medical knowledge the Brunonians were fighting against. The new movement had to show not only that Brown's methods were efficacious, but also that theory was a reliable guidepost for practice, and clinical results could be explained by Brunonian theory.

The fate of German Brunonianism took a decisive turn with the appearance on the scene of two new and powerful advocates: Andreas Röschlaub and Adalbert Friedrich Marcus (1753–1816). Far from rejecting university medicine and its standards of *Wissenschaft,* Röschlaub, a professor at the University of Bamberg, and Marcus, director of the city hospital in Bamberg, were completely committed to them. Their work on behalf of Brunonianism – Röschlaub in theory and Marcus in clinical practice – made Bamberg the center of the German medical world for a short time between 1798 and 1803. Their elaboration of Brown's principles into a complete system of medical *Wissenschaft* put Brunonianism among the leading cultural forces of the day and linked it with other powerful intellectual currents such as *Naturphilosophie.* Schelling's own opinion of Brunonianism, in fact, illustrates well the transformation given Brown's theories by Marcus and, above all, by Röschlaub. At first, Schelling had considered Brown's theory as a rather crude and mechanistic picture of life, with living things passively jerked into action by external stimuli, as a puppet is animated by pulling on its strings. Röschlaub, however, presented Brunonian physiology more dialectically as an interplay between internal substance and external force and succeeded in convincing Schelling to treat it more favorably. Schelling was completely won over to the system, and for a time he and Röschlaub became close friends and collaborators.[53]

Röschlaub's and Marcus's work gave Brunonianism a much tighter bond between theory and practice than it might otherwise have had. However, by bringing Brunonian medicine within the orbit of university scholarship and by allying it with fashionable *Wissenschaften* such as *Naturphilosophie,* they also dulled some of its radical edge. Instead of toppling the entire structure of university medicine, with its concerns for proper *Wissenschaft,* from the outside, Röschlaub and Marcus sought to integrate Brunonianism into academic medical science. To be sure, they arrayed themselves and their medical system against the established powers in university medicine, but they did so to displace those powers, not to eliminate the

---

53 On the relations between Schelling and Röschlaub, see Tsouyopoulos, *Andreas Röschlaub,* pp. 162–5.

structure. In the long run, this would prove the undoing of Brunonianism as a self-conscious, unified movement.

Like his friend Erhard, Andreas Röschlaub applied Kantian criticism to medical theory in order to set it on firm foundations and then used that theory to prove the validity of Brunonian methods of practice. Life, he argued, must have two components. First there is the peculiar organization of its material substrate, but in addition to that there must be something else, because living things routinely die even when there is no demonstrable damage to their material condition, for example in old age. These cases imply the existence of an additional factor that for some reason fails, resulting in death.[54] This factor, Röschlaub declared, has its basis "in a characteristic form and mixture of matter, or rather, in the particular orientation of the efficacy which the forces of nature receive from the characteristic form and mixture of organic matter."[55] In basing what he called the "life principle" (*Lebensprinzip*) on a characteristic form and mixture of matter, Röschlaub explicitly tied his interpretation of Brunonianism to Reil's theory of physiology, and he made use of every possible opportunity to find points of agreement between himself and Reil.[56] Although Röschlaub saw a substrate for the *Lebensprinzip* in the form and mixture of matter, he did not believe it was totally dependent on material conditions. It was something both in matter and apart from matter. Having defined the criteria for the *Lebensprinzip*, Röschlaub pronounced Brown's concept of irritability the medical theory that corresponded most satisfactorily to its requirements.

Röschlaub then drew upon the consequences of these physiological concepts to justify Brown's pathology, a discussion he spun out over three long volumes of his *Untersuchungen über Pathogenie* (Investigations on pathogenesis, 1798–1800). The details of that discussion are not particularly important here; for the most part, Röschlaub followed Brown's precepts fairly closely. His primary concern was twofold: first, to justify the Brunonian doctrine through a rigorous exposition, and second, to denounce all other competing theories as fallacious. In Röschlaub's view, Brown's central insight was the perception that pathology and physiology are the same thing, or more precisely, that pathology is a branch of physiology. An explanation of disease does not require the introduction of special agents or forces; it simply originates in the same processes that support life.

This gave Röschlaub purchase to attack the dominant humoralist pathology of the time. By the eighteenth century, of course, physicians no longer held to the specifically Galenic doctrine of the four humors, but two important residues of that pathology remained. Physicians still looked for the causes of disease in specific material agents or in certain stimuli, such as emotional affects. And further, they often were inclined to search for those causes in connection with the body's fluids,

---

54 Andreas Röschlaub, *Untersuchungen über Pathogenie oder Einleitung in die medizinische Theorie*, Teil 1 (Frankfurt, 1798), pp. 85–6.
55 Ibid., pp. 211–2.
56 Ibid., pp. 148–9, 157–8, 162–4. On Reil's theory of physiology, see Chapter 3.

especially the blood. To Röschlaub this was nonsense. At best, such changes in the fluids, if they occurred at all, were only products of the disease, not its causes. The absurdity of humoral pathology, he believed, was displayed most fully by physicians who sought the causes of disease in either physical-mechanical or chemical problems with the blood or other bodily fluids.

Many among the medical rabble . . . talk endlessly of almost nothing but corruption of this or that fluid in the case of every internal, general illness without distinction. They assume a fluid has the strangest sorts of corruptions, and, after a fluid has wandered through the most diverse paths and settled itself in here or there, they give it the most extraordinary roles to play.

"To investigate the illness more deeply," he sneered, "does not occur to them."[57] In direct opposition to humoralist doctrine, Röschlaub denied that fluids have life. They are, he maintained, external to the living parts of the body, carrying material to them and stimulating them in various ways, but not themselves capable of falling ill.

Röschlaub's systematization of Brunonianism in the *Untersuchungen* transformed Brown's rather sketchy ideas into a fully elaborated *Wissenschaft*. As important as this was for widening its appeal, Röschlaub saw clearly that a Brunonian theory of physiology and pathology alone would not suffice to revolutionize the medical profession. The truly radical possibilities offered by Brunonianism lay in its joining the theory to a completely new approach to practice. Röschlaub pointed to this potential in explaining why the medical establishment found Brown's ideas so dangerous:

For in this original work [of Brown's] it is not only a question of the overthrow of mere theoretical principles, of a mere alteration in the explanation of the phenomena of diseased organisms, as it has been up to now with most new theories. Here it is a matter of a complete revolution in . . . practical medicine just as much as in theoretical [medicine]. And, worst of all, it is a matter of demonstrating that the practical methods (*Praktik*) that have up to now been applied and taught by most physicians in the majority of internal illnesses are erroneous, unfounded, and mostly harmful.[58]

Although the *Untersuchungen über Pathogenie* laid the foundations of the Brunonian system in physiology and pathology, a companion volume by Röschlaub, *Von dem Einfluße der Brown'schen Theorie in die praktischen Heilkunde* (On the influence of the Brunonian theory in practical medicine, 1798), discussed how Brunonian theory applies to bedside practice. The first problem facing the practitioner, he wrote, is to determine whether an illness is general or local. Röschlaub stressed that this can only be made on the basis of the causes of the condition, not the symptoms, and it requires that the physician bring into consideration all the "harmful influences" that might have affected or are affecting the patient at

57 Ibid., pp. 35–6.
58 Ibid., p. 39.

present. If those influences affect the level of stimulation alone, the illness is general. If, however, the influences have changed the body's form and mixture then the disorder is local. Röschlaub cautioned his readers that any particular group of symptoms could be the product of either a local or general illness, and he illustrated this with the case of a patient having either a fever, convulsions, or diarrhea. If the physician should discover that the patient had recently been exposed to harmful influences such as too little food, thin or watery drink, loss of fluids, or "depressive affects such as fright, anxiety, or sorrow," then he could safely conclude that the malaise was general. Likewise, the existence of harmful influences such as a wound, splinter, or a strong suppuration on the patient's body would imply a local illness.[59]

Assuming that etiological considerations pointed to a general illness, the physician next had to decide whether it was sthenic or asthenic. Here again, Röschlaub warned his readers that they must rely not on symptoms but on the nature of the influences acting on the patient. To illustrate this, he presented the hypothetical case of a man falling ill who had always lived quietly, simply, and moderately, but who recently had been exposed to "lively company" and "better food and drink"; here is an obvious case of sthenia. If, however, the physician discovers that the patient had previously experienced debilitating influences such as "hidden dissatisfaction and vexation," poor nutrition, or a chill, the patient's illness would be asthenia.[60]

Taken together, Röschlaub's *Untersuchungen* and *Von dem Einfluße der Brown'schen Theorie* presented a fully developed system of Brunonian theory and practice. However even a completed system, encompassing everything from the definition of irritability to methods of diagnosis, did not finish the job facing the Brunonians. Opponents could and did argue that although Röschlaub had constructed a pretty castle of words, Brunonianism nevertheless did not work and their own methods did. Brunonianism still had to be brought to the bedside for its ultimate justification. A number of works did this, the most important of which was *Prüfung des Brownischen Systems* by Adalbert Friedrich Marcus, Röschlaub's colleague in Bamberg. As director of the city hospital, Marcus had at his disposal the facilities that would allow him to put Brunonian methods to the test, and he published the *Prüfung* proclaiming it to be the results of his "impartial" examination.

In form, Marcus' *Prüfung* closely resembled the reports from other clinics and hospitals that were appearing in the years around 1800. The reports consisted of two basic sections, each serving a distinct purpose. First, there was a general overview of the cases handled during a given time period, most commonly a three-month season. This summary included the total number of patients admitted, and of those the number who died, recovered, or remained in the institu-

59 Andreas Röschlaub, *Von dem Einfluße der Brown'schen Theorie in die praktischen Heilkunde* (Würzburg, 1798), p. 26.
60 Röschlaub, *Von dem Einfluße*, pp. 48–9.

tion.[61] Alongside a summary of the numbers and characteristics of the illnesses handled, these reports invariably included a description of the prevailing weather conditions: daily temperatures, precipitation and humidity, and wind direction. The inclusion of climatic factors reflected physicians' conviction, reaching at least as far back as Hippocrates and based on a type of humoral pathology, that the illnesses occurring in a certain area shared a generic character, and this character in turn was at least partly determined by the weather.[62]

Marcus retained this practice of reporting weather conditions in the *Prüfung*, although as a Brunonian he had no use for traditional epidemiology. Illness was a product of dynamic stimulation, pure and simple; there existed no specific disease entities that could be correlated with weather conditions. This, however, did not mean that weather had no influence of any kind on the types of illness. Brown had taught that temperature exerted a powerful influence on the total level of stimuli affecting an individual. This being the case, Marcus argued that Brown's theory suggested the occurrence of sthenia would be greater when temperatures were above normal, and he presented evidence to show how this prediction was borne out by the monthly distribution of patients in Bamberg.[63]

Marcus also used the introductory review of the hospital's cases to make an inductive argument for the efficacy of Brown's methods. The report he gave of their results with opium was particularly glowing. "Opium proved itself throughout in all illnesses of weakness as the most superior strengthening agent. It raised the patients' strength more rapidly and durably than all others."[64] At the same time, Marcus did not rest content with showing how his results testified to the correctness of Brunonian doctrine. He also used his results to attack prevailing views of pathology and therapy. His favorite target was the so-called "gastric" pathology, yet another variant of humoralism in which the material cause of disease was taken to originate and exert its primary effects in the stomach or bowels. The cause could be a putrefied bit of feces, a foreign body in the digestive

---

61 Adalbert Friedrich Marcus, *Prüfung des Brownischen Systems*, Stück 2 (Weimar, 1798) p. v. In most such reports, this section served to advertise to patrons – if not to patients, who would not have been persuaded in any case – the superior quality of the clinic's care, and judging by the impressive cure rates boasted in them, one wonders that people died of anything but old age at that time. For example, Marcus wrote that between April and June of 1798, the Bamberg hospital admitted 134 patients (including 30 remaining from the previous quarter), and of those 134, 102 were cured, 7 died, 3 were released without being cured, and 22 remained in the hospital at the end of the quarter. Assuming the numbers to be true, one explanation for the success of these hospitals is that many were loath to accept patients with truly nasty infectious diseases like smallpox, on the not-unreasonable grounds that such people could cause an epidemic within the institution's confined quarters. See Guenter B. Risse, *Hospital Life in Enlightenment Scotland* (Cambridge, 1986), p. 136.

62 This notion was based on the assumption that a given disease had a specific material cause, or miasma, originating outside the body, and that each variety of miasma was favored by a different set of environmental conditions. For a discussion of Hippocratic epidemiology in the eighteenth century, see Christian Probst, *Der Weg des ärztlichen Erkennens am Krankenbett*, Sudhoffs Archiv Beiheft 15 (Wiesbaden, 1972), pp. 10–18.

63 Marcus, *Prüfung des Brownischen Systems*, Stück 1, pp. 84–5.

64 Ibid., p. 90.

system, or incompletely digested food. Hufeland, for one, considered the digestive system especially susceptible to such irritants, with the effect that many fevers had symptoms of distension and tenderness of the abdomen, nausea and loss of appetite, and foulness of feces.[65] The fevers that seemed to provide the best evidence for gastric pathology were the typhoid-type "nervous" and "putrid" fevers, which at that time were considered quite dangerous. On the basis of the assumed affliction of the digestive system, physicians directed their therapies toward "cleaning up" the entire gastro-intestinal tract through a combination of emetics and purgatives.[66] Marcus denounced the widespread use of this method, saying results at Bamberg proved that it was exceedingly harmful.

When the older anti-gastric method was applied to nervous and putrid fevers, the patients declined into a severe weakness, and several died. The rest could only be saved with great effort, and in all cases the convalescence was extremely slow. But when the strengthening method was applied to nervous and putrid fevers from the beginning, not only did the gastric symptoms disappear, but healing occurred just as rapidly as recovery, with no danger of relapses.[67]

This ringing endorsement was repeated in a later issue, when Marcus declared they had given up using the gastric method completely. "Not one single time did we find it necessary to resort to emetics or purgatives."[68]

Marcus also noted that they had not observed crises in any of their cases of fever. "Critical evacuations (*Ausleerungen*) were not observed; on the contrary the patients were in the greatest danger when diarrhea or profuse sweating was present."[69] The absence of crisis in any of Marcus's cases knocked a crucial pillar out from under Hippocratic doctrine, for this was tantamount to saying that there was no healing power of nature working to aid recovery. Röschlaub's *Untersuchungen über Pathogenie* had repeatedly assailed the notion of an internal healing power, which he lambasted as just another occult power.[70] Now Marcus added the force of his empirical evidence to Röschlaub's theoretical argument.

The second part of each volume of Marcus's *Prüfung* consisted of a dozen or so detailed case histories chosen from the patients treated in the hospital. We have already seen how case histories performed a vital function in the type of medicine the Brunonians were trying to replace, but in Brunonianism itself case histories as such were left with little to do. As chronicles of disease, they offered nothing of value; at best they recorded only the causal influences acting on the patient and

65 Christoph Wilhelm Hufeland, *Ideen über Pathogenie* (Jena, 1795), p. 38.
66 This therapeutic approach is described in Risse, *Hospital Life in Enlightenment Scotland*, pp. 177–82. Also useful is Lester S. King, *The Medical World of the Eighteenth Century* (Chicago, 1958), pp. 297–325.
67 Marcus, *Prüfung*, Stück 1, pp. 88–9.
68 Ibid., Stück 2, p. viii.
69 Ibid., Stück 1, p. 89.
70 Röschlaub, *Untersuchungen*, Teil 1, pp. 196–8.

the triumph of the Brunonian doctor's accurate diagnosis and successful treatment. The advantage of case histories for Marcus was that they illustrated those very successes far more vividly and convincingly than any summary description, and he applied them skillfully to this rhetorical purpose. Marcus also applied individual case histories to the didactic mission of reiterating the particular Brunonian teachings confirmed by the case, thereby transforming them into fables depicting the triumph and efficacy of Brunonian theory. He took special care to select a good number of cases showing the deleterious effects of patients having received gastric treatments from an assortment of unenlightened healers before being admitted to the Bamberg hospital. In one stubbornly difficult early case, Marcus himself even ventured a gastric treatment on a patient.[71] As always, the patient became worse before recovering eventually under the proper Brunonian methods, and Marcus blithely tallied it up as still another example of how hopelessly inadequate the method of gastric treatment was. Over the four volumes of the *Prüfung*, Marcus did not credit the gastric method with having worked in one single case.

The work of Marcus and Röschlaub at Bamberg represented the high-water mark of German Brunonianism. They demonstrated that Brunonianism was far more than just an outpouring of resentment from a pack of young ideologues and older cranks like Weikard. In their hands it came as close as it ever would to being the complete and seamless union of theory and practice. By joining theory to practice, Marcus and Röschlaub opened the door to a radically new form of medical practice. Marcus's *Prüfung* presented narratives of control; its lesson was that disease could be cured through domination. The prescriptions for operation of the Bamberg hospital regulated everything in the patients' environment down to the smallest detail, extending even to housing sthenic patients in cool rooms and asthenic patients in warm ones, and preparing and administering meals in strict accordance with Brunonian precepts.[72] Just as importantly, Brunonian medicine cast a dramatically new light on the patient and, by implication, on the doctor's relationship with patients. By the precepts of Brunonian theory, the individual patient shriveled down to nothing more than a substrate for the reception of external stimuli. The patient was drained of individuality, becoming instead a walking embodiment of the universal processes that constitute life.

---

71 Marcus, *Prüfung*, Stück 1, pp. 116–21.
72 In this respect it is noteworthy that the American physician Benjamin Rush (1745–1813), who denied unequivocally any healing power of nature and advocated strenuous therapeutic interventions by medical practitioners, had studied at Edinburgh and was influenced by Brunonian doctrine. On one occasion, Rush declared: "Always treat nature in a sick room as you would a noisy dog or cat[;] drive her out at the door & lock it upon her." For a comprehensive discussion of therapeutic doctrine in early nineteenth-century America, see John Harley Warner, *The Therapeutic Perspective: Medical Practice, Knowledge, and Identity in America, 1820–1885* (Cambridge, Mass., 1986), pp. 11–36, quoted from Rush on p. 18.

CONCLUSION: WHITHER BRUNONIANISM?

It only remains to explain what happened to the Brunonian revolution. If the bright days at Bamberg in the years right around 1800 signalled the dawning of a new medical age, what happened to it? Did Brunonianism succeed in revolutionizing German medical theory and practice? If by this question we mean did Brunonianism produce major transformations of German medical theory and practice, then the movement would have to be judged a success. It forged a far tighter link between pathology and physiology than any that had existed previously, and this had important consequences for the medical *Wissenschaften* of the 1810s. Brunonianism also profoundly altered the conception of disease held even by its staunchest opponents. Readers who did not know anything about Hufeland before cracking open the first volume of his *System der practischen Heilkunde* in 1800 would likely get the impression that Hufeland was a Brunonian. Gone from the theoretical section was the concept, presented in Hufeland's previous monograph on pathology, the *Ideen über Pathogenie*, of a *Lebenskraft* which by its action canceled the normal operation of physico-mechanical and chemical forces. Now the talk was all of external stimuli and irritability. The very word, *Lebenskraft*, had dropped out of sight completely. In the practical section, the reader would have found row upon row of diseases placed under the general headings of sthenia and asthenia – Hufeland even found it appropriate to create a category of indirect asthenia.[73] So readily did Hufeland incorporate Brunonian doctrines into his medical picture that he once even had to defend himself in writing against a reviewer's charge that he had been strongly influenced by Brunonianism.[74] Hecker too was confronted by similar charges. One lingering legacy of Brunonianism after its disappearance as an organized movement was the tendency of German physicians to emphasize illness as a dynamic problem affecting the entire organism, rather than a localized and material affliction. For this reason many Germans were conspicuously unreceptive to the pathological anatomy of Bichat and his successors in France.

If, however, we ask if Brunonianism succeeded in creating a unified medical theory and practice, then the answer would have to be no. It failed to revolutionize university medicine, and theory and practice went their separate ways in the medical faculties of the Restoration period. Hufeland, Hecker, and the other foes of Brunonianism could so effortlessly and almost unconsciously incorporate Brunonian methods of practice into their own medical kits because the methods themselves had never been the issue for them. It was the claim for the *exclusive*

---

73 Christoph Wilhelm Hufeland, *System der practischen Heilkunde*, Bd. 1, 2nd ed. (Jena, 1818), pp. 264–5.

74 Among other things, Hufeland complained that he had come up with his ideas of illness "long" before anyone had heard of Brown. "It shows little philosophical knowledge of the state of *Wissenschaft*, . . . and even less patriotism when one attributes even German accomplishments to the English account, as appears to be fashionable these days. . . ." *Medicinisch-chirurgische Zeitung* 24 May 1798, pp. 287–8, quoted on p. 288.

efficacy of those methods, based in Brunonianism being a philosophical *Wissenschaft* of medicine, which they had opposed. So they adopted much of the Brunonians' therapeutic approach while rejecting the systematic basis for those methods.

The failure of Brunonianism to establish itself over the long run as a *Wissenschaft* of medical practice can be traced to a number of other factors, some of them institutional and others intellectual. One of them was the inability of its advocates to separate themselves sufficiently from traditional medicine. Marcus and Röschlaub retained the medical language of their predecessors, thereby binding themselves as well to the world view contained in that language, however much they attempted to escape it. The cases reported in Marcus's *Prüfung*, for example, were not endless repetitions of "Geschichte einer Asthenie," (because the Bamberg clinic handled scant numbers of sthenic cases), but talked instead about dropsies, nervous fevers, pneumonias, and colics. This retention of the symptomatic characterization of diseases caused opponents to suspect that what Brunonian physicians really did, in spite of their loud proclamations to the contrary, was first to diagnose a disease symptomatically like everyone else, and then designate it as a sthenic or asthenic illness on the basis of the first diagnosis. As one critic pointed out, Brown himself certainly had not scrupled at ordering illnesses according to the common nosologies and then further classifying them as sthenias or asthenias.[75] Obviously, the revolutionary claims of Brunonian medicine would be greatly attenuated if the supposedly fundamental categories of sthenia and asthenia turned out to depend on symptomatic diagnoses, with all their nasty intrusions of disease's manifestation in unique individuals.

Furthermore, Röschlaub added to his own difficulties by tinkering incessantly with the theory to such an extent that no one could ever be entirely sure just what it claimed. His most frequent reply to critics was that they misunderstood what he had said, proceeding then to clarify his meaning while modifying his stance. As a result of these constant changes, Röschlaub came to accept some role for the healing power of Nature in illnesses. And most surprising of all, his shifting position eventually brought him to arguing (as if he had come up with the idea!) that medical practice could not be mere applied theory, but required teaching by example and experience at the bedside.[76] Given these shifts by one of the movement's leading spokesmen, observers might be forgiven for losing their place in the argument.

Other developments may also have played a role in the failure of the Brunonian revolution. One of these was the attack launched by Schelling and other *Naturphilosophen* on Röschlaub and Brunonianism. The causes of this surprising falling-

---

75 *Allgemeine Literatur-Zeitung*, 29 November 1799, pp. 537–8.
76 Andreas Röschlaub, *Lehrbuch der Nosologie* (Bamberg, 1802), pp. 49–50. On Röschlaub's new claims for medical practice, see Tsouyopoulos, *Andreas Röschlaub*, p. 139ff, which, however, fails to point out that this represents a departure from Röschlaub's earlier views, as expressed in *Von dem Einfluße der Brown'schen Theorie*.

out have never been clear. Rivalry for leadership of the new medical sciences may have had a hand in it,[77] but a more likely explanation is a parting of ways. Schelling and the medical *Naturphilosophen* ultimately came to view the physiological theory of Brunonianism as too narrow, and its view of the individual as too passive. It was also a matter of different goals. Röschlaub's physiology extended only far enough to provide a sufficient grounding for pathology and therapeutics. The *Naturphilosophen*, meanwhile, did not think of physiology as a mere handmaiden of practice; they wanted to study the processes of the living world for their own sake. In any case, the attack by the *Naturphilosophen* weakened the claims of Brunonianism to being a philosophical *Wissenschaft*. The quarrel between Röschlaub and the *Naturphilosophen* attracted considerable attention from contemporaries including Hufeland, who seemed to find no irony in praising the *Naturphilosophen* for "shattering these false idols."[78]

Finally, Brunonianism became a victim of the larger political transformations that were beginning to take place in Central Europe. Medical enrollments declined precipitously immediately after 1800, as the French armies began occupying large areas of Germany. Numerous universities either closed down or were reorganized during those years, including Bamberg, which became a surgical academy after the ecclesiastical principality of Bamberg was dissolved along with the Holy Roman Empire and its territories given over to Bavaria.[79] Not until peace was finally restored in 1815 would enrollments begin to recover. And by the time they did, Brunonianism was a specter of the past, while the movement for a unified medical theory and practice had fragmented into several distinct enterprises.

77 Nelly Tsouyopoulos, "Der Streit zwischen Friedrich Wilhelm Joseph Schelling und Andreas Röschlaub über die Grundlagen der Medizin," *Medizinhistorisches Journal* 13 (1978): 229–46. In Tsouyopoulos' view, Schelling realized that Röschlaub was going to succeed in reforming medicine without subordinating medical practice to *Naturphilosophie* and attacked Röschlaub out of jealousy. However, this explanation, even if it could account for Schelling's own actions, does not extend to why other *Naturphilosophen* joined the criticism. Schelling's jealousy may have had a role, but other factors must also have contributed.

78 *Journal der practischen Heilkunde* 27 (1808): 131.

79 For an account of the checkered career of the medical school in Bamberg after 1803, see P. Boehmer, *Die medizinische Schulen Bambergs in der ersten Hälfte des 19. Jahrhunderts* (med. Diss., Erlangen-Nürnberg, 1970).

6

German academic medicine during the reform era

Revolutions do not conform to a single historical pattern. Some follow a logic of development that builds to a radical denouement, while others may incorporate moments of radicalism, but never reach a climactic resolution. Instead, they simply lose energy gradually, like a hurricane whose force is spent by traveling over land. Beyond any question, the Brunonian revolution resembled the second kind. As the first years of the nineteenth century slipped by, the energy and rancor of the debate over Brunonianism diminished noticeably. This was so much the case that by 1811, when Andreas Röschlaub published a letter in the *Journal der practischen Heilkunde* declaring in effect that he no longer held to the principles of Brunonianism, the gesture had little dramatic impact. Hufeland, the editor of the *Journal,* permitted himself a smug, self-congratulatory observation to mark the occasion, but the moment passed largely unnoticed.[1]

Although the final act of the Brunonian revolution may have played before a nearly empty house, its impact on German medical theory and practice was substantial. At least for the short term, the most significant product of the controversies over Brunonianism was the construction of a stout wall between theory and practice. The great majority of physicians who wrote on practice after 1810 continued to speak of it in terms of a *Kunst* characterized by the physician's creative synthesis of judgment, experience, and talent. Meanwhile, non-clinical members of medical faculties enjoyed the freedom to pursue their interests in a setting largely unencumbered by considerations of how their research might inform or threaten practical doctrines. Nor were university faculties alone in acknowledging the separation of theory and practice. In 1811, the editors of the *Allgemeine medizinische Annalen* decided that henceforth they would publish the monthly as two separate issues, an *Annalen der Heilkunde* containing materials of theoretical interest, and an *Annalen der Heilkunst* aimed at practitioners.

If the aftermath of the Brunonian controversy encouraged theorists and practitioners to stay out of each other's way, such inclinations received ample reinforce-

---

1 For Röschlaub's letter, see *Journal der practischen Heilkunde* 32, no. 1 (1811): 9–21. Hufeland's reply was printed in the next issue, pp. 3–29.

ment from the development of university medical faculties after 1800. Led by reforms initiated by Baden at Heidelberg and Bavaria at Würzburg and Landshut (the former University of Ingolstadt), the universities of German-speaking Europe were restructured in several ways. New statutes carried on the project begun in the preceding century of subordinating the universities more effectively to government will. In a few cases, states also attempted – futilely, as it turned out – to reform university practices by shaking up faculty structures. Finally, governments began founding new institutes for teaching and research shortly after the turn of the century, a program of institutional expansion that would accelerate greatly as the decades passed.

These transformations constituted one aspect of a larger series of reforms through which German states remade themselves in the early nineteenth century. The breakup of the Holy Roman Empire and the reconfiguration by Napoleon of the political map of Central Europe gave states a chance to assert new political authority over their lands and remake government bureaucracies into effective organs of policy-making and administration. In many cases, the reform programs were breathtakingly comprehensive, reaching into every obscure corner of society. University reform certainly figured into these programs, but so too did regulation of the medical profession (along with other healers) and the creation of a new apparatus for distributing medical care among the rural peasantry and the urban poor.

The irony of these twin reforms of the universities and the medical profession is that in some important respects they furthered an already existing separation of medical faculties from the rest of the profession, instead of promoting their reconciliation. One reason for this is that the avowedly nonutilitarian ideology of *Bildung* received its most emphatic articulation after 1800, and became a ready tool for defending a sphere of inner freedom against political authority. In essence, *Bildung* was the dialectical twin of "the State" raising itself to self-consciousness; the more state governments animated and extended themselves in the advancement of the common good, the more loudly did the educated middle class (as both agents of power and its objects) proclaim its freedom from objective determination by external forces.

As influential as this ideology was as a justification for university reform, the cultivation of *Bildung* through *Wissenschaft* was not the only reason for promoting research in the reorganized universities. What was perhaps still more compelling to state governments was the fact that research and its publication could add luster to a state's reputation as a center of profound scholarly inquiry. In an era when Germans exchanged cosmopolitan for nationalistic sensibilities, the universities became tokens in an elaborate game of cultural politics.[2] States such as Prussia and

2 On the growth of nationalism in this period, see James J. Sheehan, "State and Nationality in the Napoleonic Period," in *The State of Germany: The National Idea in the Making, Unmaking and Remaking of a Modern Nation-State*, ed. John Breuilly (New York, 1992), pp. 47–59; and Friedrich Meinecke, *Cosmopolitanism and the Modern State*, trans. Robert B. Kimber, with introduction by Felix Gilbert (Princeton, N.J., 1970).

Bavaria competed for recognition in the public sphere as the leaders of a politically fragmented German nation, and the eminence of their institutions, among the most prominent of which were the universities, added authority to those claims. The effect of this new cultural politics was to make the advancement of knowledge through research a *sine qua non* for academic success. Those professors who achieved a measure of prominence through their literary activity reaped a rich harvest from their labors in the form of increased salaries and the expansion of research facilities.

Taken together, these developments encouraged the emergence of the professoriate as a specific social and occupational subgroup. Drawn out between the competing demands of *Wissenschaft* and social practice, the medical profession became in effect two different occupations, one pursuing research in academic institutions, the other filling roles as district and town medical officers and bedside healers. As we shall see, this situation created quite distinct senses of professional identity in the two groups. For the researchers, we can see the formation of a disciplinary identity, the acknowledgement among a community of researchers of two things: first, that they are a community, and second, that they set themselves up as the arbiters of truth and merit in their own subject domain.[3] Medical practitioners, on the other hand, developed their sense of professional identity in terms of their problematic relationship with an ever-more intrusive state. For my present purposes, it is neither possible nor desirable to give equal treatment to the two emerging sides of the profession. Because this is a book about "academic medicine," my primary concern is to describe the institutional evolution of university medical faculties. My presentation of the other side of the story amounts to a provisional sketch for a more detailed examination of the relationship between the medical faculties and the larger profession.

To a great extent, the structural changes in university medicine and the medical profession that have been alluded to here were products of the larger political transformations that were reshaping Europe in the years surrounding 1800. Thus we will proceed from the outside inward, that is from the larger political environment toward the medical faculties and profession themselves. The path we will be

3 My quite pragmatic definition of a "discipline" draws upon Karl Hufbauer, *The Formation of the German Chemical Community (1720–1795)* (Berkeley and Los Angeles, 1982), p. 1, where a "community" is defined as a group in which "members regard one another as important peers, as primary arbiters of truth and merit." For a more theoretically comprehensive treatment of scientific disciplines, see Rudolf Stichweh, *Zur Entstehung des modernen Systems wissenschaftlicher Disziplinen: Physik in Deutschland 1740–1890* (Frankfurt, 1984). See also R. Steven Turner, "The Great Transition and Social Patterns of German Science," *Minerva* 25 (1987): 56–76, which uses the occasion of a review of Stichweh's book to mount a broader inquiry into the patterns of disciplinary development in Germany; and Kathryn M. Olesko, "Commentary: On Institutes, Investigations, and Scientific Training," in *The Investigative Enterprise: Experimental Physiology in Nineteenth-Century Medicine*, ed. William Coleman and Frederic L. Holmes (Berkeley and Los Angeles, 1988), pp. 295–332. The tension pointed to here between disciplinary and pedagogical/practical imperatives in university education has also been highlighted by Gert Schubring with reference to the natural sciences seminar at Bonn during the first half of the nineteenth century. See Schubring, "The Rise and Decline of the Bonn Natural Sciences Seminar," in *Science in Germany: The Intersection of Institutional and Intellectual Issues*, ed. Kathryn M. Olesko, *Osiris*, 2nd ser. 5 (1989): 57–93.

taking is broadly chronological as well as causal, reflecting my belief that the political and institutional reforms implemented during the first decade of the nineteenth century set the conditions for disciplinary and professional developments described at the end of the chapter. The appropriate starting point, therefore, is the redrawing of the political landscape that began in 1803.

THE END OF THE OLD REICH

No one who participated in the vituperative conflict over Brunonianism at the end of the 1790s would have suspected that their struggle would soon shrink before the larger transformations that would remake Central Europe. The Treaty of Lunéville, signed in 1801 by the Holy Roman Emperor, Francis II, confirmed French control over territories on the left bank of the Rhine stretching from Switzerland to the Netherlands, and made provisions for those princes of the Empire who had lost territory to the French to receive compensation elsewhere. The final disposition of lands, incorporated in the *Reichsdeputationshauptschluß* of 1803, made dramatic changes in the political composition of the Empire. Gone were most of the ecclesiastical territories that had constituted the majority of Catholic states. Wiped off the map too were the preponderance of imperial free cities and lands belonging to the Imperial Knights. The territories belonging to these sovereignties were redistributed among a number of other states, in some cases producing dramatic changes. Baden, which in 1789 had consisted of two small principalities (Protestant Baden-Durlach and Catholic Baden-Baden) covering some 3,500 sq. km. united in the person of its prince, had by 1810 quadrupled to 15,000 sq. km. and about one million inhabitants.[4] Moreover, in contrast to the numerous scattered enclaves that had belonged to Baden before the Revolution, in 1810 the new Grand Duchy consisted of a single continuous territory. Other south German states, such as Bavaria and Württemberg, also grew considerably.[5]

The breakup of the Holy Roman Empire did more than redraw the political map of Europe; it also broke apart the complex system of traditional rights and privileges that had defined political and social life under the old regime. The creation of new, geographically unified polities in places such as Baden and Bavaria cleared the ground for those states to remake themselves politically and administratively as well. Thus, no sooner had Baden acquired its new lands in 1803 than did the grand duke's principal minister, Johann Friedrich Brauer (1754–1813), begin developing a set of organizational edicts intended to integrate the new lands into the duchy. The main thrust of these edicts was an attempt to level and "rationalize" the dense thicket of legally privileged social groups, institutions,

---

4 Gerhard Köbler, *Historisches Lexikon der deutschen Länder* (Munich, 1988), pp. 27–8.
5 For useful summaries of the complicated political and diplomatic developments of the period, see Hajo Holborn, *A History of Modern Germany 1648–1840* (Princeton, 1982), pp. 355–85; and James J. Sheehan, *German History 1770–1866* (Oxford, 1989), pp. 218–310.

and corporations that had characterized the old regime. Towns and communities (*Gemeinde*) were subjected to the state's administrative authority, while another edict stripped away the rights of political sovereignty previously exercised by members of the aristocracy. In effect, these nobles were made citizens of Baden, although they continued to enjoy certain privileges, such as the right to retain a portion of the taxes they collected on their lands. By attempting to define an idea of citizenship that made all inhabitants of Baden directly subordinate to the state itself, Brauer's aim was to eliminate those structures that had formerly mediated between the duchy's subjects and the state's ultimate political authority.[6]

A similar story of administrative and political reform could be told for Bavaria, which also was rewarded in the reshuffling of territory that took place in 1803. Under the energetic leadership of Maximilian von Montgelas (1759–1838), the Bavarian administration was transformed into a salaried and highly centralized bureaucracy, while the Bavarian Constitution of 1808 made the king and the Wittelsbach dynasty into organs of the state. The kind of friction between princely autocracy and bureaucratic administration that had characterized affairs in Brandenburg-Prussia and other states during the eighteenth century was done away with by curtailing the king's authority to make law without the concurrence of his ministers. Montgelas took on old regime religious institutions as well, and secularized a number of cloisters and monasteries holding feudal privileges. Their properties were confiscated, their libraries carted off to establish the wonderful *Staatsbibliothek* in Munich, and their peasants offered the chance to extinguish their feudal obligations (a step actually taken by only a small minority before 1848). To a lesser extent, several of the nobility's traditional privileges likewise came under attack, including its exclusive claims on the higher levels of civil service, and towns were subordinated directly to state government.[7]

Although Baden and Bavaria represented the most dramatic instances of political and administrative reform, other states, such as Württemberg, Hesse-Darmstadt, and Nassau undertook similar programs.[8] As is well known, Prussia too began a reform era in the wake of its military collapse and subsequent political dismemberment in 1807. Arising as they did in an atmosphere of crisis and defeat, Prussia's reforms were unique in some respects. As we shall see, the political crisis certainly influenced Prussian discussions of higher education after 1807 and figured promi-

6 On Brauer and his work, see Willy Andreas, *Geschichte der badischen Verwaltungsorganisation und Verfassung in den Jahren 1802–1818*, Bd. 1, "Der Aufbau des Staates im Zusammenhang der allgemeinen Politik" (Leipzig, 1913), pp. 38ff. As Andreas points out (p. 62n), the first organizational edict was actually published before the conclusion of the *Reichsdeputationshauptschluß*. For a summary of the edicts and their impact, see Lloyd E. Lee, *The Politics of Harmony: Civil Service, Liberalism and Social Reform in Baden, 1800–1850* (Newark, Dela., 1980), pp. 21–30.

7 See Eberhard Weis, "Die Begründung des modernen bayerischen Staates unter König Max I. (1799–1825)," in *Handbuch der bayerischen Geschichte*, ed. Max Spindler, Bd. 4 (Munich, 1979), pp. 38–60.

8 For a broad survey of the reforms, see Franz-Ludwig Knemeyer, *Regierungs- und Verwaltungsreformen in Deutschland zu Beginn des 19. Jahrhunderts* (Cologne, 1970). A detailed case study is Eckhardt Treichel, *Der Primat der Bürokratie: Bürokratischer Staat und bürokratische Elite im Herzogtum Nassau 1806–1866* (Stuttgart, 1991).

nently in the organization of the new university of Berlin. Yet despite the peculiarities of the Prussian situation, its reforms shared with other states the broad goal of creating an administrative apparatus capable of exercising real authority over social and economic life.[9]

As part of these activities, higher education – including medical education – came to the center of attention. In Baden, Brauer's comprehensive thirteenth edict addressed schooling at all levels, from primary schools up through the University of Heidelberg itself. Indeed the very placement of the university together with other schools in a single edict represented an extension of ministerial authority over an institution that had enjoyed a considerable degree of autonomy in the old regime. To be frank, the university was not in a position to do anything but welcome the changes, because its financial situation was horrendous. Like most other universities, Heidelberg's endowment consisted of the income derived from specified properties, which furnished both its liquid capital and the payments in kind that composed a portion of professors' salaries. But the majority of these properties and their incomes had been lost when the French army occupied the portion of the Palatinate on the left bank of the Rhine in 1792. Believing the situation to be only temporary, however, Heidelberg continued to operate with a deficit budget. By 1798, such practices had rewarded the university with a debt of some 79,000 fl (*Gulden*) and brought it to the threshold of bankruptcy.[10]

When Baden took charge of its impoverished stepchild in 1803, the government recognized that the only way the university could remain viable was for the government to take over its operating expenses. Consequently, Brauer recommended that the duchy appropriate 40,000 fl annually for salaries and maintenance of the university's facilities, such as the library, botanical garden, and anatomy

9 The distinctiveness of the Prussian reform movement and its continuity with earlier developments has for years been a subject of scholarly disagreement. For Hans Rosenberg, the reform period beginning in 1807 marked the culmination of a long process of "replacing the absolute monarch and his cabinet by the ministerial bureaucracy as the chief holder of positive political power...." See Rosenberg, *Bureaucracy, Autocracy and Authority: The Prussian Experience, 1660–1815* (Boston, 1958), p. 206. For Thomas Nipperdey, on the other hand, the shattering experience of Napoleonic hegemony in Central Europe proved the decisive break not only for Prussia, but for all of Germany. "In the beginning," he intoned at the outset of his survey of nineteenth-century German history, "was Napoleon." Nipperdey treated Prussian reforms separately from those initiated elsewhere, but his emphasis was on the exemplary character of the Prussian case. Thomas Nipperdey, *Deutsche Geschichte 1800–1866* (Munich, 1983), pp. 33–79. Eberhard Weis, meanwhile, underscored the distinctiveness of Bavaria's reform program compared to Prussia's, going so far as to claim that the centralizing tendency of Montgelas' reforms was exactly the opposite of the Prussian program. See Weis, "Die Begründung des modernen bayerischen Staates," pp. 48–9.

10 On the university's financial situation in the 1790s, see E. Winkelmann, "Die Universität Heidelberg in den letzten Jahren der pfalzbairischen Regierung," *Zeitschrift für die Geschichte des Oberrheins* 36 (1883): 63–80. To get some idea of how much money 78,000 fl was, consider that in 1803 Brauer's plans for the university envisioned having six full professors in the reorganized medical faculty, who together would be paid a total of 5,500 fl annually, along with specified quantities of grain. Richard August Keller, *Geschichte der Universität Heidelberg im ersten Jahrzehnt nach der Reorganisation durch Karl Friedrich (1803–1813)*, Heidelberger Abhandlungen zur mittleren und neueren Geschichte, Heft 40 (Heidelberg, 1913), p. 37.

theater. That would allow income from the university's remaining properties to be applied to retiring its debt.[11] Such aid came at an obvious cost, however, for the thirteenth edict also specified that university affairs were to come under the direct supervision of the duchy's privy council, an unmistakable indication of the university's subordinate status in Baden's new administrative apparatus.[12]

Montgelas proved himself no less anxious to integrate higher education into Bavaria's new administrative apparatus. Although revised statutes for Ingolstadt had been published as recently as 1799, the new situation in which Bavaria found itself prompted still another set in 1804.[13] One stimulus for the new statutes was the removal of the university from Ingolstadt, a garrison town where students had regularly fallen into tumults with soldiers, to Landshut in the summer of 1801.[14] Leaving Ingolstadt also meant ridding the university of the taint of Jesuit influence that had long colored it, and breaking the university's status as a legally privileged corporation. The academic Senate, to which the 1799 statutes had given a hand in administering the university's funds and properties, was reduced in the 1804 statutes to an advisory council and surrogate parent for the university's students, those ever-suspect troublemakers who so occupied the energies of administrators in Bavaria and elsewhere. Real power over university governance was given in the 1804 statutes to a university curator, who functioned as part of the ministry of religious affairs.[15] Other more symbolic acts of subordination came as well. The university's official seal was sawed through with a file, and replaced with the Bavarian coat of arms. Professors were prohibited from wearing traditional academic regalia on ceremonial occasions, in favor of the civil service uniforms previously prescribed to them in 1800.[16]

The incorporation of universities into the administrative structures of Baden and Bavaria settled their position externally; internal reorganization followed hard on its heels. Each government saw as one of its first tasks the dismantling of the

---

11 Eduard Winkelmann, *Urkendenbuch der Universität Heidelberg*, Bd. 1 (Heidelberg, 1886), pp. 440–50; and Franz Schneider, *Geschichte der Universität Heidelberg im ersten Jahrzehnt nach der Reorganisation durch Karl Friedrich (1803–1813)*, Heidelberger Abhandlungen zur mittleren und neueren Geschichte, Heft 38 (Heidelberg, 1913), pp. 204–7.

12 Winkelmann, *Urkundenbuch*, p. 449.

13 For the 1799 statutes, see Georg Karl Mayr, *Sammlung der Churpfalz-Baierischen allgemeinen und besondern Landes-Verordnungen von Sr. Churfürstl. Durchlaut Maximilian Joseph IV,* Bd. 1 (Munich, 1800), pp. 289–304. For the 1804 statutes, see *Churpfalzbaierisches Regierungsblatt* (1804), cols. 443–54, 464–70, 495–502, 522–6, 555–6.

14 Munich had also been considered a possible destination, but that idea had been squelched by the Elector, Maximilian Joseph IV, who not unreasonably wished not to have a horde of rowdy students disrupting the peace of his capital. Laetitia Boehm, "Das akademische Bildungswesen in seiner organisatorischen Entwicklung (1800–1920)," in *Handbuch*, Bd. 4.2, p. 998.

15 On clerical influence in Ingolstadt after the elimination of the Jesuit order, see Winfried Müller, *Universität und Orden* (Berlin, 1986). After 1810, university affairs came under the supervision of the reorganized ministry of the interior. *Königlich-Baierisches Regierungsblatt*, Stück 52, 10 October 1810, cols. 889–99.

16 On the new administrative structures, see Boehm, "Das akademische Bildungswesen," pp. 998–1004; and Karl von Prantl, *Geschichte der Ludwigs-Maximilians-Universität in Ingolstadt, Landshut, München*, Bd. 1 (1968 repr. of Munich, 1872), pp. 697–705.

existing faculty structure and its replacement with one more attuned to the contemporary shape of knowledge and – what for the governments amounted to much the same thing – more responsive to state needs. The first such move was made at the University of Würzburg, which Bavaria acquired late in 1802. In a set of "*Organisationsakte*" published in October of 1803, the traditional faculty structure was wiped away in favor of a division into two classes of general and particular sciences, each of which was further divided into four sections. The general sciences comprised philosophy, mathematics and physical science, historical sciences, and finally a section for "fine arts and sciences," which included philology, literary history, rhetoric, and related subjects. The class of "particular sciences" were divided between sections for "education of teachers of popular religion," jurisprudence, administrative sciences and cameralism, and medicine. The new and thoroughly secularized character of the formerly Jesuit university was underscored not only by that quintessentially bureaucratic label pasted over the theological faculty, but also by the inclusion of professors to teach Protestant theology. Moreover, as would be the case subsequently at the University of Landshut, the faculty Senate in Würzburg was stripped of its former administrative power and reduced to an advisory and disciplinary board.[17] The government of Baden moved in a similar direction. In the thirteenth organizational edict of 1803, Heidelberg's faculty was divided between five "sections": ecclesiastical (*kirchliche*), constitutional (*staatsrechtliche*), medical (*ärztliche*), economical (*staatswirthschaftliche*), and general (*allgemeine*). Prescribed topics for each section placed an unmistakable emphasis on practical application of knowledge, especially applications of interest to the government. Thus among the topics prominently mentioned for the medical section was veterinary medicine, while alongside the more traditional topics in the "general section," such as metaphysics and natural history, there was also geography and the history of commerce.[18]

Although the restructuring of university faculties had no effect over the long term,[19] it reveals an interesting and not completely harmonious mixture of motivations. Both states expected their universities to produce a corps of well-trained experts for service as bureaucrats, educators and physicians. But at the same time, they were clearly uneasy with the kinds of expertise that had traditionally been embodied in the universities. Of course, such uneasiness and even outright suspi-

---

17 See Franz Xaver Wegele, *Geschichte der Universität Wirzburg* Teil 2 (Würzburg, 1882), pp. 467–81, for a reprint of the 1803 *Organisationsakte*.

18 Winkelmann, *Urkundenbuch*, Bd. 1, pp. 442–3.

19 In 1806, control over Würzburg passed from Bavaria to the Grand Duchy of Tuscany, which was far less interested than Bavaria in educational reform. It simply retained the old faculty structure, and by the time Bavaria regained control of Würzburg in 1814, emulation of French institutional models had become considerably less fashionable. See Werner Engelhorn, "Der bayerische Staat und die Universität Würzburg im frühen 19. Jahrhundert," in *Vierhundert Jahre Universität Würzburg*, ed. Peter Baumgart (Neustadt/Aisch, 1982), pp. 129–78, for a discussion of Würzburg's changing status. In Heidelberg, the new *staatswissenschaftliche* section was organized, but the other measures regarding participation in faculty business (discussed immediately below) seem never to have been implemented.

cion had appeared as well during the eighteenth century (indeed, in Bavaria as early as the seventeenth century), and it was embodied, among other ways, in the creation of independent *collegia medica*. But the measures taken immediately after 1800 seemed to be an attempt not just to check the excesses of university faculties, but to alter them fundamentally. In this respect, Baden's thirteenth organizational edict attempted to break down traditional faculty collegiality in a unique and illustrative way. It did not dismantle the faculties outright, preferring instead to leave them charged with conferring degrees and granting permissions to teach as private lecturers. But the new regulations attempted to dilute faculty corporatism by bringing outsiders into the process. Consequently, the law faculty was described as consisting of the professors of the constitutional section, plus the two professors (one Protestant and one Catholic) of canon law from the ecclesiastical section, as well as those teachers in the economical section "who perhaps have learned a sufficient amount of one or another branch of law thereby to be matriculated (*inscribirt*) in this faculty." Similarly, the medical faculty was to be composed of the professors in the medical section, along with members of the economical section "who have qualified themselves to teach in this subject."[20]

In many ways, the reform programs implemented in Baden and Bavaria continued the utilitarian thrust of Enlightenment university reform. Emphasis was placed on education for practical application of knowledge, and career training was given unmistakable priority over general education in the arts or philosophy.[21] For this reason, the South German reforms might appear to have been entirely unconnected with the reforms of higher education that began in Brandenburg-Prussia after 1800, which stressed universities as institutions for education of the whole person, not factories for producing cogs for the state machinery. Certainly it has seemed that way to legions of university historians, who have marked the establishment of the University of Berlin in 1810 as an epochal moment in the history of higher education in Germany.[22] To be sure, one should not discount the political, ideological and cultural environment in which Berlin was organized, which differed substantially from the situation in Baden and Bavaria. These differences

20 Winkelmann, *Urkundenbuch*, Bd. 1, p. 445.
21 See the discussion of university reforms in Chapter 2.
22 An influential interpreter of Berlin's pivotal role in the birth of the "modern" university has been Helmut Schelsky, *Einsamkeit und Freiheit: Idee und Gestalt der deutschen Universität und ihrer Reformen*, 2nd ed. (Düsseldorf, 1971), esp. pp. 48–50. A view more like the one presented here is offered by Charles McClelland, who treats Berlin and the South German reforms together. McClelland acknowledges that different impulses drove the reforms, but he considers their outcomes to have been broadly similar. See Charles E. McClelland, *State, Society and University in Germany, 1700–1914* (Cambridge, 1980), chap. 4. The standard history of Berlin remains Max Lenz, *Geschichte der Königlichen Friedrich-Wilhelms-Universität Berlin*, 4 vols. (Halle, 1910–18); see also R. Steven Turner, "Universitäten," in *Handbuch der deutschen Bildungsgeschichte*, ed. Karl-Ernst Jeismann and Peter Lundgreen, Bd. 3 1800–70, "Von der Neuordnung Deutschlands bis zur Gründung des Deutschen Reiches" (Munich, 1987), pp. 221–49, esp. 221–7 on Berlin; and Ulrich Mühlack, "Die Universitäten im Zeichen von Neuhumanismus und Idealismus: Berlin," in *Beiträge zu Problemen deutscher Universitätsgründungen der frühen Neuzeit*, ed. Peter Baumgart and Notker Hammerstein, Wolfenbütteler Forschungen, Bd. 4 (Nendeln/Liechtenstein, 1978), pp. 299–340.

alone merit the recounting of Berlin's story, to which we shall turn below. But in the end what will be stressed is not Berlin's uniqueness in comparison with her sister universities, but her similarities.

By the final decade of the eighteenth century, universities had fallen into rather low repute among some Prussians. Pedagogical reformers derided the pedantry and lack of utility in university curricula, while government ministers fumed at their inability to assert administrative control over them.[23] This prompted some voices to be raised, the most prominent of which belonged to Julius von Massow, the Prussian Minister with responsibility for religious and educational affairs, who called for the abolition of the universities and their replacement with more specialized training schools of the kind France had organized in recent years.[24] These scattered and desultory plans for reform of higher education took a dramatic turn in 1807, in the wake of Prussia's overwhelming military defeat at the hands of the French army. By the terms of the Treaty of Tilsit, Prussia was stripped of all its possessions west of the Elbe River and forced to endure occupations by French troops along the Oder. The lost territories included the University of Halle, which had been Prussia's leading university in the eighteenth century. The shattering blow to Prussia's sense of itself as a great power prompted a flurry of self-recriminations and reform programs directed by Karl von Stein and, somewhat later, by Karl von Hardenberg. The loss of Halle also gave new impetus to the idea of founding a university in Berlin.

The task of organizing the new university fell to Karl Friedrich Beyme (1765–1832), chief of the Prussian civil cabinet, who solicited suggestions from a number of scholars on how the new institution should be organized. Among the memoranda he received, those from Johann Gottlieb Fichte and Friedrich Schleiermacher mounted strong arguments for a new vision of university education.[25] Neither wanted to see Berlin become an institution for cultivating and disseminating knowledge useful for government or commerce. They wanted nothing to do with the kind of thinking that had animated university reform in the preceding century, and the reforms implemented more recently in Bavaria and Baden. Instead, each writer urged that the university's central task be the cultivation of a spirit of *Wissenschaft* in students. Fichte described the university as a "school for

---

23 This literature is surveyed in René König, *Vom Wesen der deutschen Universität,* repr. ed. (Darmstadt, 1970), pp. 22–7. In my view, the extent of this criticism has been greatly exaggerated by historians, and has been used to argue for the existence of a "crisis" in the universities at the end of the eighteenth century.

24 Massow acknowledged that the universities could not be replaced with specialized schools in the near future. Until such time as preparations could be made, he concluded, "we will have to tolerate the abnormal (*anormalen*) universities." On Massow's plans, see Lenz, *Geschichte der Universität Berlin,* Bd. 1, pp. 36–9, quoted on p. 38.

25 Johann Gottlieb Fichte, "Deduzierter Plan einer zu Berlin zu errichtenden höhern Lehranstalt, die in gehöriger Verbindung mit einer Akademie der Wissenschaft stehe" (1807); and Friedrich Schleiermacher, "Gelegentliche Gedanken über Universitäten im deutschen Sinn, nebst einem Anhang über eine neu zu errichtende Universität" (1808). Both in Wilhelm Weischedel (ed.), *Idee und Wirklichkeit einer Universität: Dokumente zur Geschichte der Friedrich-Wilhelms-Universität zu Berlin* (Berlin, 1960), pp. 30–192.

the scholarly use of the understanding," by which he meant to underscore the necessity of allowing students to grasp freely the principles of *Wissenschaft*, in order that they may apply such principles actively and self-consciously. In Fichte's view, therefore, what students learn is not a particular body of doctrine, but "the art of learning in general."[26] For his part, Schleiermacher gave universities the mission of awakening in students the "idea of *Wissenschaft*," and directing them to their particular region of intellectual endeavor. The university, he explained, must see to it that students learn "to become conscious in every thought of the basic principles of *Wissenschaft*," thereby developing for themselves "the ability to investigate, discover, and present" new knowledge.[27]

What is noteworthy in both Fichte's and Schleiermacher's vision of university education is the prominence given to the active pursuit of knowledge. It was no longer the mere fund of knowledge that distinguished the scholar; in this new sense of *Wissenschaft*, the *Gelehrter* must yield to the lonely seeker of truth, whose renunciation of all worldly ambition underscored the spiritually cleansing function of his quest. Needless to say, such a vision did not coexist easily with the professional faculties of law, theology, and medicine, with their disagreeable whiff of careerism. For this reason, both Fichte and Schleiermacher located the university's true center of gravity in the philosophical faculty and in the discipline of philosophy itself.[28]

In Schleiermacher's memorandum, the point of departure had been the opposition of interests between scholarly academies and the state, and this theme would be taken up by Wilhelm von Humboldt (1767–1835), who was appointed chief of the Interior Ministry's section of religion and public instruction (with responsibility for the universities) in 1809. Humboldt insisted that university education be for the private *Mensch* and not for the public *Staatsbürger*, and the medium for such an education was to be the student's immersion in *Wissenschaft*. Only in the free pursuit of *Wissenschaft*, Humboldt believed, and especially through study of the culture of ancient Greece, can a student cultivate the virtue and aesthetic sensibility that marks him as truly free. Drawing upon themes sounded earlier by Kant and Schiller, Humboldt defined an ideal environment for academic study, one unencumbered by concern for practical application and protected from external coercion, where the private individual can freely develop his humanity to the greatest possible extent.

Such was the grandiose vision that Humboldt brought to office in 1809, as planning for the university of Berlin entered its decisive phase. It was a peculiar idea of higher education for a government minister to use as the guiding principle for an expensive new institution, but these were no ordinary times. And then again, Humboldt was a peculiar person. Born into the aristocracy, an unambitious and almost unwilling servant of the state, Humboldt became perhaps the most

26 Fichte, "Deduzierter Plan," p. 34.
27 Schleiermacher, "Gelegentliche Gedanken," p. 123.
28 Fichte, "Deduzierter Plan," pp. 41–3, 49–51; Schleiermacher, "Gelegentliche Gedanken," pp. 141–6.

prominent exponent of that very middle-class ideology of *Bildung*.[29] The irony inherent in Humboldt's embrace of *Bildung* becomes all the more pointed when we consider, as La Vopa has pointed out, that Humboldt's inherited title and wealth dispensed him from the requirements of assuming a professional identity and pursuing a career. Thus only he was in a position to *be* the very man his ideology was enshrining.[30] Those bourgeois teachers, jurists, and physicians who shared his vision would have to make their peace with worldly needs some other way.

In pushing the king into giving final approval to the new university, Humboldt painted his pet themes of *Wissenschaft* and *Bildung* on a national canvas. His formal request, dated 24 July 1804, remained silent on the pragmatic benefits to be expected from a new university, playing instead on Prussia's self-appointed place at the head of the German nation. Even in such unsettled times, he observed, the king had "not lost track of the important point of national education and development *(National-Erziehung und Bildung)*."[31] Far from diminishing, the trust previously placed in Prussia for "real enlightenment and higher spiritual cultivation" by the rest of Germany had only grown in the wake of its recent, unfortunate circumstances. This meant that Prussia would continue "to maintain the first rank in Germany and to exercise the most decisive influence on its intellectual and moral direction." Only an institution such as the new university of Berlin, he concluded, would give Prussia the means of fulfilling its cultural vocation and permitting its influence "to extend beyond the boundaries of the State."[32]

29 On the ideology of *Bildung* and Humboldt's articulation of it, see Schelsky, *Einsamkeit und Freiheit*, p. 55ff; David Sorkin, "Wilhelm von Humboldt: The Theory and Practice of Self-Formation *(Bildung)*, 1791–1810," *Journal of the History of Ideas* 44 (1983): 55–73; Rudolf Vierhaus, "Bildung," in *Geschichtliche Grundbegriffe: Historisches Lexikon zur politisch-sozialen Sprache in Deutschland*, ed. Otto Brunner, Werner Conze, and Reinhart Koselleck, Bd. 1 (Stuttgart, 1972), pp. 508–51; and W. H. Bruford, *The German Tradition of Self-Cultivation: 'Bildung' from Humboldt to Thomas Mann* (Cambridge, 1975), pp. 1–28. Prior to his appointment in the Interior Ministry, Humboldt had been the Prussian ambassador in Rome, where he had been happily indulging his passion for classical antiquity. He returned to Berlin in October 1808 for what he thought was only a temporary vacation, and there learned that he was to be appointed to his new post. After putting up some resistance to the idea, he finally capitulated in March of 1809.
30 Anthony J. La Vopa, "Specialists Against Specialization: Hellenism as Professional Ideology in German Classical Studies," in *German Professions, 1800–1950*, ed. Geoffrey Cocks and Konrad H. Jarausch (Oxford, 1990), pp. 27–45.
31 The distinctive role of the nation in mediating Humboldt's concept of *Bildung* has been underscored by Sorkin, "Wilhelm von Humboldt." There is some uncertainty over whether this request or an earlier one, dated 23 May 1809, was the one that actually reached the king. Lenz claims *(Geschichte der Universität Berlin*, Bd. 1, p. 211) the earlier request received royal approval on 30 May. However, Bruno Gebhardt, the editor of Humboldt's official writings, claims the May request was never submitted. See *Humboldts Gesammelte Schriften*, vol. 10 (Berlin, 1903), p. 139. For my purposes, the actual date matters little, since both the May and July versions invoked Prussia's cultural leadership in virtually the same language. For the text of the May version, see pp. 139–45.
32 "Antrag auf Errichtung der Universität Berlin. 24. Juli 1809," in *Humboldts Gesammelte Schriften*, Bd. 10, pp. 148–54. Humboldt had not been alone in placing the question of the new university in a national/cultural context. Schleiermacher's 1807 memorandum had also observed that the boundaries of scholarship were properly those of the language region, and not of an individual state. Fichte's own ardent nationalism in the wake of 1807, meanwhile, is well known.

There is no telling what effect Humboldt's rhetoric ultimately had, but the idea of a "national university" extending Prussia's cultural leadership over all of Central Europe must have been flattering, particularly at a time when Prussia still bore the weight of French political domination. Yet far from being unique, Prussia's use of its university in a program of *Kulturpolitik* had already been anticipated several times over. There was of course Göttingen from the eighteenth century, although that university had been founded less in the spirit of exerting cultural leadership over the German nation than because, as one planner put it, all the other electors of the Empire had one. Still, the glamour that radiated from Göttingen and the reputation its scholars had acquired among the public provided a model of how universities might fill a larger cultural role.[33]

By the early nineteenth century, more direct examples for the Berlin planners were actions taken at Würzburg, Landshut, and Heidelberg in the half dozen years before Berlin opened. From the moment Bavaria assumed control of Würzburg and committed itself to making the university "flourish," it interpreted that task to mean recruiting the most prominent scholars it could find. One of its first targets was Heidelberg, from which the Bavarians attempted in vain to lure two faculty members. More successful was Würzburg's raid on the University of Jena, which had been sinking steadily in morale and student numbers ever since the government of Saxe-Weimar had clamped down hard against what it perceived to be student Jacobinism, and especially because Fichte, a prominent democrat, had been driven out in 1799 over his alleged atheism. From Jena the Bavarians lured a number of professors, including most importantly Friedrich Schelling, just the sort of person whose notoriety would proclaim that Würzburg had become a university to be taken seriously.[34]

Baden too decided to court prominent scholars, though not without some initial hesitation. Brauer, who was all too aware of the burden being assumed by the government in taking control of the university and trying to attract new personnel to it, tried navigating a course between establishing Heidelberg as a local institution devoted primarily to professional training, and giving it a national reputation. He suggested that prominent people be called only for the principal subjects in each discipline, while leaving other areas to more middling and inexpensive talents. Those plans were scuppered, however, by the Bavarians' energetic efforts on behalf of nearby Würzburg, which not only threatened to overshadow the changes made at Heidelberg, but also to empty Baden's new

---

33 Emil Franz Rössler, *Die Gründung der Universität Göttingen* (1987 repr. of Göttingen, 1855), p. 3; Notker Hammerstein, "Die Universitätsgründungen im Zeichen der Aufklärung," in *Beiträge zu Problemen deutscher Universitätsgründungen*, ed. Baumgart and Hammerstein, pp. 263–98.

34 For brief treatments of Würzburg's entry into the academic marketplace, see Wegele, *Geschichte der Universität Wirzburg* Bd.1, pp. 493–4; and Engelhorn, "Der bayerische Staat und die Universität Würzburg," pp. 135–7. For a description of the situation in Jena, see *Alma Mater Jenensis*, ed. Siegfried Schmidt (Weimar, 1983), pp. 162–7. Schelling's own situation and motivations for leaving Jena are presented in Horst Fuhrmans (ed.), *F. W. J. Schelling: Briefe und Dokumente*, Bd. 1 1775–1809 (Bonn, 1962), pp. 209–16.

university of some of its more well-regarded professors. Brauer's own doubts notwithstanding, the government of Baden plunged into the new game of academic recruitment. Prussia too would play for high stakes, both with Berlin and with the new university of Bonn, which opened in 1818.[35]

It is not obvious why universities such as Heidelberg and Würzburg, which were ostensibly dedicated to training professionals and civil servants, would require famous faculty members. To be sure, the "academic mercantilism" of Göttingen continued to provide an example of a sort. University reformers – some of them, anyway – continued to believe that a university could make money by drawing large numbers of paying customers. But there are two grounds for questioning just how compelling Göttingen's influence was. First, although Göttingen's prominence had represented a powerful argument for hiring famous professors, even in the eighteenth century it had not prompted universal emulation. Some states had been content to let their universities continue as institutions for training future professionals and civil servants, without much concern for their public acclaim.[36] Second, even if economic arguments continued to support such policies after 1800, their illusoriness soon became obvious. To take just one case, total faculty salaries at Würzburg ballooned from just over 17,000 fl in 1803 to 47,000 fl in 1806, whereas student enrollments swelled temporarily to 432 in 1803 and 335 in 1804, but then returned to their previous average of a little over 100.[37] Whatever reasons states might have for chasing after prominent scholars, enrichment of the treasury from student fees would not long remain one of them.

In searching for reasons why universities should become so important in state *Kulturpolitik,* and indeed why states should even conceive of pursuing a program of *Kulturpolitik,* one must return to the development of the public sphere. Through it Germany was posited as a geographical space unified culturally, if not politically, and individual states attempted to cut a favorable figure before "the public" as one way of asserting their place on the crowded political stage. Although this sense of national identity grew out of the effects of the French Revolution, the formation of a literary public sphere was an indispensable condition for it. And there is little question that the "public" was an important audience in the calculations of university reformers. Humboldt clearly believed this, as the petition cited above demonstrates, as did jurist Karl von Savigny, who urged the government of Baden

35 Schneider, "Geschichte der Universität Heidelberg," pp. 60–9. For an excellent account of the organization of Bonn, see Christian Renger, *Die Gründung und Einrichtung der Universität Bonn und die Berufungspolitik des Kultusministers Altenstein* (Bonn, 1982).

36 On Göttingen and academic mercantilism, see Chapter 2. For a later application of the same thinking, see the 1802 memorandum by Johann Jacob Engel describing the possibility of a new university in Berlin in Weischedel, *Idee und Wirklichkeit einer Universität,* pp. 3–10.

37 Engelhorn, "Der bayerische Staat und die Universität Würzburg," p. 144. For enrollments at Würzburg, see Franz Eulenberg, "Die Frequenz der deutschen Universitäten von ihrer Gründung bis zur Gegenwart," *Abhandlungen der philologisch-historischen Klasse der königlich sächsischen Gesellschaft der Wissenschaften* 24, no.2 (1906): 299.

to move rapidly in filling Heidelberg's faculty roster. Savigny drove his point home by claiming that favorable public attention, which was currently directed at what was going on at Heidelberg, would soon fade in the absence of positive action.[38]

Thus, despite their apparent contrasts in rhetoric and intended mission, the South German universities and Berlin came to resemble each other rather more than either their organizers or later apologists might have cared to acknowledge. For all the talk of utilitarianism, faculty members were recruited to Heidelberg, Würzburg, and Landshut using the same criteria and for the same reasons as they were for Prussia, and in both cases universities became an integral element of their states' external *Kulturpolitik*. The pursuit of prominent faculty members was not, of course, intended as a rejection of the university's practical mission in professional education. But it was clear from the outset that making a reputation was expected along with effective teaching.[39] Meanwhile Berlin, notwithstanding the conviction of Schleiermacher, Fichte, and Humboldt that the "real" university resided in the philosophical faculty, would attract large numbers of professional students who might fashion themselves as men of *Bildung*, but who would also go out and make careers in the professions or civil service.

Whether located in the North or the South, the reorganized universities found themselves assigned two distinct tasks: the cultivation of knowledge and the training of professional practitioners. Although university apologists throughout the nineteenth century hailed the mutually supportive functions of teaching and research, their life together was (and still is) not an entirely comfortable one. In classical philology, for example, the university curriculum increasingly emphasized the carrying out of research into the minutiae of Hellenic and Roman antiquity. The result was that students gained technical research expertise at the expense of an overall appreciation of classical culture that had been the original justification for teaching philology.[40] In medicine, the pairing of teaching and research would similarly create problems, but the consequences would be different. The practice of philology, after all, was basically identical with university philology itself; it did not occupy a distinct social realm of practice. Not so with medicine. In its research mission, the goal of university medicine was the study of organic nature, while the goal of medical therapy as a form of social practice was the care of patients and the healing of sickness. Therefore, perhaps more than any other academic discipline, medicine manifested the tensions implicit in the nineteenth-century universities.

38 Cited in Schneider, "Geschichte der Universität Heidelberg," pp. 104–7.
39 Brauer's original plans for the University of Heidelberg included a sum of money – roughly the equivalent of a junior professor's annual salary – set aside in each section as a premium to encourage literary diligence. Keller, "Geschichte der Universität Heidelberg," pp. 35–8.
40 La Vopa, "Specialists Against Specialization"; and Anthony Grafton, "Polyhistor into *Philolog*: Notes on the Transformation of Classical Scholarship, 1780–1850," *History of Universities* 3 (1983): 159–92.

THE REFORMED MEDICAL FACULTIES

It should come as no surprise that external reorganization of the universities was accompanied by internal restructuring as well. In part, as we have seen, the restructuring was intentional, reflecting ministerial resolve to eliminate old forms of faculty behavior and promote topics, such as cameralism, that governments wanted to see taught. Governments also set out to improve the physical facilities at many universities, or to construct new institutes, such as stationary clinics for medical teaching. But in part too the reorganization was thrust on governments by those professors they wanted to bring in to make their schools "flourish." It took but a short while for governments to learn that the greatly enhanced competition for prestigious faculty would cost them dearly, both in terms of salary and facilities. This would prove particularly to be the case with the medical faculties, which required anatomical theaters, teaching clinics, botanical gardens and chemical laboratories. Consequently rising institutional costs were likely to manifest themselves first and most forcefully there.

Baden swallowed this lesson early on. One of its earliest recruits for Heidelberg was Samuel Thomas Sömmerring (1755–1830), in 1803 arguably the most famous anatomist in Central Europe. Sömmerring evinced some interest in making the move, but after seeing the decrepit condition of Heidelberg's facilities for anatomy, which were more than a century old, he rejected the offer.[41] Baden also attempted to secure Friedrich Hildebrandt, who for a number of years had been a member of the excellent medical faculty in Erlangen, to teach physiology. Hildebrandt was inclined to come, although he wanted his position broadened to include the chairs of chemistry and experimental physics (the latter in the philosophical faculty). The government readily assented to this request, and when negotiations with Sömmerring collapsed, Hildebrandt was offered anatomy as well, which he agreed to take on for the time being. All appeared to be going smoothly. But Prussia, which had recently taken over Erlangen as part of its acquisition of Ansbach-Bayreuth, decided it wanted to retain Hildebrandt, and eventually he turned down Baden's offer.[42]

Heidelberg finally succeeded with its third major recruit, Jacob Fidelis Ackermann (1766–1815). A former student of Sömmerring's at Mainz, Ackermann was offered a position on his mentor's recommendation to teach anatomy and physiology. Ackermann accepted the call, but demanded a salary of 3,000 fl, a hefty amount, considering that Brauer's original plan for the medical faculty had foreseen a top salary of 1,200 fl. Yet the realities of the situation rapidly made themselves manifest, and the government acceded to Ackermann's demand. After

41 On Sömmerring and Heidelberg, see Schneider, "Geschichte der Universität Heidelberg," pp. 80–1.
42 Ibid., p. 81ff.

securing release from his position in Jena, Ackermann arrived to begin teaching in 1805.[43]

Baden's experiences with Heidelberg would be repeated many times over in the coming years, especially at those universities chosen by their governments for special attention: Heidelberg, Würzburg, Landshut, Tübingen, Berlin, and Bonn. By late 1817, when Prussia began organizing the University of Bonn in its newly acquired Rhine territories, the stakes had become very high indeed and the game so popular that the mere rumor of a new university sufficed to unleash a blizzard of applications in the office of Karl vom Stein zum Altenstein (1770–1840), the head of the new ministry of religion and education.[44] From Heidelberg, the Prussians attempted to lure away Friedrich Tiedemann (1781–1861), the renowned comparative anatomist. Reports of political unrest in Baden gave the Prussians cause to hope that Tiedemann and others could be pried away from Heidelberg, but Tiedemann's price was high: he asked about plans for the anatomy theater in Bonn, including how much money would be available annually for its operation. Tiedemann also asked about the quality of the anatomical and zoological collections in Bonn, and about who else would be named to the faculty. Finally, he mentioned that he would not think of coming for less than 2,000 Rthlr, and made specific inquiries about the widows' and orphans' pension at Bonn, a matter of special interest motivated by concern for his six children.[45]

In the end, Tiedemann remained in Heidelberg, but the extent and nature of his demands were fast becoming the norm by 1818. Of course such leverage could not be wielded by every professor, and for every Tiedemann there was a Johann C. F. Harless (1773–1853), who was called to Bonn from Erlangen to teach pathology, therapeutics, and medical history. Although Altenstein turned away Harless's attempts to secure additional compensation for moving expenses, an appointment as director of the university clinic, and a student fellowship for his son, he came nevertheless.[46] Yet the bargaining position of academic recruits was a strong one, especially with respect to salary and facilities for teaching and research. One last example from Bonn will illustrate this. After negotiations with Tiedemann had fallen through, attention next turned to August Carl Mayer

43 Eberhard Stübler, *Geschichte der medizinischen Fakultät der Universität Heidelberg 1386–1925* (Heidelberg, 1926), p. 186.
44 Renger, *Die Gründung und Einrichtung der Universität Bonn*, p. 96.
45 GStA Merseburg Rep. 76 Vᵃ Sekt. 3 Tit. IV Nr. 1 Vol. II, fol. 144–5, letter dated 5 August 1818, from Tiedemann to the Berlin anatomist Karl Asmund Rudolphi, who was acting as Altenstein's representative in negotiating Tiedemann's appointment. As Renger reports, the tardiness of Tiedemann's response to the letter of appointment at Bonn, in which he avoided making a firm commitment, caused Rudolphi to suspect that Tiedemann was using the call to Bonn to play off Prussia against Baden, and perhaps other states as well, to improve his circumstances. See Renger, *Die Gründung und Einrichtung der Universität Bonn*, pp. 164–5.
46 GStA Merseburg Rep. 76 Vᵃ Sekt. 3 Tit. IV Nr. 1 Vol. II, fols. 119–23, 283–5. Harless had been appointed to Bonn at the behest of the Prussian chancellor Hardenberg against Altenstein's wishes, which perhaps disposed Altenstein not to grant Harless any more than he had to. See Renger, *Die Gründung und Einrichtung der Universität Bonn*, pp. 75–7.

(1787–1865), professor of anatomy and physiology in Bern. Initially, Mayer was offered both the professorship of anatomy and the position of anatomical prosector (head laboratory instructor), but he refused the latter, describing a prosector's work as merely "mechanical" and not "scientific," and therefore unworthy of him. Mayer then described his larger scientific vision, including his intention of conducting research in experimental physiology, for which he claimed there was a "real need" in Germany. This so impressed Altenstein that in his letter appointing Mayer to the professorship of anatomy and physiology he added on top of Mayer's salary (1,000 Rthlr) an extra 300 Rthlr for conduct of his experiments. The only stipulation was that Mayer send in an annual report describing his results.[47]

As the preceding discussion has suggested, the expansion of facilities for teaching and research was a matter of great concern to university administrators. Yet all this ministerial initiative and largesse had limits both budgetary and political, a circumstance that contributed to making the early nineteenth-century medical faculties more continuous with their eighteenth-century predecessors than has been hitherto recognized. In Heidelberg, a former Dominican cloister was purchased with the expectation that it would house a new anatomy theater and botany collection on the ground floor, a stationary clinic on the first floor, and an obstetrical clinic on the second floor. After some 15,000 fl worth of rebuilding – payment for which the laborers had to wait years in some cases – the building was ready. But the clinic could not be put in operation. The Heidelberg city government had offered 2,000 fl for support of eighteen beds in exchange for the clinic's care of the city's poor, but the city's own finances were in such bad shape that it could not uphold its end of the contract. Nor did the government of Baden have the resources to support the clinic. For the short term, Heidelberg made do with a polyclinic, directed by the anatomist Ackermann, whose interests lay more in medical therapeutics than in anatomy. The polyclinic received 600 fl annually from the state government, but the demands on its services caused it to pile up a sizeable debt with local apothecaries. Meanwhile, Ackermann's repeated efforts to secure funding for a stationary clinic were fruitless. Only under Ackermann's successor, Johann W. H. Conradi (1780–1861), would a stationary clinic finally be opened in the former Dominican cloister.[48]

Along with the financial obstacles encountered at Heidelberg, communities sometimes put up surprisingly tenacious political resistance to state-sponsored university reforms, offering another illustration of the limits of state power. Such was the situation at Landshut where, because the university was being moved to a new location, everything had to be built anew. The temporary establishment of a university clinic in one of Landshut's hospitals created enormous tension between the city and the university, with the city objecting to the fact that one of its hospitals had been, in its view, expropriated and its poor relief funds drained away

47 GStA Merseburg, Rep. 76 V^{a}· Sekt. 3 Tit. IV Nr. 1 Vol. IV, fols. 328–31.
48 Schneider, "Geschichte der Universität Heidelberg," pp. 132–44; Stübler, "Geschichte der medizin-
    ischen Fakultät," pp. 196–214.

for the university's use. The university attempted to mobilize direct public support for the clinic by publishing a pamphlet describing the incalculable benefits that would accrue to Landshut by having a modern hospital within its walls, the equivalent – so the pamphlet proclaimed – to anything found in Munich or Vienna.[49] However, such attempts at public relations left the city's Poor Commission unmoved, and it continued to stand in the way. This prompted the university to retaliate by charging the Poor Commission with misappropriation of funds.[50] This happy state of affairs was undoubtedly worsened by the attitude taken toward the locals by Andreas Röschlaub, the new university clinic's director, who suggested that three of Landshut's six hospitals be closed and their lands sold, with the proceeds from the sales used to fund construction of a new university hospital.[51] In any case, funds for the clinic were scarce, and by 1806 its debt burden had become so intractable that it was ordered closed until its finances could be straightened out.[52]

The establishment of new facilities for research and teaching, to the extent that it could go forward, was paralleled by another kind of reorganization in medical faculties as well as the entire university: the redefinition of professors' teaching responsibilities. The exchange of one set of courses for another as a professor moved up the faculty hierarchy (*Aufrücken*) was definitively eliminated at nearly all of the universities where it had remained in practice, in favor of a system whereby a professor remained within a more or less narrowly defined orbit of subjects throughout his career.[53] Even at the University of Leipzig, which remained largely unreformed before 1830, there were founded several new and more specialized positions, among them clinical medicine, chemistry, obstetrics, and forensic medicine and medical police, to accompany the traditional chairs of physiology and pathology, therapeutics and materia medica, surgery, and anatomy.[54]

One conspicuous product of this shuffling of positions was the separation of

49 *An die Bürgerschaft zu Landshut über Einrichtung eines Krankenhaus* (Landshut, 1802).
50 Bayer. Hauptstaatsarch. München, MInn 23680, vols. 1–3. These volumes contain documents relating to the entire dispute between 1802 and 1807, and also contain copies of the pamphlets published by both sides.
51 Röschlaub's memorandum is contained in ibid., vol. 2.
52 Ibid., vol. 3. Relations with the locals were not so strained everywhere, as demonstrated by a contract made in 1819 between the Bonn city government and the university clinic's medical and surgical directors, Friedrich Nasse (1778–1851) and Philipp Franz von Walther (1781–1849). According to its various terms, the university clinic promised to assume responsibility for medical and surgical care for all of Bonn's poor citizens, in return for which the city would pay 800 Rthlr per year and 50 portions weekly from the city's soup kitchen. GStA Merseburg Rep. 76 V^a Sekt. 3 Tit. X Nr. 6 Vol. I, fols. 1–9.
53 This narrowing certainly did not proceed uniformly, as demonstrated by Heidelberg's offer of anatomy, physiology, physics, and chemistry to Friedrich Hildebrandt and Johann Fidelis Ackermann's assumption both of the chair of anatomy and physiology and leadership of the polyclinic. But these cases were very much exceptions to the general trend, and for that matter they proved exceptional at Heidelberg as well.
54 Ingrid Kästner and Achim Thom (eds.), *575 Jahre Medizinische Fakultät der Universität Leipzig* (Leipzig, 1990), pp. 22–3.

178   *The transformation of German academic medicine*

clinical subjects from theoretical subjects. By 1818, when Bonn opened, it was scarcely possible to find a professor anywhere whose teaching spanned both areas.[55] Curiously, Bonn did have one such professor, Friedrich Nasse, who taught both clinical medicine and comparative anatomy. But the combination represented by Nasse was virtually unique; much more typical was the situation of Johann Friedrich Meckel the Younger (1781–1833) at Halle. Born into one of Germany's premier medical families, Meckel was the son of Philipp F. T. Meckel (1755–1803), professor of anatomy, surgery, and obstetrics at Halle, and the grandson of Johann Friedrich Meckel the Elder (1714–74), who had held an identical position in the Royal Academy of Sciences in Berlin. After university studies at Halle and Göttingen, Meckel returned to Halle in 1802 to defend his doctoral dissertation, a study of developmental abnormalities of the heart. He received an appointment as extraordinary professor at Halle in 1805, two years after his father's death, but he did not remain there long, choosing instead to take off for Vienna, where he spent some time studying with Johann Peter Frank, and then for Paris. In Paris, he studied with the comparative anatomist Georges Cuvier, and enjoyed access to the enormous natural history collections that were at Cuvier's disposal. Although Meckel's postgraduate tour had been arranged to give him advanced training in both clinical medicine and comparative anatomy, it rapidly became apparent that the latter had taken hold of him more powerfully. Meckel returned to Halle late in 1806, shortly after its occupation by French troops and the closing of the university. When Halle reopened in 1808 following its incorporation into the Kingdom of Westphalia, Meckel assumed his father's former chair, the professorship of anatomy, pathological anatomy, surgery, and obstetrics. Unlike his father, however, he soon gave up responsibility for the two clinical subjects in order to concentrate better on his anatomical teaching and physiological research.[56]

The details of Meckel's biography are instructive, both for the separation of anatomy from surgery and obstetrics that he initiated at Halle and for his attachment of anatomy to broader physiological questions of form and function. We will return to this research program below; here it merits notice that the same association of anatomy with physiology was going on elsewhere in Germany. Friedrich Tiedemann, born in the same year as Meckel and also a beneficiary of having studied at Cuvier's elbow, held a similar position at Heidelberg, as did Karl Asmund Rudolphi in Berlin and Ignaz Döllinger in Würzburg. Döllinger's case is interesting because he took over anatomy in 1805 as an expansion of his original appointment in pathology and physiology, prevailing in the face of opposition from colleagues who did not want to see a "theoretician" such as Döllinger given

---

55 The argument here is based on study of lecture catalogues for the period 1810-1825 from the following universities: Berlin, Bonn, Erlangen, Freiburg, Göttingen, Halle, Heidelberg, Landshut, Leipzig and Tübingen. Missing from this list are Giessen, Greifswald, Jena, Königsberg and Marburg.
56 Rudolf Beneke, *Johann Friedrich Meckel der Jüngere* (Halle, 1934), p. 35.

control over the "practical" subject of anatomy.[57] Alongside these positions at Halle, Heidelberg, Berlin and Würzburg, by 1820 anatomy was being taught by someone other than the professor of surgery at Bonn, Breslau, Freiburg, Göttingen, Königsberg, Landshut, Leipzig, and Tübingen.[58]

Taken together, the changes made in the medical faculties of the early nineteenth century certainly gave them a distinctively new appearance. The expectation that professors would both teach and publish original research was perhaps the most important novelty, and it was linked to another characteristic of the new faculties, the competition for prestigious scholars. Although precedents for both could certainly be found in the eighteenth century, it would be hard to deny the pervasiveness and vigor of the phenomenon after 1800. The institutional expansion of the faculties, by contrast, was more modest. Ambition for new facilities often outstripped the resources available for them, and in various cases the establishment of institutes stumbled against the same barriers that had confronted them in earlier decades.[59]

These institutional changes, however, did not immediately translate into dramatic curricular novelty. The medical faculties may have been increasingly populated with famous, well paid and full-time professors, who taught and conducted research in new facilities. But what they taught looked much like what had been taught to those students' fathers and even to their grandfathers. Teaching in the theoretical subjects was largely doctrinal, not experimental, although at some universities those doctrines might include *Naturphilosophie*, a variety of theory that earlier generations would not have recognized, to say the least. For its part, clinical teaching emphasized the same collection of bedside experience that had been the cornerstone of the theory of medical practice for centuries. What was new in the medical curriculum was an ongoing concern for the proper balance between the theoretical and practical portions of the medical curriculum, and a continuing debate over the relationship between the two. Few physicians still subscribed to

---

57 Johannes Friedrich, *Ignaz von Döllinger*, Teil 1, Von dem Geburt bis zum Ministerium Abel 1799–1837 (Munich, 1899), p. 40. The biography is not of Döllinger the anatomist, but of his son Ignaz von Döllinger, a famous theologian. However it also includes an extensive discussion of the father. The transfer of anatomy from its former connection with surgery to its new link with physiology was also noted by Hans-Heinz Eulner, *Die Entwicklung der medizinischen Spezialfächer an den Universitäten des deutschen Sprachgebiets* (Stuttgart, 1970), p. 48.

58 This list is compiled from university lecture catalogues published between 1818 and 1820. This does not mean that the professor of surgery *never* taught anatomy. At Göttingen, in fact, Conrad J. H. Langenbeck (1776–1851) was appointed professor of anatomy and surgery in 1814. But Göttingen also had Johann Friedrich Blumenbach (1752–1840), who regularly lectured on comparative anatomy and physiology.

59 Even Berlin suffered from local rivalries. The medical faculty was supposed to have free use of the Charité hospital for clinical teaching in medicine and surgery, but the Charité clinics were under the direction of the faculty of the Collegium Medico-Chirurgicum, a school for military surgeons. The university professors complained repeatedly about the inaccessibility of the Charité clinics for their students. See GStA Merseburg Rep. 76 Vᵃ Sekt. 2 Tit. IV Nr. 5 Vol. III, fols. 3, 47; and Tit. X Nr. 3 Vol. I, fols. 164–70.

the kind of theory-driven practice advocated by the Brunonians, but the disappearance of Brunonianism did not signal a widely agreed-upon solution to the problem. Quite to the contrary, the respective places of theory and practice in medicine remained a contentious issue in the 1810s.

THEORY AND PRACTICE IN MEDICAL TEACHING

"Theory in general is the act of knowing (*das Erkennen*) as the basis of an action," wrote the Würzburg anatomist Ignaz Döllinger in 1806. "How can any action have reliability that [is] not determined or based on some knowledge (*irgend eine Erkentniß*)?"[60] With these rapid strokes, Döllinger sketched the commonly held relationship between theory and practice. Yet as Döllinger himself recognized, such a simple portrait belied a more complicated interaction. In antiquity, he observed, the connection between theory and practice had been an immediate one; Hippocratic medical theory had been derived directly from bedside experience and had consisted of rules that guided practice. But more recently attempts had been made to construct general theories that did not necessarily depend on the sickbed for their empirical content. After all, Döllinger pointed out, the organism is more than what it is in sickness;

therefore one must know more about [the organism] than one learns from its diseased condition and from the connections of medicaments to it, and before one hopes to make judgments about particular circumstances and relationships, one must know the entirety (*das Ganze*), because the particular conditions and relationships, in so far as they are conditions of an organism, can only be appropriate to the nature of the entirety.[61]

Döllinger's apology for an independently grounded science of physiology was one familiar to his contemporaries, for it posited a relationship between the theory of the organism and illness that Brunonianism had made its guiding principle and that many (though not all) of Döllinger's contemporaries shared. According to this principle, pathology was understood as a branch of physiology, and, what is crucial, only a science of physiology grounded on general principles and in possession of secure empirical knowledge would eventually be adequate to developing a science of medical practice: "Accordingly, the establishment of medical theory can take place only through knowledge of the nature of the organism, and only by means of such a general theory of the human organism can it be determined what disease is, how the causes [of disease] work, what relationship medicaments have to particular illnesses, and therefore how illnesses must be handled."[62]

Such optimistic programmatic statements were not unusual, but they always

---

60 Ignaz Döllinger, "Ueber den jetzigen Zustand der Physiologie," *Jahrbücher der Medicin als Wissenschaft* 1 (1806): 119–42, quoted on p. 119.
61 Ibid., p. 122.
62 Ibid., pp. 122–3.

pointed to a unification of theory and practice that barely glimmered somewhere on the furthest horizon.[63] For the present, however, the actual relation between theory and practice in medical teaching was a distinctly uncomfortable one, and made all the more difficult by the unpleasant memories of the rancor over Brunonianism. The institutional developments taking place in various universities during the 1810s only made things worse. As members of the larger university, medical faculties were supposed to cultivate knowledge for its own sake, penetrate ever more deeply into the secrets of life, and awaken the spirit of *Wissenschaft* in students. But as educators of aspiring physicians, they were charged with providing students with the tools they would need for carrying out a particular kind of social practice. The obvious question was, what did cultivation of *Wissenschaft* have to do with practice? The obvious answer was that no one was sure.[64]

One way among many that such uncertainties manifested themselves was in textbooks covering key subjects such as pathology. Just as in the eighteenth century, pathology after 1800 continued to be the subject that defined the realm of medicine proper as separate from physiology. Yet the nature of that demarcation was highly variable. Döllinger's view of pathology as a branch of physiology differed considerably from that offered in Johann W. H. Conradi's highly successful *Grundriß der Pathologie und Therapie* (Outline of pathology and therapeutics). In many respects, Conradi handled pathology in a manner that strikingly resembled the standard pathology textbooks of the preceding century. To be sure, among his fundamental categories he gave a prominent position to diseased changes of the vital force, including quantitative changes in a Brunonian sense. But many of Conradi's categories were virtually indistinguishable from older ones used by Boerhaave or Gaub: faulty conjunction of the solid parts (either too rigid or too flaccid); infirmity of the vessels; defects in bodily fluids (abundance, shortage, altered properties); excess production of mucous; black-bilious thickening of the fluids; watery thinning of the blood; acidity of fluids, caused by foreign substances; tendency of fluids toward putrefaction, and so on.[65]

A conception of pathology more in keeping with Döllinger's was Karl Friedrich Burdach's (1776–1847) *Handbuch der Pathologie* (1808). For Burdach, an adequate treatment of pathology required that it be brought under a systematic framework. The one Burdach chose was a synthesis of Brunonianism and *Naturphilosophie* that

63 Similar sentiments were expressed in a pamphlet by the Greifswald professor Ludwig Caspar Mende, *Ueber den wissenschaftliche Unterricht in der Medizin* (n.p., n.d.), pp. 8–9. The copy I saw is in GStA Merseburg Rep. 76 Vᵃ Sekt. 7 Tit. X Nr. 3 Vol. I.

64 For a comprehensive survey of the theory of medical practice during this period, see Volker Hess, *Von der semiotischen zur diagnostischen Medizin: Die Entstehung der klinischen Methode zwischen 1750 und 1850* (med. Diss., Freie Universität Berlin, 1992), esp. pp. 171–92. Hess emphasizes the number of physicians in the 1810s who rejected medical systems in favor of a return to the traditional doctrines of semiotics as a guide to bedside practice.

65 Johann Wilhelm Heinrich Conradi, *Grundriß der Pathologie und Therapie zum Gebrauch bei seinen Vorlesungen entworfen*, Band 1, 2nd ed. (Marburg, 1817), pp. 94–186. Compare this with Boerhaave's pathology, as described in Chapter 3, and in Lester S. King, *The Medical World of the Eighteenth Century* (Huntington, N.Y., 1971), pp. 59–93.

defined life as a "circle of diverse things that is perfected in itself and defined through itself (*einen in sich vollendeten, durch sich bestimmten, Kreis mannigfaltiger Dinge*)."[66] He claimed that life has two sides, a dynamic, growing side and a physical side manifested in a particular structure. This duality implied for Burdach, as it did for the Brunonian Röschlaub, two types of illness. The first type was "abnormalities of irritability," and the second "abnormalities of structure (*Bildung*)."

Clearly, therefore, when Conradi and Burdach used the word "pathology," they meant by it two very different things. Conradi considered it to be a survey of the diverse problems that can befall a living being, the purpose of which was to provide a working guide to interpreting the phenomena that confront a practitioner at the bedside. For Burdach, pathology was that branch of medical theory that comprehended the occurrence of illness within a general definition of life. He would have agreed with Conradi that pathology must address itself to the concrete phenomena involved with illness, but to Burdach its primary importance lay in explaining those phenomena in terms of the general theory, rather than in their applicability to clinical practice. In a sense, the struggles that took place in medical education during the 1810s and 1820s came down to the question of whose definition – Conradi's or Burdach's – would become the guiding one.

The disagreement embodied in Conradi's and Burdach's textbooks took concrete form in the competition between Christoph Wilhelm Hufeland and Johann Christian Reil for the dominant position in the new medical faculty at Berlin. As early as 1807, when memoranda were being solicited by Karl Friedrich Beyme on the proposed university, Reil and Hufeland offered contrasting visions of the medical faculty. Reil's memorandum largely reiterated views he had expounded in his 1804 book on medical reform in Prussia, the *Pepinieren zum Unterricht ärztlicher Routiniers als Bedürfnisse des Staats nach seiner Lage wie sie ist*. He continued to insist that the first duty of universities was to awaken the idea of *Wissenschaft* in medical students. This, he claimed, depends on finding professors who embody the idea. "Above all," he urged, "the apostles of utility must be banished from the universities to the industrial schools, because they lack entirely any sense for *Wissenschaft*. They value *Wissenschaft* not for its own sake as the pure image of objective universal Reason, but rather because it is useful for building houses, tilling fields, and stimulating commerce."[67] Reil also emphasized the importance of studying natural sciences without any particular reference to their applicability in medical practice. He complained that German universities customarily confine this study too narrowly to medical topics, which prevents the full development and cultivation of *Wissenschaft* in students.[68]

Hufeland, meanwhile, envisioned the university's medical faculty as the continuation of the previously established Collegium Medico-Chirurgicum in Berlin.

66 Karl Friedrich Burdach, *Handbuch der Pathologie* (Leipzig, 1808), p. 15.
67 Reprinted in Lenz, *Geschichte der Universität Berlin*, Bd. 4, pp. 50–67, quoted on pp. 51–2.
68 Ibid., pp. 52–3.

Far from sharing Reil's advocacy of the distinctiveness of university education, Hufeland believed the new medical faculty would serve the same end that the Collegium had served: the education of accomplished medical practitioners. Thus Hufeland assumed the Collegium's professors could simply be transferred to the new faculty, where they would frame its statutes and develop its curriculum. Hufeland further hoped to see students of Prussia's school for military surgeons, the *Pepinière*, attend classes at the university in those subjects appropriate for their craft. In this way too he discounted the uniqueness of university education.[69]

Reil's vision of medical education received decisive support from Wilhelm von Humboldt when he took over planning for the new university. One difficulty confronting Humboldt was the ambiguous division of responsibility for medical education between two offices in the Interior Ministry: the *Obermedicinalrath*, which supervised Prussia's medical system, ran the Collegium Medico-Chirurgicum, and regulated licensing, and Humboldt's own Section of Religion and Public Education. Of particular importance was the vexing question of whether the *Obermedicinalrath* would have any influence over the appointment of university medical professors. In this case, Humboldt's deeply held belief in the value of *Bildung* dovetailed nicely with the imperatives of bureaucratic aggrandisement.[70]

Expressly taking his cue from Reil's *Pepinieren*, Humboldt divided institutions for medical education into three groups. The first, of course, were the universities, which offer "theoretical instruction in connection with the entire range of *Wissenschaft*"; the second group were "medical-practical institutes" that allowed continued training after the completion of university studies; and finally, there were "medical specialty schools." Of this third class, the specialty schools, Humboldt distinguished two types: *wissenschaftliche* specialty schools, "of the sort that exists in Paris and, unfortunately, also in Berlin for some time past," and empirical ones for students not intended for higher education. Humboldt placed the Berlin *Pepinière* in this latter group, while rejecting the very idea of *wissenschaftliche* specialty schools out of hand, calling them "pernicious."[71]

Between the universities and medical-practical institutes, Humboldt envisioned a division of labor between the Section of Religion and Public Instruction, which would administer the universities, and the *Obermedicinalrath*, which would control the *Pepinière*. In no uncertain terms, he warned that any degree of interference by the medical authorities in the affairs of the university would have the most

69 See Hufeland's 1807 memorandum in Weischedel, *Idee und Wirklichkeit*, pp. 16–27.

70 For a more extensive discussion of Humboldt's plans for medical education, see Richard L. Kremer, "Between *Wissenschaft* and Praxis: Experimental Medicine and the Prussian State, 1807-1848," in *"Einsamkeit und Freiheit" neu besichtigt: Universitätsreformen und Disziplinenbildung in Preussen als Modell für Wissenschaftspolitik im Europa des 19. Jahrhunderts*, ed. Gert Schubring (Stuttgart, 1991), pp. 156–61.

71 Wilhelm von Humboldt, "Ueber die Organisation des Medizinalwesens," *Humboldts Gesammelte Schriften*, Bd. 13, p. 258. The reference to the *wissenschaftliche* specialty school in Berlin was to the Collegium medico-chirurgicum.

damaging consequences. Such meddling, he wrote, "would be manifestly contrary to the goals of general medical education."[72]

Hufeland might be forgiven for feeling aggrieved that he had been circumvented by Humboldt in favor of Reil, whose way of thinking was far more congenial to Humboldt than was Hufeland's.[73] After the university opened, Reil and Hufeland continued to get in each other's way. Among other points of disagreement, they clashed over the traditional requirement that students write and defend a doctoral dissertation. Hufeland objected to the control exercised by Reil over his students' dissertations. Because they were far more Reil's product than the students', Hufeland argued, they showed nothing of those students' capacities as future physicians. More fundamentally still, Hufeland objected to the content of those dissertations:

The chief goal of medicine is eternal – healing. And so too must an inaugural dissertation demonstrate to the world, beyond the writer's general capabilities and education, that he has achieved the knowledge necessary for healing. Now I ask, what sort of idea would the world get of our teaching institutions if it received from them nothing but dissertations on comparative anatomy? It would believe that we educate truly good anatomists and researchers, but not good physicians.[74]

The ill feelings between Reil and Hufeland even spilled over to their students, with Hufeland's cohort declaring that they would chase away any of Reil's followers whom they found in the vicinity of their own master.[75]

Reil's death in 1813 gave Hufeland a priceless opportunity to insure that his own vision for the faculty would be the one that prevailed. And to Hufeland's credit, he did not waste it. For Reil's replacement as the other professor of clinical medicine, Hufeland urged the appointment of the Breslau professor Karl August Wilhelm Berends (1759–1826), of whom he wrote, "He is a clinical teacher like no other known to me, educated as a true Hippocratic. He builds solely on the basis of experience and a thorough study of classical literature, he is free from any passion for systems and zealotry, and he is an accomplished Latinist and has an exceptional talent for teaching."[76] In other words, Hufeland wanted someone as much like himself as he could find, someone who would not challenge the supremacy of Hippocratic medicine in the Berlin clinics. Despite strenuous objections raised by Berlin's anatomist, Karl Asmund Rudolphi, that Berends enjoyed "absolutely no literary reputation" and that he had done little to advance *Wissenschaft*, Berends received the appointment.[77]

72 Ibid., p. 257.
73 Humboldt also wanted Reil to be head of the *wissenschaftliche Deputation*, an influential board within the *Obermedicinalrath* with control over licensing examinations, among other things. See Lenz, *Geschichte der Universität Berlin*, Bd. 1, pp. 200–1. Humboldt's request that Reil be appointed professor at the new university and chief of the *wissenschaftliche Deputation* is contained in *Humboldts Gesammelte Schriften*, Bd. 10, pp. 224–6.
74 Lenz, *Geschichte der Universität Berlin*, Bd. 1, pp. 376–9, quoted on 378.
75 Ibid., p. 343.
76 Quoted in ibid., p. 546.
77 GStA Merseburg Rep. 76 Vᵃ Sekt. 2 Tit. IV Nr. 5 Vol. III, fols. 52–4.

The conflict that took place in the Berlin medical faculty over the place of theory and practice in the curriculum was the most dramatic instance of such disagreements, but it was certainly not the only one. Disputes arose at Heidelberg, Bonn, and Freiburg over the appropriateness of *Naturphilosophie* in medical teaching. At Bonn, the conflict even reached to the highest levels of the Prussian government.[78] Together they bore witness to the conflicting missions that university education was being called upon to fill in the nineteenth century, as well as divisions within the medical profession itself. Later on, in the 1830s and 1840s, medical educators would learn how to use medicine's research mission in a more positive way, by immersing students in laboratory techniques. If such training did not help the aspiring physicians become better practitioners, at least it helped confer upon them the status of men of science. But of course even these modifications did not and could not address the more fundamental ambiguities of function that characterized medical education throughout the nineteenth century.[79]

THE CRYSTALLIZATION OF SEPARATE DISCIPLINARY AND PROFESSIONAL IDENTITIES

One thing that made the ideology of *Bildung* attractive to those responsible for running Prussia and other German states was the way its promised cultivation of internal freedom would in some unspecified way make the possessor of *Bildung* a more useful citizen. The cultivated man, it was assumed, would be able to understand and accept his proper function in the society and the state.[80] The same

---

78　On Heidelberg, see Eduard Seidler, "Die Entwicklung naturwissenschaftlichen Denkens in der Medizin zur Zeit der Heidelberger Romantik," *Sudhoffs Archiv* 47 (1963): 43–58; and idem, "Heidelberger Medizin in Aufklärung und Romantik," in Wilhelm Doerr, *Semper Apertus: Sechshundert Jahre Ruprecht-Karls-Universität Heidelberg 1386–1986*, Bd. 2 (Berlin, 1985), pp. 132–44. On Freiburg, see Ernst Georg Kurz, "Die Freiburger medizinische Fakultät und die Romantik," *Münchener Beiträge zur Geschichte und Literatur der Naturwissenschaften und Medizin* 17 (1929): 1–85. At Bonn, the Prussian Chancellor Karl von Hardenberg "approved" the appointment of a well-known *Naturphilosoph*, Heidelberg botanist Franz Joseph Schelver, to a chair of *Naturphilosophie*, although Altenstein, the Minister of Education, had not requested such approval and did not wish to have Schelver at Bonn. Altenstein blocked Hardenberg's ploy simply by burying Hardenburg's approval in the files and ignoring it. Renger, *Die Gründung und Einrichtung der Universität Bonn*, pp. 179–81.

79　Arleen Tuchman, "Experimental Physiology, Medical Reform, and the Politics of Education at the University of Heidelberg: A Case Study," *Bulletin of the History of Medicine* 61 (1987): 203–15; and idem, *Science, Medicine, and the State in Germany: The Case of Baden, 1815–1871* (Oxford, 1993), pp. 54–71; and Lynn K. Nyhart, *Biology Takes Form: Animal Morphology and the German Universities, 1800–1900* (Chicago, 1995). Similar ambiguities would beset American medical education too, as discussed in Gerald L. Geison, "Divided We Stand: Physiologists and Clinicians in the American Context," in *The Therapeutic Revolution: Essays in the Social History of American Medicine*, ed. Morris J. Vogel and Charles Rosenberg (Philadelphia, 1979), pp. 67–90; and John Harley Warner, "Ideals of Science and Their Discontents in Late Nineteenth-Century American Medicine," *Isis* 82 (1991): 454–78.

80　Vierhaus, "Bildung."

held true for a medical profession composed of such men of *Bildung*; it too would simultaneously maintain a sphere of intellectual freedom sheltered from external restraint, and fill a needed role in society.

No doubt eighteenth-century physicians would have recognized this division too, if not in all its dialectical irony, and without the sense of centrality to professional identity with which their nineteenth-century descendants saw it. What had dramatically changed, however, was the profession's institutional structure. In contrast to the eighteenth-century profession, where occupational boundaries between university professors and other healers were considerably less distinct, the evolution of the universities in the years following 1800 had made it possible for academically centered theoreticians to be separated from nonacademic practitioners. Doctors of medicine though they were, individual physicians outside the university gradually lost their ability to participate in the judgment of what constituted medical truth. To explore this development in all its ramifications would be the topic for another book. Yet it might not be out of place here to illustrate the significance of this separation by looking briefly at two novel developments during the 1810s. The first development concerns the emergence of animal morphology as the research program of a self-conscious community of largely university-based researchers. The second development, which took place at the profession's external boundary, consisted of an increasingly urgent examination of the physician's proper relationship with and obligations toward the state.

Let us turn first to the "internal" development, the emergence of animal morphology as a research discipline. Morphology – the study of the laws of organic form – was a characteristically German science, if not a uniquely German one. To be sure, the comparative anatomy upon which it built was derived in large measure from French practitioners, as E. S. Russell pointed out many years ago.[81] But it took the Germans to add their own twist to Georges Cuvier's basically static view of the harmonious composition of living beings. They took the position that organic form could best be understood sequentially through its development in embryos and immature individuals. And it was a characteristically Germanic faith in the unity and intelligibility of being, a faith articulated in *Naturphilosophie*, that encouraged the morphologists' search for transcendental laws of form.

The contents of this research program have been described elsewhere, and will not be repeated here.[82] More relevant to our purposes is how the morphologist-anatomists conceived of that program in relation to other branches of medicine. Meckel's own research agenda for the topic provides a good example. Pathological anatomy, Meckel observed as early as 1805, had usually been studied in one of two ways. It had consisted either of a catalogue of an organ's possible deviations

---

81 E. S. Russell, *Form and Function: A Contribution to the History of Animal Morphology* (repr. ed. Chicago, 1982), pp. 89–90.
82 Nyhart, *Biology Takes Form*; and Timothy Lenoir, *The Strategy of Life: Teleology and Mechanics in Nineteenth-Century German Biology* (Dordrecht, 1982).

from its normal form and mixture, without regard for the impaired or defective processes by which the deviation occurred, or it had laid primary weight on the processes, appending a merely supplemental description of the anatomical changes undergone by the organ. In either case, pathological anatomy had studied the degenerative changes of organs that were at one time healthy and normal, an inquiry driven by medical practitioners' desire to know what changes were produced by diseases in the body. Although such goals may be laudable, Meckel argued that the subject need not be restricted to serving clinical needs; it could also serve a "higher interest." This interest, he continued, consisted of "the developmental history of the organ under normal circumstances," along with "the harmonization of various organs and systems with each other."[83] Meckel was particularly intrigued by what he believed were pronounced similarities between the congenital deformities of an organ and the normal forms of that same organ in lower animals.[84]

Meckel's claims of a "higher viewpoint" for anatomical studies beyond their service to clinical medicine was echoed by Karl Friedrich Burdach who, in cooperation with Karl Ernst von Baer (1792–1876), made the anatomical institute at Königsberg one of Germany's most productive centers of morphological research. In an essay commemorating the opening of his institute in 1817, Burdach underscored the scientific value of morphology. It was true, he conceded, that morphology could contribute to the understanding of disease, because disease is an organic process and all such processes are "bound to a specific existence in space."[85] But, he added later, as important as the goal of preserving human life is, "the theory of human form achieves a higher signification and development only when it is understood and handled independently of this goal."[86] Burdach thus appropriated what by 1817 had become the standard language for cultivation of *Wissenschaft* to carve out a niche for morphology.

The striking thing about morphology as represented by Meckel and Burdach is how much it contrasts with the goals for physiology set out by Reil in 1795 in the *Archiv für die Physiologie.* Reil, it will be recalled, had begun the *Archiv* with the intention of bringing physiology closer to the rest of medicine. Yet despite his best intentions, Reil's own journal demonstrated a clear movement toward the study of organic function in terms of its connection with form and a movement away from matters of interest to clinicians. Volume seven of the *Archiv* (1807), which saw the Tübingen professor J. H. F. Autenrieth (1773–1835) brought aboard as co-

83 Johann Friedrich Meckel, "Ueber die Bildungsfehler des Herzens," *Archiv für die Physiologie* 6 (1805): 549–51. Meckel's vision of pathological anatomy differed substantially from the more clinically oriented views of researchers in France and Great Britain. See Russell Maulitz, *Morbid Appearances: The Anatomy of Pathology in the Early Nineteenth Century* (Cambridge, 1987).

84 Meckel, "Ueber die Bildungsfehler des Herzens," pp. 606–10. This became the basis for what became known as the Meckel-Serres law, the idea that embryonic development recapitulates an organism's position on the ladder of nature in relation to other animals. See Johann Friedrich Meckel, *Handbuch der pathologischen Anatomie*, Bd. 1, (Leipzig, 1812), pp. 44–9.

85 Karl Friedrich Burdach, *Ueber die Aufgabe der Morphologie* (Leipzig, 1817), pp. 1–2.

86 Ibid., p. 5.

editor, clearly displayed the move toward framing physiology in terms of the study of form. The editors showed the way, with Autenrieth contributing an essay on the differences in form between men and women, and Reil publishing a comparative study on the structure and function of the sympathetic and central nervous systems.[87] Following Reil's death in 1813, Meckel began editing a journal that would become the successor to Reil's *Archiv*, the *Deutsches Archiv für die Physiologie*. Meckel intended the *Deutsches Archiv*, in contrast to the earlier journal, to be strictly a forum for presentation of new empirical research. It contained no book reviews and only a scattering of theoretical essays. The *Deutsches Archiv* was also larger and more richly produced than its predecessor. It regularly included engraved plates, some even hand-colored, as opposed to the sparser illustration that had characterized Reil's *Archiv*. Most significant, however, was the claim made on the title page of the *Deutsches Archiv* proclaiming it to be the collaborative work of a board that included most of the leading names in German physiology. Thus Meckel's journal proclaimed the existence of a self-conscious disciplinary community, a community that Reil had not only never conceived of when he launched the journal in 1795, but was in fact directly contrary to his original aspirations for physiology.[88]

While Meckel and his compatriots were formulating their research program for morphology and defending it against the constraints of practice, physicians outside the universities faced completely different problems at the profession's "external" boundary. One difficulty was that government intervention in medical affairs, which eighteenth-century physicians had supported (if at times somewhat ambivalently) as a way of raising their own profile in the civil service, threatened to become after 1800 an ever more burdensome supervision and regulation of practice. A second problem concerned the profession's social position. Viewing their profession as a learned one, physicians resented being regulated in a manner like other trades, an insult to their gentlemanly status that was reinforced by what they regarded as the insecure and undignified way they earned their incomes. This prompted a torrent of complaints about physicians' impoverished financial situation, and led them to formulate plans for more stable incomes without surrendering their independence completely to state service.

What brought these issues into focus during the first quarter of the nineteenth century was the elaboration of the medical system in a number of states. Motivated by continuing concerns for the quality of medical care among the general popula-

---

87 J. H. F. Autenrieth, "Bemerkungen über die Verschiedenheit beyder Geschlechter und ihre Zeugungsorgane," *Archiv für die Physiologie* 7 (1807): 1–139; and Johann Christian Reil, "Ueber die Eigenschaften des Ganglien-Systems und sein Verhältniß zum Cerebral-System," *Archiv für die Physiologie* 7 (1807): 189–254.

88 For another example of a disciplinary community coalescing around a journal, see Hufbauer, *The Formation of the German Chemical Community*. For a more extensive discussion of the evolution of the *Archiv für die Physiologie* and the *Deutches Archiv*, see Thomas H. Broman, "J. C. Reil and the 'Journalization' of Physiology," in *The Literary Structure of Scientific Argument*, ed. Peter Dear (Philadelphia, 1991), pp. 13–42.

tion, states such as Prussia and Bavaria tinkered with creation of different classes of medical personnel as a way of better distributing practitioners over their lands. As had been the case with Christoph Ludwig Hoffmann's plans for Münster and Hesse-Kassel in the eighteenth century and Reil's recommendations in the *Pepinieren*, the idea was to produce a corps of qualified second-tier healers who would attend to the basic health needs of the rural peasantry and urban lower classes, but who would not compete directly with the fully educated doctors of medicine. Physicians often supported such efforts, since the creation of these healers was coupled with strengthened proscriptions against quackery and unlicensed practice, although some questioned whether the public was being helped by the establishment of healers who lacked the academic credentials of university-educated doctors.[89]

In a number of states, better care for the poor overlapped with governments' desire for closer control of the health care system in the articulation of increasingly elaborate regulatory structures. In Württemberg, the entire kingdom was divided into twelve administrative regions (*Landvogteien*), each with a physician appointed to direct medical affairs in the region. His specific duties were: to submit annual reports on the illnesses in the *Landvogtei*; to supervise and examine all medical personnel; to conduct biennial visitations of each district (*Oberamt*) within his jurisdiction, where he was to check up on surgeons and midwives in the *Oberamt*; inspect apothecary shops; and finally, to insure that the official *Oberamtsarzt* was fulfilling his own duties. The sixty-four *Oberamtsärzte* in turn were charged with supervising other medical personnel within the district; providing medical aid free of charge to the poor and to hospitals and other public institutions; and conducting medical-forensic inquiries.[90]

The Duchy of Nassau, located to the north and east of the confluence of the Rhine and Main rivers, went one step further and incorporated virtually all physicians – along with a large number of other healers – into the civil service. According to an edict issued in 1818, one medical officer was appointed to each of the duchy's twenty-eight districts, along with an assistant, a district apothecary, and a district midwife. These medical personnel were required to reside in their districts, although they did not have to restrict their practice to the district. The Nassau edict also eliminated the traditional division between physicians and surgeons in favor of a requirement that anyone wishing to practice surgery in the

---

89 On the medical system in Bavaria, see *Königlich-Baierisches Regierungsblatt*, Stück 40 (1808), cols. 1,701–11. For a discussion of Prussia's 1825 reform plan, see Huerkamp, *Der Aufstieg der Ärzte*, pp. 45–50. For reservations about such plans, see "Einige Bemerkungen über die Einführung der sogenannten Landärzte," *Allgemeine medicinische Annalen*, Zweite Abtheilung (1812), cols. 163–175, and the discussion of reactions to Reil's *Pepinieren* in Chapter 4.

90 These regulations were formulated in 1807 and 1808. See Lorenz Friedrich Hezel, *Repertorium der Policey-Gesetze des Königreichs Württemberg*, 9 vols. (Ellwangen, 1814–1827), esp. vol. 1, pp. 31–7, and vol. 3, pp. 183–99, 380–96. For discussion of Württemberg's system, see Annette Drees, *Die Ärzte auf dem Weg zu Prestige und Wohlstand: Sozialgeschichte der württembergischen Ärzte im 19. Jahrhundert* (Münster, 1988), pp. 33–8.

future would have to be a university-educated doctor of medicine. Surgeons currently in practice were allowed to continue with their craft, and many received appointment as district assistants.[91]

Such finely grained regulation of the medical system increased the number of positions in state service open to physicians, but it also burdened the profession with an oppressive blanket of regulatory directives. Even private physicians in Württemberg and elsewhere were ordered to care for impoverished supplicants when official medical aid was unavailable, and physicians in private practice were also required to conform to various schedules of fees, limitations on where they practiced, and other mandates conjured up by ever-productive governments.[92] Government intervention in the health care system made life difficult for private practitioners in still another way: Because physicians in civil service were allowed to maintain private practices as a way of augmenting their regular salaries, the expansion of medical positions in the civil service opened up a new source of competition for the private share of the healing market.

The issue of income ensnared private physicians in an embarrassing dilemma. On the one hand, they believed they were not receiving the income that was their due, a situation arising from the state's meddling in the fees they could charge and from competition from other healers (among them physicians employed by the state). On the other hand, their sense of themselves as men of *Bildung* and *Wissenschaft* and of what it meant to belong to a profession made it difficult, if not impossible, to complain directly about their incomes. Consequently their discussion of medicine as an occupation tended to be veiled and elliptical. For example, one commentator observed that medicine, as the "freest of all arts," maintains its special dignity principally because "the thought of exercising it for any mere pecuniary gain is repugnant to the feelings of every right thinking physician."[93] Another writer pointed out that physicians may not receive the earnings rightfully due them, but the true healing artist practices his art for its own sake, and not for any gain. The physician who looks at medicine this way and strives constantly toward its perfection, the writer concluded, will lack neither love for his art nor people around him who appreciate it and reward him for it.[94]

In contrast to these indirect and romanticized complaints about physicians' status, Friedrich Nasse's 1823 monograph on medical reform, *Von der Stellung der Aerzte im Staate* (On the place of physicians in the state), did not shrink from a more blunt assessment. Physicians have sunk so low in the view of the state, Nasse complained, that governments treat them just as they would any other tradesmen. The physician is privileged by the state to carry on his business, and like other

---

91 Treichel, *Der Primat der Bürokratie*, pp. 229–31.
92 Charles E. McClelland, *The German Experience of Professionalization* (Cambridge, 1991), p. 39.
93 "Über Contracte zwischen Ärzte und Kranken," *Allgemeine medizinische Annalen*, Zweite Abtheilung (1812), col. 463–72, quoted in col. 463.
94 "Ueber Dank und Undank gegen die Ärzte," *Allgemeine medizinische Annalen* (1810), cols. 1,129–40.

tradesmen he is dependent for his livelihood on patients. That patients necessarily become a mere object of income to the physician is the necessary outcome of this situation.[95] Interestingly enough, Nasse did not see the profession's declining status as the result of the physician's avarice, but as the cause of it. Only after physicians had lost the honor they had once enjoyed, he argued, did they begin treating their profession as a trade.[96]

Much of Nasse's book was devoted to cataloguing the evils that arise from medicine's status as a trade: manipulation of patients, competition between colleagues, lack of incentive for cultivation of *Wissenschaft,* and a host of others. But toward the end he began considering what could be done to remedy the situation. Nasse rejected the idea of making all doctors civil servants, saying that doing so and giving them a salary appropriate to their work would place an intolerable burden on the tax structure. He also worried that state payment – either full or partial – for medical care would open the door to state control of bedside practice.[97]

Instead of allowing the State to be the anchor for medicine's status and income, Nasse came up with the novel and revealing idea of using medical societies as agencies for billing patients. After all, Nasse noted, it is really the entire profession that cures a patient, when one takes into account that an individual physician draws on other physicians for his formal education and bedside knowledge. Why not therefore have patients pay the profession? Each physician would be required to join a medical society, to which he would send in monthly reports on the cases he treated, and the society would then bill patients, with adjustments made for the patient's ability to pay. Physicians would then draw their salaries from the societies, based on their activities in both treatment and prevention of illnesses, contributions to scientific research, and so on.[98]

Nasse's plan obviously was hopelessly unrealistic, and it did not enjoy a favorable reception in the medical press. What makes it interesting, however, is not its feasibility but instead its vision of the profession. Like so many of his contemporaries (not to mention later generations of physicians), Nasse held to a vision of professionalism that attempted to preserve a profession's freedom against the regulatory encroachments of state government. Just like other men of *Bildung,* physicians did not cherish the vision of themselves as mere cogs in the apparatus of government. Nasse's response was not to deny the state any legitimate role in medicine's business; to my knowledge, no physician writing at the time did that. Instead, Nasse believed that the profession's freedom and dignity could be preserved (or more precisely, reestablished) by creating an internal regulatory structure to oversee the crucial matters of fees and incomes. In a manner that has become the anthem of countless professions since Nasse's time, self-regulation would be

95 Friedrich Nasse, *Von der Stellung der Aerzte im Staate* (Leipzig, 1823), p. 20.
96 Ibid., pp. 12–18.
97 Ibid., pp. 322–36.
98 Ibid., pp. 360–79.

the means of answering simultaneously the interests of state, society, *and* the profession.

CONCLUSION: THE REFORM ERA AND ACADEMIC MEDICINE

It cannot be denied that there is a satisfying thoroughness to the changes that took place in Germany after 1803. The dissolution of the Holy Roman Empire, the partial leveling of the tangled legal and political system that had prevailed in the Empire, the reform of state bureaucracies and of course the reorganization of the universities all attest to a transformation that was much more than superficial. For this reason alone, the stories of the professionalization of German medicine and the rise of modern German science have been written as nineteenth-century phenomena.

And yet something important is lost when we fail to pay attention to the continuities of the story. It makes a difference, for example, that universities in Germany were continuous with institutions of the old regime, and not closed down as they were in France. German universities were not so radically transformed that they became mere instruments of the state, grinding out teachers, doctors, and other functionaries like so much sausage. Instead they acted both as loci for a particular portion of German culture as well as institutions for the formation of a social elite. In both respects, universities carried on functions they had performed in the eighteenth century and earlier. Even the ideology of *Bildung,* which occupied so central a position in the identity of the nineteenth-century educated middle class, had been clearly articulated well before 1800 and represented a modification of the earlier scholarly ideal of *Gelehrsamkeit.*

The same point can be made, of course, for physicians. It merits repeating here that the changes we have been examining did not involve trading in the costume of an outmoded, scholastic, practically inefficacious profession for the white laboratory coat that characterizes the scientifically trained expert practitioner. Instead, the former identity based on gentlemanly learnedness was complemented by a new sense of professionalism based on the socially progressive uses of knowledge. I say "complemented" deliberately, for if in some respects the two identities produced antagonistic confrontations, in a larger sense they shaped and defined each other. *Bildung* arose out of the confrontation with practice and was distinguished from *Gelehrsamkeit* precisely on the basis of its explicit insistence on an interior space of personal freedom, a space where the external constraints of social practice cannot penetrate. Practice, meanwhile, was ultimately redefined as scientific practice, a practice that supposedly "embodies" or "applies" theory in its concrete choices and actions. That the precise contours of the relationship between theory and practice became an immensely contentious issue in the period should come as no surprise, for it reflected the ambiguities inherent in the medical profession itself.

CONCLUSION: DISCIPLINES, PROFESSIONS, AND THE PUBLIC SPHERE

The emergence of the professoriate as a full-time career during the early years of the nineteenth century marked a signal change in the social organization of German intellectual life, which would have enormous consequences over the long term. In the first place, it would lead to the recruitment of students directly into the professorial ranks, creating in medical faculties a cadre of "physicians" whose attachment to the practice of medicine was uncertain. By mid-century, medical students like Carl Gegenbaur, Ernst Haeckel and Emil Du Bois-Reymond could take an M.D. without seriously intending to make a career as practitioners. Such career goals would have been virtually inconceivable in 1750, and were remarkable even in 1800. Secondly, these new professors would begin trading older forms of academic scholarship for the production of research more akin to our sense of the word: empirical discoveries meant to enrich the store of knowledge. While such research would eventually find its way into medical curricula, it was not conducted necessarily with pedagogical aims in mind, and much of what had once counted as scholarship in the eighteenth century (such as writing textbooks) no longer carried the same prestige. Of course, this is not to imply that empirical research had been unknown to eighteenth-century scholars, only to explain that the weight of research effort had shifted and that the environment for it – both institutional and cultural – had changed considerably.

What is remarkable in this transformation is the fact that the medical profession retained a veneer of professional unity at all. The emergence of specialized research disciplines such as comparative anatomy and physiological chemistry more or less within the profession did not cause it to fragment. It is tempting, though of course also futile, to speculate on what would have happened had the recommendations of a Massow or a Hufeland been taken more seriously in Prussia, and medical research had been moved out of the university environment. What consequences would there have been for physicians as a professional group? It is at least conceivable that such a move would have created a separate cohort of medical theorists while reducing physicians to the status of Routiniers, those practicing "automata" described by Reil. Things did not turn out that way, as we know, and every

physician, whether a research oncologist, cardiovascular surgeon or family practitioner, retains to this day the same title to professional status.

Although in one sense this has been a story of the "professionalization" of
German medicine, I have broken off the narrative at a point where most historians
have thought it barely worth taking up. As a story of professionalization, then,
mine is an odd one. The only people who can be said to have professionalized in
this story are those communities of university-based researchers represented by
Meckel, Döllinger, and the other animal morphologists.[1] They are the ones who
defined themselves as a separate community, established journals as organs of
communication, set themselves up as judges of each other's work and carved out
full-time occupational niches. The larger community of physicians, by contrast,
did not professionalize much beyond where it had been in 1750. Their situation
was certainly not stagnant, as indicated by the increasing levels of bureaucratic
regulation and the evolution in physicians' sense of themselves from *Gelehrter* to
men of *Bildung* and *Wissenschaft*. Yet by the usual standards of what it means to be
a "modern" profession – monopolization of practice and autonomous regulation
of professional affairs, for example – German physicians in 1820 little resembled
their twentieth-century medical descendants.

Be that as it may, I would argue that in one respect the German medical
profession by 1820 had acquired a crucial characteristic of modern professionalism,
and that is what I described in the introduction as the "discourse of theory and
practice."[2] An early version of that discourse first appeared in the context of
Enlightenment reforms of education, when it was claimed that the legitimacy of
knowledge acquired through formal education depended on its ability to guide
social practice in commerce, public health, or other domains. From the other
direction too, practice was to be reformed by being grounded on general scientific
principles. This goal saw its implementation in the provision of advanced medical
education to surgeons, which would encompass study of the theoretical disciplines
alongside the techniques of surgical practice. And needless to say, Brunonianism
represented the most complete expression of this idea.

Having seen how this discourse of theory and practice took form, a couple of
questions can now be posed. First, how novel in fact was it? I certainly do not
want to claim too much here. We are talking about medicine, after all, which for
centuries before 1800 had concerned itself both with formulating a philosophical
comprehension of its subject and with developing effective therapies. Obviously
physicians had proceeded from the conviction that theory had some relevance to
practice, a point made repeatedly in the Hippocratic Corpus and in countless
writings thereafter. Yet the intellectual environment in which medicine was
practiced and philosophized about allowed for clear distinctions between the
two. According to Aristotle, for example, knowledge could be divided between

1 I certainly do not want to suggest that the morphologists were the only such group.
2 See Introduction.

theoretical knowledge (*theoria*), practical knowledge (*praxis*), and productive knowledge (*techne*). *Theoria* consisted of contemplation of the eternal verities, manifested in pursuits such as astronomy, natural philosophy and mathematics. *Praxis,* meanwhile, denoted the goal-directed, normative kind of knowledge represented most essentially for Aristotle by politics. *Techne,* finally, was also goal-oriented like *praxis,* but differed from it in being directed not toward the creation of political and social norms, but instead toward artifacts for human use.

Now, Aristotle and other ancient writers acknowledged that these three kinds of knowledge ramified and overlapped with each other. In particular, medicine represented a domain of significant overlap. Celsus, who lived in the first century a.d., described medicine as a kind of *techne* (because health was an "artifact" of human effort), but a *techne* linked to *theoria.* Yet the links between the three kinds of knowledge described by Aristotle and Celsus were largely circumstantial, instead of thoroughgoing or systematic. This led them in most cases to treat the three as different. In the same treatise in which Celsus offered the preceding characterization of medical knowledge, for example, he also denied that theorizing belongs to the practice of the art.[3]

The ancient three-fold configuration of knowledge, in which theory and practice were held as distinct forms of cognition, has blurred considerably, although traces of it remain today. In his 1968 essay "Technical Progress and Social Life-World," for example, Jürgen Habermas argued that the modern structure of knowledge has become largely a binary one, a duality implied in the famous "two cultures problem" addressed by C. P. Snow and Aldous Huxley. Habermas described these two kinds as the "action-oriented self-understanding of social groups," which generates a cosmos of values and meaning that provides normative guides to social action, and the "technically exploitable knowledge" provided by the sciences. In themselves these two realms of knowledge, the one intimately immersed in the experiential matrix of the "life-world" (the echoes of Husserl's phenomenology here are unmistakable), the other in a contextless universe of fact, have little to do with each other. Knowledge of, say, molecular genetics in itself has no relevance for our life experiences. Only when that knowledge is given a technological import, when it is exploited and becomes a tool for control, does it acquire relevance.[4]

Habermas's point in describing these two kinds of knowledge was to criticize the way that scientific/technical knowledge has come to supersede that other form of practical knowledge, but this is not the only lesson to be drawn. In fact, there is an instructive correspondence between this version of the two cultures and the situation in German medicine in the early nineteenth century. The Brunonians, of course, represented the technological alternative. To them, medical

---

3 My discussion of theory and practice in Aristotle and Celsus is based on Nicholas Lobkowicz, *Theory and Practice: History of a Concept from Aristotle to Marx* (Notre Dame, Ind., 1967), pp. 35–46.
4 Jürgen Habermas, "Technical Progress and Social Life-World," in idem, *Toward a Rational Society,* trans. Jeremy J. Shapiro (Boston, 1970), pp. 50–61.

theory took its "meaning" from its capacity for application and control. Those physicians who opposed Brunonianism in effect rejected an instrumentalist vision of medical science. The anti-Brunonians readily assented to the cultivation of theory, insofar as theory could aid in elaborating a vision of what the world is and how it works. But their practice was self-consciously a practice embedded in the social milieu of the life-world; it was a practice that constructed meaning out of everyday experience by eschewing the totalizing – and especially the decontextualizing – claims of scientific theory. Thus, whereas the Brunonians saw an intimate interdependence between theory and practice, their opponents insistently held them apart.

Therefore, it should be evident that the early nineteenth century presented a considerable departure from the ancient categories of *theoria, praxis,* and *techne.*[5] For some, such as the Brunonians, theory became the basis for a generally valid technical knowledge. For others, medicine represented a mixed form of *praxis* played out on a field filled with doctors and patients in normative communication and acting in well defined social circumstances. Even the opponents of the Brunonians would not have rejected medicine's ancient association with *techne* as a product of human artifice – illustrated if nowhere else by their description of it as a *Kunst* – but their conception of medical practice and their active promotion of medical Enlightenment made it no less a kind of *praxis.*

However, the modern relationship between theory and practice is not exhausted in theory's application to practice.[6] For it requires additionally an understanding of theory as valuable not merely for its instrumental benefits, but also as something to be cultivated for its own sake, as the manifestation of "the human spirit" or "the quest for knowledge." Theory thus retains an important residue of its ancient characteristic as insight into the changeless nature of things, and this lends theory its twin aspect as instrumental guide for technical control and source of *Bildung*. To my mind, this duality is essential to modern professionalism. Here we should recall that Brunonianism became an important cultural phenomenon not only because of its proffered union of theory and practice and the democratizing possibilities implicit therein, but also because of its links with *Naturphilosophie* and Jena Romanticism. Brunonian medicine articulated a dialectical view of life and illness that fit in nicely with Schelling's own program and the interests of a larger community of avant-garde intellectuals. Not coincidentally, when the adherents

---

5 I am not claiming that nothing at all had happened in the intervening two millennia to alter the balance between these kinds of knowledge, or even that the Aristotelian division had exerted any kind of regulative influence over the partitioning of knowledge, medical or otherwise, during that time. Nevertheless, insofar as Aristotle's writing maintained some kind of authority for European scholars up through the seventeenth century, his partitioning of knowledge would have remained relevant to discussions of theory and practice.

6 In case it is not evident from the context, medical "practice" in the modern era has little in common with the ancient understanding of *praxis*. This migration of the meaning of practice away from its etymological root and toward the idea of theoretically grounded technical control became the object of vigorous criticism by Habermas and by Herbert Marcuse in *One Dimensional Man*.

of *Naturphilosophie* turned on the Brunonians and began attacking their theory, the movement lost much of its appeal.

Yet if theory retains value as an end in and of itself, for contemporary professions such as medicine it must be the right kind of theory. One thing that distinguishes a profession like medicine today from other pursuits, such as history or social theory, is that medicine largely shuts out meta-theory from its professional identity. That is, physicians do not routinely ponder questions such as the possibility of medical knowledge, what it means to have "instrumental knowledge," and the social conditions of professionalism. In contrast to students of history and literary criticism, who are incessantly inundated by meta-theoretical conundrums as part of their training, medical students encounter at most a few discussions of ethical matters, many of which are pragmatically centered on questions of professional conduct.

This was certainly not the case in the early nineteenth century, when *Naturphilosophie* broached the meta-theoretical option not only in medicine, but in the entire realm of science. Indeed Fichte had already opened this meta-theoretical portal, something he realized himself, as indicated by the title of his great work: *Wissenschaftslehre* (Theory of science). The Jena Romantics perceived it too, and hailed the *Wissenschaftslehre* as "simultaneously philosophy and philosophy of philosophy." Then they and the *Naturphilosophen* went Fichte one better by pushing the foundations of meta-theoretical criticism to a still deeper level. For at least a couple of decades, the question of whether *Naturphilosophie* belonged within academic medicine was hotly contested, and this debate greatly complicated the relationship between theory and practice.

Ultimately, meta-theoretical programs such as *Naturphilosophie* were excluded from academic medicine. How and why this happened would be the subject of another book. Yet we should recognize that, however foreordained the outcome looks from our side of the event, in the first decade of the nineteenth century it was by no means a settled question. The exclusion of *Naturphilosophie* was certainly not the defining moment of the modern medical profession in Germany; I doubt whether any one event would qualify as this threshold. But it did help to establish the contours of the relationship between theory and practice in medicine. So long as it avoided undermining its own epistemological and methodological underpinnings, medical theory would be accorded the twin qualities of "insight into the nature of things" and "guide for practical control." Not just physicians but a large number of professional experts today continue to plant their flags on this very ground.

A second question concerning the discourse of theory and practice is a comparative one: what relevance does my story have for the history of medicine in Europe? In the first place, as I have said before, I am not presenting my story as if the entire discursive formation of modern medicine could be traced back to a single Germanic source. Quite to the contrary, my years of work in the quiet historiographic backwater of eighteenth-century Germany have convinced me how remarkably different were the social, institutional and political environments for science and medicine in Britain, France and Germany, to name only three nations. If the Germans found the discourse of theory and practice to be a matter of some urgency in the years around 1800, there is no reason to suppose that the British or the French or anyone else would have felt the same urgency, or would have responded to it in the same way. Of course, this argument about the distinctiveness of medicine in Britain, France, and Germany cuts both ways: if I cannot use it to argue for Germany as the birthplace of modern medicine, it should also call into question similar and much more widely held claims for the Paris clinic.[7]

The final question raised by the emergence of theory-practice discourse is perhaps the most important of all, and it is the question that has been suspended since the introduction: what is the connection between this discourse and the public sphere, that space of cultural exchange opened by the appearance of a civil society situated between the intimate domain of the family and the state? Their simultaneous appearance, one would like to argue, surely was not coincidental, yet the matter turns out to be a complex issue. Nevertheless, I do not want to dismiss the matter without presenting at least a tentative explanation of how they might have been connected in 1800, and suggesting why the connection continues to be important today. What follows therefore is the first framing of an account that I hope to develop more satisfactorily in the future.

Part of the problem in understanding the relationship between theory-practice discourse and the public sphere stems from the fact that Habermas's original discussion of the eighteenth-century public sphere paid no attention to the role of scientific knowledge in constituting the public sphere. Nor did he suggest what epistemological status was accorded by contemporaries to judgments reached by the public exercising its critical function. Did natural philosophy, for example, furnish a model of secure, objective knowledge that judgments reached by the public would attempt to emulate? Kant for one seemed to think there was a connection, for he made Newtonian mechanics the object of his inquiry in the *Critique of Pure Reason*. In doing so, he attempted not only to offer a sufficient

---

7 Erwin Ackerknecht's vision of the Paris clinics in the early nineteenth century as the source of a progressive medical epistemology that was ultimately superseded by German "laboratory" medicine after 1850 has proven remarkably durable. See his *Medicine at the Paris Hospital, 1794–1848* (Baltimore, 1967). In part, the reason for this durability is its continuity with what generations of German medical historians and polemicists have written about Germany and France. When Karl Wunderlich called for the implementation of what he called "physiological medicine" in 1841, for example, he explicitly held up the Paris clinics, along with the Vienna clinics in which he had been educated, as models of clinical practice. Yet Wunderlich's polemics and the similarly polemical medical histories produced in the late nineteenth century by Julius Pagel and Johann Hermann Baas, among others, must be interpreted in light of the situation of the German profession, and not simply as instances of direct French "influence." See Karl Wunderlich, *Wien und Paris* (Stuttgart, 1841), and idem, *Geschichte der Medizin* (Stuttgart, 1859); Johann Hermann Baas, *Die geschichtliche Entwicklung des ärztlichen Standes und der medicinischen Wissenschaften* (Berlin, 1896); and Julius Pagel, *Einführung in die Geschichte der Medizin* (Berlin, 1898).

epistemological grounding for Newton's physics, but also to produce a more general method of philosophical/critical inquiry.

In asking about the connection between the public sphere and theory-practice discourses, it is important that we make the question as historically specific as possible. This is all the more necessary as recent treatments of the public sphere in various national contexts have located it in different institutions, such as coffee houses or salons. Habermas's own description set up the English public sphere as a model and made the coffee houses of London its point of origin; the public sphere in other national contexts thus became variants on the English "model."[8] But it seems to me that institutions such as coffee houses and salons, where the interlocutors could converse directly with each other and often could know each other, would establish those interlocutors as "the public" (both in their own minds and in the eyes of contemporaries writing about the public) in a different way than would the exchanges featured in literary media such as periodicals. In making this distinction, I am not denying that coffee houses and salons were legitimate institutions of the public sphere. Rather, I am saying that such public spaces, along with the cultural dominance exerted by the national capitals of London and Paris, gave the English and French public spheres a distinctive structure that set them apart from Germany, which contained a number of dispersed cultural centers. Precisely because Germany had no single dominant center, its public sphere was much more significantly constituted through its print media. One consequence of this situation may have been that the German public was a far more idealized construction than was the case in Britain or France. In a real sense, the German "public" was structured – indeed, one might even say called into existence – by the discursive conventions of its print media, for example in the way that periodicals allowed readers and writers to exchange roles and by the kinds of authorial voices they fostered. With such considerations in mind, then, we can return to the question of what might have been the connection between the German public sphere and theory/practice discourses in professionalization.

Let us begin with the specific historical case and ask how the late eighteenth-century German public might have comprehended the nature of its own judgments. The public invoked for example by Kant in the *Critique of Pure Reason,* or by Reil in the *Archiv für die Physiologie,* or by Hecker in the *Journal der Erfindungen,* did not appear to be a kind of universal debating society, in which decisions would be reached by majority vote after an airing of the pros and cons of an issue. Instead, I believe the authority of public judgments was based on the conviction that the public sphere was the cultural embodiment of Reason itself. As such, the

8 Jürgen Habermas, *The Structural Transformation of the Public Sphere: An Inquiry into a Category of Bourgeois Society,* trans. Thomas Burger, with the assistance of Frederick Lawrence (Cambridge, Mass., 1989), pp. 57–73. On English coffee houses, see Steve Pincus, " 'Coffee Politicians Does Create': Coffeehouses and Restoration Political Culture," *The Journal of Modern History* 67 (1995): 807–34; and on French salons, Dena Goodman, *The Republic of Letters: A Cultural History of the French Enlightenment* (Ithaca, N.Y., 1994).

give-and-take of critical debate and reflection by an enlightened public (and the qualifier is an important one) was itself the sufficient condition for the eventual overcoming of all partiality and prejudice. Thus if a writer chose to enter the public sphere by taking up the pen – a literary critic writing about a play, for example – that writer's voice was presented as the voice of any reasonable person, or, more precisely, of all such people. Debate between participants in the public sphere was not shrugged off by readers and the disputants themselves as an endless wrangle leading nowhere, but instead as necessary stages on the road to the final resolution of a problem. That final stage, distant as it may be, would not be reached by exhausting one's opponents or by coercing them into silence, but by making the truth of the matter self-evident. The public sphere therefore was conceived of first and last as the arena in which Reason would make itself present in cultural exchange.[9]

Now if the public sphere was indeed understood in this way at the end of the eighteenth century, then I think it becomes plain that the public would have little means of digesting knowledge claims based on experience that is necessarily subjective or that requires special competence to be understood. Recall here the debate between Hufeland and Erhard over medical knowledge. Hufeland's vision of medical knowledge was deeply subjective and dependent on the accumulation of particular kinds of direct experience. For this reason, he attempted to declare the public incapable of judging medicine because of its lack of experience with medical practice (except of course as patients, which apparently did not count for much). Erhard, by contrast, deliberately attacked Hufeland's claims to privileged knowledge and sought to drag medicine before the public tribunal, realizing, I suspect, that in such a court Hufeland's case would be hopeless because it would be incomprehensible. In the same way, the link between theory and practice presented by Brunonianism was based on statements that were as thoroughly objective and accessible to public standards of critical judgment as they could be. The scientific theory on which Brunonianism was based, the modes of its application in practice, indeed even the patient as a concrete person were emptied of all subjective content and became passive objects of theoretical understanding and therapeutic control.

However, at this point we come to an intriguing paradox. It has been the contention of this book that the discourse of theory linked to practice is a defining feature of modern professionalism, but our consideration of the debate between Hufeland and Erhard suggests that the public in the 1790s would discount or reject claims to privileged knowledge. If the claim to possession of a scientifically valid expert knowledge is essential to modern professionalism, then how could the public sphere have played any role whatsoever in the formulation or validation of

9 Roger Chartier offers similar comments about the function of the public sphere, as displayed in Kant's essay, "What Is Enlightenment?" See "The Public Sphere and Public Opinion," in Roger Chartier, *The Cultural Origins of the French Revolution*, trans. Lydia G. Cochrane (Durham, N.C., 1991), pp. 20–37.

claims that are by definition beyond its comprehension? To make the point another way: as long as the public was credited by people such as Erhard with having a role in validating medical knowledge, then how could medicine ever become a privileged professional domain?[10]

The answer, I think, has to do with how professions such as medicine have made use of scientific knowledge since 1800. Let us suppose that my account of how knowledge claims were evaluated by the public sphere is correct, and that in 1800 nearly all knowledge that could legitimately claim to be such was available to critical judgment by the public.[11] What happens then over the course of the nineteenth and twentieth centuries is a gradual sequestration of chunks of knowledge within regions of narrowly professional discourse. At the same time, however – and this is crucial – that knowledge is not thereby given up as belonging to the secret incantations of some weird, if also practically efficacious, cult, but continues to appear to the public as open and scientific.

Although properly speaking not a "profession," the development of the community of morphologists described in chapter six provides a good example of what I am talking about. Meckel's *Deutsches Archiv für die Physiologie* differed from Reil's earlier *Archiv* precisely in the stance it took toward the public and in how it defined its audience. Meckel's journal no longer saw itself engaged in the public task of criticizing physiology. Instead, the *Deutsches Archiv* invoked a community of scientists engaged with a common set of problems and, most importantly, a community of judges of each other's work. Meckel did not explicitly tell the nonspecialist readers/writers of the *Deutsches Archiv* that their opinions no longer counted for anything. He did not need to, because anyone who could participate in the work of the *Deutsches Archiv* would necessarily do so on terms defined by the journal itself. Otherwise their work simply would not be published.

What qualified someone to participate in the work of the *Deutsches Archiv* and other disciplinary communities? It was not a set of secret handshakes or passwords, nor the spiritual enlightenment that had once qualified adepts for alchemical and cabalistic studies. Instead, the qualifications for participation consisted of mastery of research practices and knowledge of the discipline's language and theoretical concerns. And that of course is the key to the authority of scientific knowledge in

---

10 For the purposes of this argument, it does not matter that already in 1795 there was a good deal of medical knowledge that would have been inaccessible to the public. So long as writers such as Erhard could speak *as if* medical knowledge belonged before the public tribunal, then ultimate authority over medical knowledge did not belong exclusively to physicians.

11 I say "nearly" because some kinds of scientific knowledge, such as the physics of an Euler or a Bernoulli, would obviously not be very accessible to the public, although it would be recognized as legitimately scientific. However, the existence of such examples does not bear on my argument. First, it could be noted that books on mechanics and other abstruse subjects were reviewed in the general literary reviews, as if they were just as liable to public scrutiny as the latest drama by Schiller. More fundamentally, however, these sciences manifested that "contextless world of fact" alluded to by Habermas in his discussion of the two-cultures problem. So long as they remained abstract constructions of physical reality, such work would not have any significance for the public sphere.

the modern world, and of the professional practices that claim to be based on it.[12] Scientific knowledge is universally accessible in principle but recondite in practice. In principle, the public *could* judge the work of Meckel and his compatriots, because that research presented itself as objective, disinterested, and sharing in all the other normative principles that guide scientific practice. The public had only to familiarize itself with the terminology and learn the laboratory practices on which morphology was based and it too would judge it as valid knowledge.

Much of what I have said here about the recondite nature of scientific practice will not be new to historians of science, but my point is to emphasize the important role played by the public sphere in the growth of the authority of science. Even though animal morphology and countless other disciplines effectively began to withdraw large regions of scientific knowledge from the public sphere almost as soon as it formed and to establish problem domains largely defined and regulated by themselves alone, they did so while maintaining the public sphere as an ideological shell. As a consequence, when scientific experts today tell us what to think about something like teen-age alcoholism or the genetic basis of homosexuality, they speak not as prophets – a Daniel or an Isaiah inspired with a unique vision – nor as Delphic oracles. They speak for *us*; that is, they speak for anyone sufficiently apprised of the facts to formulate a scientific comprehension of the matter. To be sure, there is an infinite regress here, because only "competent judges" (i.e., experts themselves) are qualified to certify when someone is "sufficiently apprised" of the facts to judge them adequately. Therefore, whenever experts attempt to ground their authority as scientific practitioners on some objective source outside of themselves, it turns out that they are the only ones who can locate that source. But what keeps the whole system going is the ideological remnant of the public sphere.

No doubt this sketch of the relationship between theory/practice discourses and the public sphere suffers from all manner of defects. Yet I hope that it has been sufficiently plausible in its main contours to suggest how much might be gained from a better understanding of the relationship. The benefits of such an understanding go beyond the historical events I have recounted here. More importantly, an understanding of the relationship between theory/practice discourse and the public sphere would allow a more critical insight into the rise of the modern professions in the last two centuries and ultimately into the phenomenon of professionalism today.

12 This is not to say that professional practices are uniquely validated by the theoretical knowledge that is claimed to undergird them; their efficacy obviously contributes too. Physicians therefore can claim authority for their practices both because they command scientific knowledge and because they do heal the sick. Both elements, however, are essential.

INDEX

Absolute, The, 93–4
academic resort, *see* Göttingen (university)
Academy of Useful Sciences (Erfurt), 68
Ackerknecht, Erwin H., 103n
Ackermann, Jacob Fidelis, 174–5, 176
aesthetics, 95
Allgemeine deutsche Bibliothek, 74
Allgemeine Literatur-Zeitung, 74, 98, 145, 147
Allgemeine medizinische Annalen, 123, 159
Almanach für Aerzte und Nichtärzte, 84–5
Altdorf (university), 49, 59, 61, 66
Altenstein, Karl vom Stein zum, 175, 176, 185n
Althoff, Friedrich, 42n
anatomy, 28, 30, 36, 136, 176; in Berlin, 53–4;
    comparative, 184, 186; demonstrations by
    M.D. candidates, 46, 53; provision of ca-
    davers, 29; relationship with clinical sub-
    jects, 178–9, 187; separation from sur-
    gery, 178–9; student dissections in, 34,
    46; *see also* morphology, animal
Ansbach-Bayreuth (principality), 54, 65–6, 174
Apothecaries Act, 9
apothecaries and pharmacy, 19, 21–2, 25, 27n,
    38, 52–3, 189
Archiv für die Physiologie, see Reil, Johann Chris-
    tian
Aristotle, 194–5
Der Arzt, eine medicinische Wochenschrift, 18, 109
Athenaeum, 94, 98
Aufklärung, see Enlightenment
Aufrücken, see medical faculties
Autenrieth, Johann H. F., 187–8
avant-garde, 97–9
Avicenna, 76

Baar (landgravate), 25
Baas, Johann Hermann, 198n
Baden, 24, 160, 176; administrative reforms,
    162–3; faculty recruitment policies, 171–
    3, 174–5; political reorganization in 1803,
    162; university reforms, 164–7

Baer, Karl Ernst von, 187
Baldinger, Ernst Gottfried, 31, 39; *Biographien
    jetztlebender Aerzte*, 27n; clinic in Göt-
    tingen, 64; concept of medical education,
    30; on Hippocratic medicine, 141; as
    medical journalist, 84–5
Bamberg (principality), 38, 158
Bamberg (university), 59, 149, 158
barbers, 19, 21, 25, 38, 53
bathkeepers, 19, 25
Baumer, Johann Wilhelm, 63
Bavaria, 25n, 26n, 33, 158, 160, 161, 162; faculty
    recruitment policies, 171; political and
    administrative reforms, 163; origins of *col-
    legium medicum*, 52; university reforms,
    165–7
Benzel, Anselm Franz von, 50
Berends, Karl A. W., 184
Berlin (university), 9, 122, 175, 178; appointment
    of Reil's successor, 184; competition be-
    tween Hufeland and Reil, 182–4; found-
    ing, 168–70; plans for medical faculty,
    182–4; and Prussian *Kulturpolitik*, 172
Beyme, Karl Friedrich, 168, 182
Bichat, Xavier, 156
Bildung, 73, 119, 173, 191, 196; and anti-utilitari-
    anism, 97, 160; and citizenship, 185–6;
    general characteristics, 71–2; Humboldt's
    advocacy of, 169–70; neo-classicism and,
    140; origins, 71; relationship with social
    practice, 192
Bildungsbürgertum, 4
Bildungstrieb, 81
Blackbourn, David, 3
Blumenbach, Johann Friedrich, 81
Boerhaave, Hermann, 18, 31, 83, 181; *Aphorismi
    de cognoscendis et curandis morbis*, 15; clini-
    cal teaching, 15, 62–3; eighteenth-
    century reputation, 13–16; *Institutiones
    medicae*, 14; and Newtonianism, 80; physi-
    ology and pathology of, 76–80

Boerner, Friedrich, 15–17, 27n, 31, 126
Bonaparte, Napoleon, 99, 160, 164n
Bonn (university), 172, 175, 177n, 178, 179, 185
botany, 28–9, 30, 36
Brandenburg-Onolzbach, 31n
Brandenburg-Prussia, 4, 120, 121, 160, 174; criticism of universities, 68, 168; faculty recruitment policies, 172; *Kulturpolitik,* 170–1, 173; organization of University of Bonn, 175–6; origins of *collegium medicum,* 52–4; planning for University of Berlin 167, 168–70, 182–4; political and administrative reforms after 1807, 163–4; *see also* Collegium medico-chirurgicum (Berlin)
Brauer, Johann Friedrich, 162–3, 164, 171–2
Braunschweig-Wolfenbüttel, 54, 67
Brendel, Johann Gottfried, 63
Breslau (university), 179
Brown, John, 129, 143–4, 145; *see also* Brunonianism
Brunonianism, 9, 11–12, 83, 159, 180, 181, 194; attack on Hippocratic medicine, 150–1, 154; Bamberg hospital and, 152–5; basic doctrines, 143–4, 150–1; etiology, 151–2; introduction into Germany, 129–30, 144n; and *Naturphilosophie,* 129–30, 149, 157–8, 196–7; reasons for disappearance, 157–8; revolutionary rhetoric in, 144–6; as unity of theory and practice, 144, 149, 155, 196; as *Wissenschaft,* 148–50; *see also* pathology; therapeutics
Brunschwig, Henri, 99
Burdach, Karl Friedrich, 181–2, 187

cameralism, 46–8
case histories, 132, 138–9, 154–5
Celsus, 195
charlatans, 3, 19, 189
chemistry, 28–9, 30, 36, 87–8, 177
civil service, 22, 44, 50; ideals of, 40; physicians and, 24–6, 58, 67, 124–25, 189–90
Clement XIII, Pope, 58
clergy, 27n, 44, 46, 51; as rural medical practitioners, 107–8; similarities with medical profession, 102–3, 106–7, 108; status of, 107, 108
clinical instruction, 29, 36, 43, 46, 53; ambulatory clinics and hospitals, 14, 104, 122–5; availability in mid-eighteenth century, 30–1; introduction of, 60–1; patronage and, 66; and poor relief, 61–2, 176–7; *see also* medical practice; public health; therapeutics
Clinton, Hillary Rodham, 1
Cobb, James Dennis, 42n
coffee houses, 199

Coleman, William, 91
collegia medica, 43, 52–4, 55–9, 60
Collegium Carolinum (Kassel), 48n, 57
Collegium Carolinum (Braunschweig), 48n
Collegium medico-chirurgicum (Berlin), 53–4, 67, 68, 182–3
Cologne (university), 39
Conradi, Johann W. H., 176, 181–2
Cook, Harold, 7
court physician, 22, 33
crisis, healing, *see* Hippocrates and Hippocratic medicine
Cullen, William, 84, 143
Cuvier, Georges, 178, 186

Dalberg, Karl von, 45, 47
Deutsches Archiv für die Physiologie, 188, 201
disciplines, medical and scientific, 161, 186–8, 194, 201–2
dissertations, 32, 184; *see also* medical education, disputations and promotions
district doctor, *see* Physicus
Döllinger, Ignaz, 178–9, 180–1
Du Bois-Reymond, Emil, 193
Duisburg (university), 13, 69n
dyskrasia, 79

Eley, Geoff, 3
Engelberger, Joseph Daniel, 25
England, *see* Great Britain
Enlightenment, 67, 72, 85, 103; authoritarian and egalitarian tensions, 136; concepts of merit, 69–70; as ideology of social progress, 43–4, 73, 108; utilitarian value of knowledge, 9–11, 167; *see also* medical advice literature
epidemiology, 153
Erfurt (university), 31, 38; clinical instruction at, 63; eighteenth-century reform plans for, 45, 47; emulation of Göttingen, 48; medical enrollments, 28, 69n; publicity for, 49, 50
Erhard, Johann Benjamin, 131–3, 134–6, 144, 150, 200–1
Erlangen (university), 31, 54, 110, 175; anatomical demonstrations, 45; clinical instruction, 59–60, 65–6; *Erlangische Anzeigen,* 50; founding of, 48; medical enrollments, 28, 69n; publicity for, 49
etiology, *see* pathology; therapeutics

Faculté de Médecine (Paris), 60
fevers, 114–15, 154
Fichte, Johann Gottlieb, 173, 197; and *Bildung,* 97; departure from Jena, 171; memorandum on proposed university in Berlin, 168–9; philosophical doctrines, 92–3

forensic medicine, 29, 36, 177
Foucault, Michel, 4n, 10, 115n
France, 8, 192, 198, 199
Francis II, Holy Roman Emperor, 162
Francke, August Hermann, 62
Frank, Johann Peter, 38n, 61–2, 108, 114–15, 178
Frankfurt an der Oder (university), 28, 40, 47
Freiburg (university), 23–4, 69n, 179, 185
Freidson, Eliot, 3, 6
French, Roger, 115n
French Revolution, 2–3, 9, 130, 146, 148
Frevert, Ute, 4–6
Friedrich II, King of Brandenburg-Prussia, 46, 54
Friedrich Wilhelm I, King of Brandenburg-Prussia, 53
Fulda (university), 28
Fürstenberg (principality), 24

Galen, 79, 141
Gaub, Hieronymus David, 82, 83, 181
Gedike, Friedrich, 31n
Gegenbauer, Carl, 193
Gelehrsamkeit, see physicians, scholarly ideal
Gelehrtenstand, 7
Gelfand, Toby, 9, 103n
gentility, *see* professions
Germany, *see* Holy Roman Empire
Giessen (university), 17, 23, 31, 40, 63
Girtanner, Christoph, 144n
Gmelin, Johann Friedrich, 40
Gmelin, Maria Veronica, 40
Gmelin, Samuel Gottlieb, 40
Goethe, Johann Wolfgang, 129
Goldhagen, Johann Friedrich, 86
Görres, Joseph, 95–6
Göttingen (city), 48, 49
Göttingen (university), 29n, 38, 81, 105, 124, 171, 179; academic mercantilism and, 172; anatomical demonstrations, 45–6n; attractiveness for students, 48–9; clinical instruction, 59–60, 62, 63–5; founding of, 44, 47–8; *Göttingische Zeitungen von gelehrten Sachen*, 50; medical enrollments, 28, 69n; publicity for, 49; recruitment of faculty, 37
Goubert, Jean-Pierre 4n
grand tour, 16
Great Britain, 6, 9, 198, 199
Greece, ancient, *see* neo-classicism
Greifswald (university), 29n, 46, 55, 59
Gruner, Christian Gottfried, 69, 84–5, 107
guilds, 21, 67

Habermas, Jürgen, 11–12, 195, 196n; *see also* public sphere

Haeckel, Ernst, 193
Halle (city), 62
Halle (university), 16, 44, 50, 86, 168; clinical instruction, 31, 59–60, 62–3, 64–5; examinations, 32n; introduction of cameralism, 47; Meckel's separation of anatomy from clinical subjects, 178; medical enrollment, 28
Haller, Albrecht von, 13–4, 29n, 80–1
Hardenberg, Karl von, 168, 185n
Harless, Johann C. F., 175
Hecker, August Friedrich, 117, 142, 146, 156; criticism of medical systems, 84–5, 113–14; as historian of medicine, 139–40; *Journal der Erfindungen, Theorien, und Widersprüche*, 84–5; as medical journalist, 84–5
Heidelberg (city), 176
Heidelberg (university), 30, 37n, 160, 178, 185; and Baden's *Kulturpolitik*, 171–2, 173; establishment of university clinic, 176; financial problems in 1800, 164–5; medical enrollments, 28, 69n; recruitments for medical faculty, 174–5; reorganization of faculty structure in 1803, 166–7
Heim, Ernst Ludwig, 106
Herz, Marcus, 118, 119
Hess, Ludwig von, 39, 41
Hess, Volker, 181n
Hesse-Darmstadt, 163
Hesse-Kassel (principality), 57, 64, 67, 70
Hildebrandt, Friedrich, 110–11, 112–13, 125, 174
Hildesheim (principality), 54
Himly, Karl Gustav, 124
Hippocrates and Hippocratic medicine, 109, 153, 180, 184, 194; *Airs, Waters, Places*, 115; *Aphorisms*, 31; doctrine of crisis, 142; healing power of nature, 140, 142; and neo-classicism, 140–1; reputation among German physicians, 140–1
history of medicine, 130, 139, 142
Hoffmann, Christoph Ludwig, 51, 61, 67, 189; plans for Münster *collegium medicum*, 55–7, 68, 70; and University of Mainz, 57–9, 66
Hoffmann, Friedrich, 16
Hofmann, Christian Gottlieb, 61, 66
Holmes, Geoffrey, 6
Holy Roman Empire, 9, 158, 160, 162, 192
Horsch, Philipp Joseph, 124–5, 126
Hoven, Friedrich von, 20–1, 23
Huerkamp, Claudia, 4–5
Hufeland, Christoph Wilhelm, 109–110, 143, 146, 147, 154; biography, 104–6; and Brunonianism, 156–7, 158; on clinical instruction, 122–3; concept of life force, 111–12, 156; on diagnosis and etiology, 111–12, 156; on diagnosis and etiology,

Hufeland, Christoph Wilhelm (*cont.*)
114–15; *Journal der practischen Heilkunde,*
104, 117, 139, 159; *Makrobiotik,* 111–13;
on medical education, 121–2, 125, 184;
on medicine as a calling, 104–5, 107;
memorandum on new university in Berlin, 182–3; on public criticism of medicine, 133, 134–6, 200–1; on rural medical
practice by clergy, 108; on theory and
practice in medicine, 118, 128, 134
Humboldt, Wilhelm von, 169–70, 173, 183–4
Huxley, Aldous, 195

iatrochemistry, 76
Ingolstadt (city), 165
Ingolstadt (university), 27n–28, 52, 165; see also
Landshut (university)
institutes of medicine (*institutiones*), 14, 36
irritability, 81, 143

Jena (city), 93
Jena (university), 16, 50, 88, 105, 122; Fichte's de-
parture, 171; medical enrollments, 28,
69n; Schelling and, 98–9, 171
Jesuits, 26n, 58, 165, 166
Jones, Colin, 8
Journal der practischen Heilkunde, see Hufeland,
Christoph Wlhelm
Journal des Luxus und der Moden, 109
Jugler, Johann Heinrich, 34
Jülich and Berg (duchies), 54
Juncker, Johann, 31, 35, 62–3, 64–5
Justi, Johann von, 47
Jütte, Robert, 4

Kant, Immanuel, 71–2, 169, 199; epistemological
doctrines of, 92, 93; influence on medical
theory, 86–90, 130, 136, 150; *Kritik der
Urtheilskraft,* 95n; and philosophical criti-
cism, 74, 198–9; see also *Wissenschaft*
Karl August, Duke of Saxe-Weimar, 104, 105
Karl Eugen, Duke of Württemberg, 40
Kästner, Abraham Gotthelf, 35
Keel, Othmar, 103n
Kiel (university), 29, 33, 50, 59, 69n
Kielmeyer, Carl Friedrich, 81
Kocka, Jürgen, 4
Königsberg (university), 34, 179, 187
Kulturpolitik, 171–3

Lacoue-Labarthe, Philippe, 97
Landshut (city), 176–7
Landshut (university), 160, 173, 175, 179; administrative reorganization, 166; establishment of university clinic, 176–7; removal
from Ingolstadt, 165

Larson, James, 81
Larson, Magali Sarfatti, 1
La Vopa, Anthony, 70, 170
legal profession, 10, 27, 46, 48, 51, 170
Leiden (university), 13, 16, 17
Leipzig (university), 15, 35, 50, 59, 82, 179; med-
ical enrollments, 28; new chairs in medi-
cal faculty, 177; student expenses, 34
Le Roy, Lee Ann Hansen, 80, 87n
licensing, 1, 52–4
Lindeboom, G. A., 80
Linné, Carl von (Linnaeus), 17
literary sansculottism, *see* Brunonianism
Löber, Emanuel Christian, 16
Locke, John, 78n
Loetz, Francisca, 4n, 5
London, 199
Loudon, Irvine, 5
Ludwig, Christian Gottlieb, 82, 83
Ludwigsburg, 20–1, 23
Lunéville, Treaty of, 162

Mai, Franz Anton, 147–8
Mainz (principality), 38, 45, 57–9, 63
Mainz (university), 50, 58–9, 66
Mangold, Christoph Andreas, 30n
Marburg (university), 17, 30, 31, 57; clinical in-
struction at, 59–60, 64; publicity for, 49
Marcus, Adalbert Friedrich, 149, 152–5, 157
Marcuse, Herbert, 196n
Marland, Hilary, 5
Massow, Julius von, 68, 168
materia medica, 29
matriculation, 34
Mayer, August Carl, 175–6
Meckel, Johann Friedrich, the Younger, 178,
186–7, 201–2
Mecklenburg-Schwerin (principality), 54
medical advice literature, 18, 85, 126; and bourgeois values, 111–13; and child rearing,
109–110; as medium of medical enlightenment, 109; and moral weeklies, 109;
and the six non-naturals, 110–11
medical education, 12, 46, 103, 128; centrality of
lecturing in, 30–1; costs of, 33–5; curriculum, 28–9, 179–80; disputations and
promotions, 32–3, 34, 39, 41; Erhard's
criticism of, 136; examinations, 32, 39,
41; and *Naturphilosophie,* 119, 185; student stipends, 35; tension between teaching and research, 121–2, 173, 193–4; testimonials from professors, 31–2, 34; theory
and practice in, 29–30, 72, 119–22, 179–
82, 184–5; travel in, 16–17, 31; *see also*
clinical instruction; *Wissenschaft*
medical faculties, 13, 52, 159–60, 181; *Aufrücken,*
36–7, 177; criticism of, 29–30, 38–41, 52,

60; duties of, 38–9, 40–1, 54; enrollments, 68–9, 158; patronage and, 39–40;
recruitment of professors, 23, 37–8, 39–
40; reorganization after 1800, 174–6; separation of clinical and theoretical courses,
177–9; *see also* disciplines, medical and
scientific
medical police, 51, 61–2; *see also* public health
medical practice, 60, 181n; case histories in, 138–
9; clinics as introduction to, 123–4, 127;
entry into, 20–1; historicist epistemology
and, 138–9, 142–3; as *Kunst* or *savoir faire*,
118–19, 159; and medical systems, 113–
14, 117–18; and popular culture, 19–20;
public's competency in judging, 133–5;
relationship with medical theory, 73, 77–
80, 83, 87–90, 156–7, 158, 159; role of
experience in, 117–18, 139–40; social
conditions of, 19–22; theory of, 103,
113–17, 132–3, 134; *see also* therapeutics
medical profession, 7, 42, 59, 89, 160; as a calling, 72, 102–3, 104–8; division between
professors and practitioners, 161, 186,
193; Erhard's criticism of, 132–3, 135–6;
and expertise, 10, 18, 134–5; generational
conflict in, 145, 146–8; government regulation of, 188–92; and guilds, 21; hierarchy within, 135–6, 142, 148; *Licenciaten*,
33; and metatheory, 197; and monopolization of healing, 5, 22; origins of modern, 1–2, 4, 8–9; social status of, 24, 26,
67, 69–70, 143, 188–92; *see also* clergy;
physicians
medical societies, 191
medicalization, 4
Medicinisches Journal, 84
Meiners, Christoph, 60
midwives and midwifery, 19, 25, 38, 53, 189
modernization, 2–3
Mögling, Christian Ludwig, 17
Montgelas, Maximilian von, 163
Moran, Bruce, 8
Morgagni, Giovanni Battista, 82–3
morphology, animal, 186–8, 201
Munich, 25n
Münster (principality), 55–7, 68, 70

Nancy, Jean-Luc, 97
Nassau, 163, 189–90
Nasse, Friedrich, 177n, 178, 190–1
nationalism, 160
Naturphilosophie, 9, 108, 119, 146, 179, 181, 185;
and animal morphology, 186; attractiveness for physicians, 22–3, 97, 99–100,
101; basic doctrines of, 93–6; and *Bildung*, 97; and growth of medical disciplines, 101; historiography on, 90–2; and

Kant's philosophy, 92, 95n, 96; and medical practice, 102; as metatheory, 197; and
public sphere 75, 97–100, 101; role of language in, 91, 95–6; Romanticism and,
92, 94–5; *see also* Brunonianism, medical
education
neo-classicism, 140–2, 169
Newtonianism, 80, 100
Nipperdey, Thomas, 164n
nosology, 114–15n
Nuremburg, 23

Obermedicinalrath (Brandenburg-Prussia), 183
obstetrics, 29, 177
Oken, Lorenz, 96
opium, 144, 153; *see also* Brunonianism, popular
remedies in

Pagel, Julius, 198n
Palatinate, 31n, 54, 164
Paris (city), 103, 131, 199
pathological anatomy, 82–3, 156, 186–7
pathology, 28–9, 36, 87–8, 143, 177; Brunonian,
143–4, 150–1; Burdach's and Conradi's
concepts of, 181–2; development in eighteenth century, 82–3; and etiology, 115–
16; humoralist, Brunonian attack on,
150–1, 153–4; as link between theory and
practice, 83, 151; and mechanical philosophy, 77–80; *see also* six non-naturals;
pathological anatomy
Pelling, Margaret, 3, 5–6
Pepinière (Berlin), 183
periodicals, 6, 11, 45; criticism and, 74, 84–6;
medical, 84–6; and public sphere, 199,
201; and universities, 50
Peter the Great, Czar of Russia, 14
Pfuscher and *Pfuscherey, see* physicians, relations
with other healers
philology, 71, 173
philosophical faculty, 26, 71–2
physicians, 9, 24, 40, 193–4; and *Bildung*, 71–2,
73, 170, 190; complaints about incomes,
190–91; and Enlightenment reforms, 43–
4, 51, 67; Hoffmann's classification system for, 56–7; and public sphere, 75; reaction to utilitarian reforms, 68–72, 126–7;
relations with other healers, 21–2, 67–70,
120–2; scholarly ideal, 15–19, 70–2, 126;
social background, 27–8n; and social deference 8n, 113, 117, 120; *see also* civil service; medical profession; *Naturphilosophie;
Physicus*
Physicus, 29, 101; and *collegia medica*, 52; duties,
24–5, 45, 61; origins, 24–5; qualifications
for, 33, 56; sources of income, 25; and
university clinics, 64–6

physiology, 28, 177; and anatomy, 178–9; Brunonian, 143, 149–50; development in the eighteenth century, 75–6, 80–1, 83–4, 100; epistemological foundations, 86; experimental, 176; and medical practice, 77–80, 88–90, 180; and morphology, 187–8; and pathology, 78–80, 83–4, 87–8, 180–1; *see also* vital forces
Pietism, 44, 62
poetry, 94–5
poor relief, *see* public health
Porter, Roy, 4
practical reason, 18
pragmatic history, 137–8, 140
Prest, Wilfred, 6
private lecture courses, 34
professionalization, 2–3, 4–10, 192, 194, 202
professions, 1, 43, 191–2, 202; accessibility to poor students, 35; and *Bildung,* 170, 173, 190; gentility and, 6–7; patronage and, 7–8; and poor students, 70; and pursuit of *Wissenschaft,* 169; role in eighteenth-century reforms, 51; sociological criteria, 6n; and universities, 1–2, 7, 26; *see also* clergy; legal profession; medical profession; professionalization
prosector, anatomical, 176
Prussia, *see* Brandenburg-Prussia
public health, 43; cameralism and, 51–2; and clinical instruction, 124–5; medical care for the poor, 61–2, 65, 160; provision of healers, 55–6, 189–90
public sphere, 11–12, 100–1, 161; and avant-garde movements, 97–9; characteristics, 12n, 88–9; criticism and, 74–5, 199–201; and medicine, 84–6, 126, 135; national distinctions, 199; and university *Kulturpolitik,* 172–3; *see also* theory-practice discourse

quacks, *see* charlatans

Ramsey, Matthew, 9
Rehmann, Joseph F. X., 23–4
Reichsdeputationshauptschluss, 162
Reil, Johann Christian, 104, 122, 128, 136, 150; *Archiv für die Physiologie,* 86, 90, 187–8, 199; biography, 86; on medical education, 120, 182; memorandum on new university in Berlin, 182; and morphology, 187; *Pepinieren als Unterricht ärztlicher Routiniers,* 120–1, 182, 189; and reform of medical science, 86–8, 100
Reverby, Susan, 4
rigorosum, 32; *see also* medical education, examinations
Rinteln (university), 47, 50, 57

Roederer, Johann Georg, 63
Romanticism, 93, 94–5, 97–8, 146, 196; *see also* Naturphilosophie
Röschlaub, Andreas, 147, 155, 182; and development of Brunonian theory, 149–51, 157–8; relationship with Schelling, 158; renunciation of Brunonianism, 159; on theory and practice, 151–2; and university clinic in Landshut, 177
Rosenberg, Hans, 164n
Rosner, David, 4
Rostock (university), 54
Rousseau, Jean-Jacques, 144
routiniers, 120–1
Royal College of Physicians (London), 60
Rudolphi, Karl Asmund, 175, 178, 184
Russell, E. S., 186

salons, 199
Sander, Sabine, 4–5
Sauvages, François Boissier de, 115n
Savigny, Karl von, 172–3
Saxe-Weimar (duchy), 104, 105, 171
Saxony, 67
Schaarschmidt, August, 23
Schelling, Friedrich W. J., 74, 90, 101; and *Bildung,* 97; and Brunonianism, 149; and Fichte's philosophy, 93; *Ideen zu einer Philosophie der Natur,* 93–4; move to Würzburg, 171; as public figure, 98–9; and Romanticism, 95
Schiller, Friedrich, 97, 141n, 169
Schlegel, August Wilhelm, 93
Schlegel, Caroline, 99
Schlegel, Friedrich, 93, 95
Schleiermacher, Friedrich, 168–9, 173
Schleswig-Holstein, 38
Schmid, Carl C. E., 88–90, 136
Section of Religion and Public Instruction (Brandenburg-Prussia), 183
self-consciousness, 92–3
semiotics, medical, 78–9, 132, 140, 142, 181n
Sennert, Daniel, 76
sensibility, 81
Sigerist, Henry, 4
six non-naturals, 82, 110–11, 116
Smith, Pamela, 8
Snow, C. P., 195
social history of medicine, 3–5
Sömmerring, Samuel Thomas, 174
Sonnenfels, Joseph von, 47
Sprengel, Kurt Polykarp, 115, 139, 140–1, 142–3
Stahl, Georg Ernst, 16
Starr, Paul, 1
Steffens, Henrich, 98–9
Stein, Karl von, 168
Strack, Karl, 58

Stralsund (city), 55
Stromeyer, Johann Friedrich, 64
Sturm und Drang, 71
Stuttgart (university), 20
surgeons and surgery, 17, 19, 21, 22n; founding
     of surgical academies, 67; legal separation
     from physicians, 67–8, 189–90; regulation
     of, by physicians, 25, 38, 53; status, 67–8;
     and university medical study, 27n, 29,
     69–70, 177, 178
Swedish Pomerania, 29n, 54–5
Swieten, Gerard van, 13–15, 17, 31
Sydenham, Thomas, 78n, 141
symptoms, *see* semiotics, medical

Temkin, Owsei, 78
tentamen, 32; *see also* medical education, examina-
     tions
teutsche Merkur, Der, 131, 133, 135, 147
theory-practice discourse, 9–11; legal profession
     and, 10n; and modern professions, 10,
     202; and the public sphere, 198–202; rela-
     tionship with Aristotelian categories of
     knowledge, 194–6; *see also* medical educa-
     tion; medical practice
therapeutics, 36, 88, 177; Brunonian, 143–4,
     152–5; concepts of causation, 134; diag-
     nosis, 114–15; Erhard's criticisms, 132–3;
     etiology, 115–16, 151–2; individuality of
     patients, 113, 116–17; prognosis, 116;
     role of clinics and hospitals, 123
Thirty Years War, 24
Tieck, Ludwig, 99
Tiedemann, Friedrich, 175, 178
Tilsit, Treaty of, 168
Tissot, Samuel-Auguste, 107
town doctor, *see* Physicus
towns and communities, 20, 25, 66, 163
Trier (principality) 29n
Tsouyopoulos, Nelly, 129n, 158n
Tübingen (university), 38, 59, 175, 187; learned
     periodicals at, 50; medical enrollments at,
     28, 69n; recruitment of faculty, 37–8, 40;
     social background of medical students,
     27n
Turner, R. Steven, 7, 37, 101

universities and university education, 28, 68; ad-
     vertising for, 49–50; aristocracy and, 27,
     49; cameralist motives for reform of, 46–
     8; choice of, by students, 26, 30, 31;
     eighteenth-century "crisis" of, 42–3;
     eighteenth-century reforms of, 44–51;

emulation of Göttingen, 48–50; enroll-
     ments, 69; expansion of research, 160–1;
     introduction of practical training, 45–6;
     nineteenth-century reforms, 159–60,
     164–7, 192; requirements for entry, 26;
     role of *Wissenschaft,* 168–9, 182; secular-
     ization, 44–5, 57–8; tension between
     teaching and research, 173; *see also* camer-
     alism
Unzer, Johann August, 18, 109

Varnhagen, Johann Heinrich, 88
Vienna (city), 23
Vienna (university), 13
vital forces, 80–1, 83, 87, 100, 111
Vogel, Rudolf Augustin, 63–4
Vogel, Samuel Gottlieb, 116, 118–19, 125

Waddington, Ivan, 8n
Walker, Mack, 46
Walther, Philipp Franz von, 177
Webster, Charles, 3
Wedekind, Georg Christian, 59
Weikard, Melchior Adam, 144–5, 146, 148
Weis, Eberhard, 164n
Wendt, Friedrich, 31
Werlhoff, Paul Gottlieb von, 63
whiggism, *see Naturphilosophie,* historiography of
Wieland, Christoph Martin, 131
Windischmann, Karl J. H., 141–2
Wissenschaft, 22, 90, 102, 132, 148–9, 181, 187,
     191; Fichte's and Schleiermacher's con-
     cepts of, 168–9; historicist epistemology
     and, 130, 137, 142–3; Humboldt's con-
     cept of, 169; Kantian critical philosophy
     and, 136–7; place in medical education,
     120, 127, 181; Schmid's concept of, 89;
     see also universities and university educa-
     tion
Wittenberg (university), 35
Wolff, Christian Friedrich, 16, 17
Wunderlich, Karl, 198n
Württemberg, 33, 38, 67, 162, 189
Würzburg (principality), 38
Würzburg (university), 23, 30, 38, 50, 126, 160,
     175, 178; and Bavarian *Kulturpolitik,* 171,
     172–3; clinical instruction, 59–60, 124–5;
     enrollments after 1803, 172; reorganiza-
     tion after 1803, 166; salaries after 1803,
     172

Zeitschrift für spekulative Physik, 98
Zimmermann, Johann Georg, 14, 118

Continued from the front of the book

The science of woman: Gynecology and gender in England, 1800–1929
ORNELLA MOSCUCCI
Quality and quantity: The quest for biological regeneration in twentieth-century France   WILLIAM H. SCHNEIDER
Bilharzia: A history of imperial tropical medicine   JOHN FARLEY
Preserve your love for science: Life of William A. Hammond, American neurologist   BONNIE E. BLUSTEIN
Patients, power, and the poor in eighteenth-century Bristol   MARY E. FISSELL
AIDS and contemporary society   EDITED BY VIRGINIA BERRIDGE
AND PHILIP STRONG
Science and empire: East Coast fever in Rhodesia and the Transvaal
PAUL F. CRANEFIELD
The colonial disease: A social history of sleeping sickness in Northern Zaire, 1900–1940   MARYINEZ LYONS
Mission and method: The early nineteenth-century French public health movement   ANN F. LABERGE
Meanings of sex differences in the Middle Ages: Medicine, science, and culture
JOAN CADDEN
Public health in British India: Anglo-Indian preventive medicine, 1859–1914
MARK HARRISON
Medicine before the Plague: Practitioners and their patients in the Crown of Aragon, 1285–1345   MICHAEL R. MCVAUGH
The physical and the moral: Anthropology, physiology, and philosophical medicine in France, 1750–1850   ELIZABETH A. WILLIAMS
Charity and power in early modern Italy: Benefactors and their motives in Turine, 1541–1789   SANDRA CAVALLO
A social history of wet nursing in America: From breast to bottle
JANET GOLDEN
Charitable knowledge: Hospital pupils and practitioners in eighteenth-century London
SUSAN C. LAWRENCE

www.ingramcontent.com/pod-product-compliance
Ingram Content Group UK Ltd.
Pitfield, Milton Keynes, MK11 3LW, UK
UKHW040705180125
453697UK00010B/420

9 780521 524575